Antimicrobial Resistance and Environmental Health

Antimicrobial Resistance and Environmental Health

Guest Editor

Akebe Luther King Abia

MDPI

Basel • Beijing • Wuhan • Barcelona • Belgrade • Novi Sad • Cluj • Manchester

Guest Editor
Akebe Luther King Abia
College of Health Sciences
University of KwaZulu-Natal
Durban
South Africa

Editorial Office
MDPI AG
Grossepeteranlage 5
4052 Basel, Switzerland

This is a reprint of the Special Issue, published open access by the journal *Antibiotics* (ISSN 2079-6382), freely accessible at: www.mdpi.com/journal/antibiotics/special_issues/Anti_Environmental.

For citation purposes, cite each article independently as indicated on the article page online and using the guide below:

Lastname, A.A.; Lastname, B.B. Article Title. *Journal Name* **Year**, *Volume Number*, Page Range.

ISBN 978-3-7258-3046-6 (Hbk)
ISBN 978-3-7258-3045-9 (PDF)
https://doi.org/10.3390/books978-3-7258-3045-9

Contents

About the Editor vii

Preface ix

Yernar Amangelsin, Yuliya Semenova, Maryam Dadar, Mohamad Aljofan and Geir Bjørklund
The Impact of Tetracycline Pollution on the Aquatic Environment and Removal Strategies
Reprinted from: *Antibiotics* **2023**, *12*, 440, https://doi.org/10.3390/antibiotics12030440 1

Anca Farkas, Cristian Coman, Edina Szekeres, Adela Teban-Man, Rahela Carpa and Anca Butiuc-Keul
Molecular Typing Reveals Environmental Dispersion of Antibiotic-Resistant Enterococci under Anthropogenic Pressure
Reprinted from: *Antibiotics* **2022**, *11*, 1213, https://doi.org/10.3390/antibiotics11091213 16

Phathutshedzo Rakhalaru, Lutendo Munzhedzi, Akebe Luther King Abia, Jean Pierre Kabue, Natasha Potgieter and Afsatou Ndama Traore
Prevalence and Antimicrobial Resistance Profile of Diarrheagenic *Escherichia coli* from Fomites in Rural Households in South Africa
Reprinted from: *Antibiotics* **2023**, *12*, 1345, https://doi.org/10.3390/antibiotics12081345 35

Valentina Riva, Giovanni Patania, Francesco Riva, Lorenzo Vergani, Elena Crotti and Francesca Mapelli
Acinetobacter baylyi Strain BD413 Can Acquire an Antibiotic Resistance Gene by Natural Transformation on Lettuce Phylloplane and Enter the Endosphere
Reprinted from: *Antibiotics* **2022**, *11*, 1231, https://doi.org/10.3390/antibiotics11091231 49

Mohammad Irfan, Alhomidi Almotiri and Zeyad Abdullah AlZeyadi
Antimicrobial Resistance and -Lactamase Production in Clinically Significant Gram-Negative Bacteria Isolated from Hospital and Municipal Wastewater
Reprinted from: *Antibiotics* **2023**, *12*, 653, https://doi.org/10.3390/antibiotics12040653 64

Esther Ubani K. Fono-Tamo, Ilunga Kamika, John Barr Dewar and Kgaugelo Edward Lekota
Comparative Genomics Revealed a Potential Threat of *Aeromonas rivipollensis* G87 Strain and Its Antibiotic Resistance
Reprinted from: *Antibiotics* **2023**, *12*, 131, https://doi.org/10.3390/antibiotics12010131 74

Hanan A. Al-Sarawi, Nazima Habibi, Saif Uddin, Awadhesh N. Jha, Mohammed A. Al-Sarawi and Brett P. Lyons
Antibiotic Resistance Mediated by *Escherichia coli* in Kuwait Marine Environment as Revealed through Genomic Analysis
Reprinted from: *Antibiotics* **2023**, *12*, 1366, https://doi.org/10.3390/antibiotics12091366 88

Akebe Luther King Abia, Themba Baloyi, Afsatou N. Traore and Natasha Potgieter
The African Wastewater Resistome: Identifying Knowledge Gaps to Inform Future Research Directions
Reprinted from: *Antibiotics* **2023**, *12*, 805, https://doi.org/10.3390/antibiotics12050805 103

Ramganesh Selvarajan, Chinedu Obize, Timothy Sibanda, Akebe Luther King Abia and Haijun Long
Evolution and Emergence of Antibiotic Resistance in Given Ecosystems: Possible Strategies for Addressing the Challenge of Antibiotic Resistance
Reprinted from: *Antibiotics* **2022**, *12*, 28, https://doi.org/10.3390/antibiotics12010028 123

Paul B. L. George, Florent Rossi, Magali-Wen St-Germain, Pierre Amato, Thierry Badard and Michel G. Bergeron et al.
Antimicrobial Resistance in the Environment: Towards Elucidating the Roles of Bioaerosols in Transmission and Detection of Antibacterial Resistance Genes
Reprinted from: *Antibiotics* **2022**, *11*, 974, https://doi.org/10.3390/antibiotics11070974 . . . . . . **153**

Philip Mathew, Sujith J. Chandy, Satya Sivaraman, Jaya Ranjalkar, Hyfa Mohammed Ali and Shruthi Anna Thomas
Formulating a Community-Centric Indicator Framework to Quantify One Health Drivers of Antibiotic Resistance: A Preliminary Step towards Fostering 'Antibiotic-Smart Communities'
Reprinted from: *Antibiotics* **2024**, *13*, 63, https://doi.org/10.3390/antibiotics13010063 . . . . . . **171**

About the Editor

Akebe Luther King Abia

Akebe Luther King Abia (King) is an Applied and Environmental Microbiologist and high-impact researcher at the University of KwaZulu-Natal. He is also the Founder and CEO of the Environmental Research Foundation (ERF). His research focuses on, but is not limited to, antimicrobial resistance in the environment and how this relates to humans and animals through the One Health approach, using culture and molecular techniques, including metagenomics and whole-genome sequencing. He has over 20 years of experience as a microbiologist and is involved in many projects, including monitoring water and soil for human pathogens, especially antibiotic-resistant ones, under changing climates. King serves on several local and international organisations' boards, including as an advisory board member, editorial board member, and grant reviewer panelist. He has published over 100 journal articles, six book chapters, and three books. He has also graduated postgraduate students and mentored several others at the postgraduate and undergraduate level.

Preface

"The best time to plant a tree is 20 years ago. The second-best time is now." African proverb.

The recent 79th United Nations General Assembly (UNGA) held in September 2024 included the 2nd High-Level Meeting on Antimicrobial Resistance (AMR) which adopted the Political Declaration on AMR. The declaration acknowledged the severe threat AMR poses to global health and sustainable development, with an imperative need for immediate action. The declaration further emphasised the One Health approach, requiring all sectors, including the environment.

Although the One Health approach is re-emphasised, most research focus is on human and animal health, with environmental health needing more attention. Furthermore, most environmental studies focus on water and soil, with air and fomites in human settings not considered. Also, most studies on AMR are limited to culture-based approaches, with limited use of more advanced genomic techniques. These gaps paint an incomplete picture of the role played by the environment in AMR. Therefore, this volume provides a comprehensive update on antimicrobial resistance and environmental health. Given that human activities are the major contributors to the growing AMR threat, one chapter reviewed the impact of tetracycline pollution on AMR in the environment and its ripple effect on ecological and human health. The authors further evaluated possible remediation strategies for tetracycline-polluted environments. If not addressed, environmental antimicrobial pollution could lead to the development of new AMR traits and the evolution of already existing ones in different environmental matrices, as reviewed by another chapter in this volume. Two chapters address the presence and transmission of AMR fomites in households and vegetables in farms. Still focusing on unconventional environmental settings, one chapter provides a perspective on elucidating the role of bioaerosols on AMR transmission. Two other chapters discuss AMR in wastewater, one in clinical and community settings, and the other reviewed wastewater AMR in Africa while pointing out the knowledge gaps and suggesting a future perspective for the successful application of the wastewater-based epidemiology of AMR. Two chapters used genomic approaches to provide insight into environmental AMR, including in the marine environment. Finally, one chapter proposed a community-focused framework measuring One Health drivers of AMR as an approach to promote building "antibiotic-smart communities".

Akebe Luther King Abia
Guest Editor

antibiotics

MDPI

Review

The Impact of Tetracycline Pollution on the Aquatic Environment and Removal Strategies

Yernar Amangelsin [1], Yuliya Semenova [1], Maryam Dadar [2], Mohamad Aljofan [1,*] and Geir Bjørklund [3,*]

[1] Nazarbayev University School of Medicine, Astana 010000, Kazakhstan
[2] CONEM Iran Microbiology Research Group, Tehran 1316943551, Iran
[3] Council for Nutritional and Environmental Medicine (CONEM), 8610 Mo i Rana, Norway
* Correspondence: mohamad.aljofan@nu.edu.kz (M.A.); bjorklund@conem.org (G.B.)

Abstract: Antibacterial drugs are among the most commonly used medications in the world. Tetracycline is a widely used antibiotic for human and animal therapy due to its broad-spectrum activity, high effectiveness, and reasonable cost. The indications for treatment with tetracycline include pneumonia, bone and joint infections, infectious disorders of the skin, sexually transmitted and gastrointestinal infections. However, tetracycline has become a serious threat to the environment because of its overuse by humans and veterinarians and weak ability to degrade. Tetracycline is capable of accumulating along the food chain, causing toxicity to the microbial community, encouraging the development and spread of antibiotic resistance, creating threats to drinking and irrigation water, and disrupting microbial flora in the human intestine. It is essential to address the negative impact of tetracycline on the environment, as it causes ecological imbalance. Ineffective wastewater systems are among the main reasons for the increased antibiotic concentrations in aquatic sources. It is possible to degrade tetracycline by breaking it down into small molecules with less harmful or nonhazardous effects. A range of methods for physical, chemical, and biological degradation exists. The review will discuss the negative effects of tetracycline consumption on the aquatic environment and describe available removal methods.

Keywords: tetracycline; tetracycline consumption; aquatic environment; tetracycline pollution; oxidative stress

Citation: Amangelsin, Y.; Semenova, Y.; Dadar, M.; Aljofan, M.; Bjørklund, G. The Impact of Tetracycline Pollution on the Aquatic Environment and Removal Strategies. *Antibiotics* **2023**, *12*, 440. https://doi.org/10.3390/antibiotics12030440

Academic Editor: Akebe Luther King Abia

Received: 26 December 2022
Revised: 17 February 2023
Accepted: 20 February 2023
Published: 23 February 2023

1. Introduction

Antibacterial drugs are among the most commonly used medications in the world. Antibiotics are antibacterial medications with complex molecular compounds that can destroy or slow the growth of bacteria [1,2]. Antibiotic drugs are classified according to their mechanism of action, spectrum of activity, administration methods, and chemical structure. Antibacterial medications are used for therapeutic purposes and as growth promoters in livestock farming [3–5]. It should be noted that the usage of antibiotics is dramatically increasing each year. For example, according to Scaria et al. (2021), the worldwide consumption of antibiotics increased rapidly from 21 to approximately 35 billion daily doses between 2000 and 2015, which is almost a 65% upsurge [6].

Moreover, Klein et al. (2018) predicted that the utilization of antibacterial drugs will continue to grow to 200% by 2030 [7]. The overuse of antibiotics may cause the appearance of antibiotic resistance genes (ARGs) which have negative impacts on human health. ARGs are generated by microbial spontaneous mutations and are selected by antibiotics. This undermines a drug's antibacterial activity and makes it ineffective in killing bacteria [8,9]. As a result, ARGs can be transferred to other bacteria by horizontal transmission, affecting bacterial communities and developing their resistance to antibacterial medications. The circulation of such strains as methicillin-resistant *Staphylococcus aureus* (MRSA), *Clostridium difficile*, and multidrug resistant *Mycobacterium Tuberculosis* has already caused much harm [10].

One of the most commonly used types of antibiotics currently is tetracycline. The first medications of the tetracycline family were isolated from *Streptomyces* species in the late 1940s. Since then, tetracycline antibiotics have been commercialized owing to their clinical success. The more recent third generation of the tetracycline family demonstrates greater potency and efficacy. Tetracycline inhibits the ability of bacterial protein synthesis by attaching to the 30S ribosomal subunit of bacteria [11,12]. As stated by Fuoco (2012), due to its broad-spectrum activity, this antibiotic can suppress the activity of most Gram-positive and Gram-negative strains, protozoan parasites, including atypical organisms such as mycoplasma, chlamydia, and rickettsia [13]. Due to its low price and robust efficiency, tetracycline is now one of the most commonly used antibiotics.

The overconsumption of antibiotics such as tetracycline in human and animal therapy and livestock has become a major threat to the environment and human health [14]. Tetracycline residue has recently been discovered in a wide range of settings, including soil, surface water, marine environments, sediments, and even biota samples [15]. Tetracycline has negative effects on ecosystems, because it is capable of accumulating along the food chain and causing toxicity to the microbial community, encouraging the development and spread of antibiotic resistance [16]. In addition, tetracycline creates threats to drinking and irrigation water and causes disruption of microbial flora in the human intestine. These detrimental effects raise serious concerns about tetracycline contamination and present an emerging public health issue [17].

Monahan et al. (2022) reported that the weak ability of tetracycline to degrade could cause ecological imbalance [18]. The study highlights the significance of environmental pollution caused by tetracycline, as the outcomes severely affect human health, causing bacterial resistance. It was also stated that an ineffective wastewater treatment system is one of the main causes of antibiotic contamination of the food chain, which might adversely affect human health [19–21]. The pollution of soil and water has a drastic negative impact on soil and aquatic microflora [22,23]. This review will assess tetracycline consumption, analyze the antibiotic's negative impact on the marine environment and aquaculture, and discuss effective methods of tetracycline antibiotic removal from aquatic environments.

2. Tetracycline Consumption in Various Fields of Life

Tetracycline is one of the most commonly used types of antibiotics in the world. It has broad-spectrum activity against various bacterial infections, making it effective in human therapy and veterinary medicine [24]. The indications for treatment with tetracycline include infectious diseases such as pneumonia, bone and joint infections, infectious disorders of the skin and sexually transmitted infections, as well as gastrointestinal infections. Tetracycline is a potent agent against the so-called biothreat pathogens, such as *Bacillus anthracis*, *Yersinia pestis*, and *Francisella tularensis*, which are the causative pathogens of some of the most lethal infections. In general, tetracycline-class drugs are the first-line treatment options for many infectious diseases [25].

It was estimated that humans' daily consumption of tetracycline worldwide is 23 kg [26]. It was also reported that European countries and Switzerland use almost 2300 tons of tetracycline antibiotics for animal farming, approximately 66% of the total number of antibiotics [27]. According to the statistics provided by Xu et al. (2021), tetracycline antibiotics are the third most often used drugs in Brazil after penicillin and quinolones [28]. It is estimated that more than 2500 tons of tetracycline are consumed yearly for animal therapy in Europe [29].

Moreover, agriculture and aquaculture are some of the main fields of tetracycline consumption, as antibiotics are used for animal growth. According to Ahmad et al. (2021), 180 thousand tons of raw antibiotic materials were used in China for human treatment and farming, which is equivalent to 138 g per capita per year [30]. It was stated that 172 mg, 148 mg, and 45 mg of antibiotics per kilogram were administered to slaughtered pigs, chickens, and cows [31]. By the calculations of the study provided in pig and cattle livestock in China, it was stated that the daily antibiotic excretion of a single pig and cow is 18.2 and 4.24 mg, respectively [32]. Wozniak-Biel et al. (2018) state that poultry and livestock animal farming used 33% of total tetracycline antibiotics in Turkey [33].

Meanwhile, the USA manufactures 22,680 tons of antibiotic formulations annually, 40% of which is used for agriculture purposes [34]. As a result, tetracycline contamination has become an emerging issue for the environment and human use. Furthermore, the study by Mahamallik et al. (2015) provided another source for tetracycline contamination from the waste of pharmaceutical industries [35]. This study indicates that unutilized antibiotics are distributed to unsuitable places for waste products with no treatment procedures. Therefore, antibiotics will remain undegraded for years in soil or water sources.

Figure 1 represents the available data on consumption of tetracyclines in different parts of the world. Tetracyclines are widely used in European Union countries (2575 tons consumed annually) and Switzerland (1 ton consumed annually) [36]. Three other countries with high levels of tetracycline consumption are Russia (13,579 tons per year) [37] China (6950 tons per year) [38] and the USA (3230 tons) [39]. According to Xu et al., China alone accounts for 18% of global consumption [28]. South Korea consumes 732 tons of tetracyclines, and the UK consumes 240 tons every year [39]. These considerably large proportions of tetracyclines could be explained by the ampleness of animal livestock; therefore, tetracycline is used as a feed promoter. The negative consequences associated with excess tetracycline consumption are discussed in the following paragraphs.

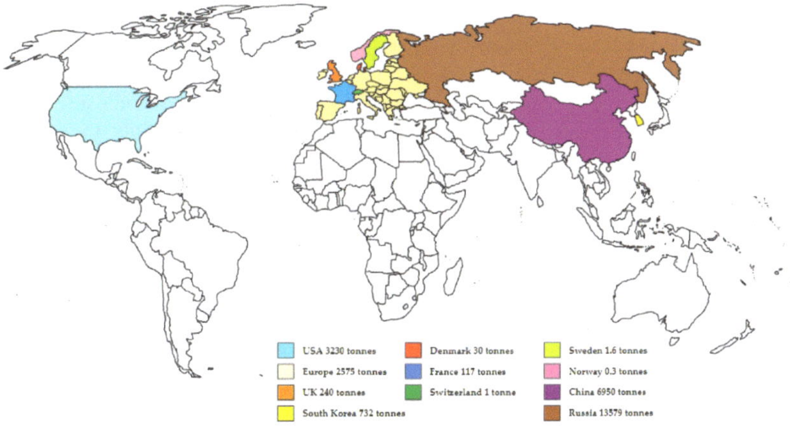

Figure 1. Tons of tetracycline consumed in different countries.

3. The Adverse Effect of Tetracycline Antibiotics on the Aquatic Environment

The most common reason for tetracycline pollution is its stability and low metabolism in human and animal organisms. As stated by Xu et al. (2021), tetracycline antibiotics cannot be fully absorbed and metabolized in the body [28]. Therefore, approximately 75% of the antibiotic is excreted in its parenteral form [40,41]. Tetracycline contamination has been identified primarily in water sources, which causes environmental pollution in the surrounding area, damaging the ecological system [42–44]. Overconsumption of this antibiotic in human and animal therapy and its utilization in agriculture as a growth promoter are among the main causes of tetracycline pollution in the aquatic environment [28].

Moreover, tetracycline is also used in aquaculture for fish feeding. It can be assumed that approximately 80% of utilized antibiotics in aquaculture will be freed in the aquatic environment [45]. It has been estimated that the concentration of tetracycline antibiotics is high in rivers due to pharmaceutical manufacturing, its usage in hospitals, and facilities for animal management [46,47]. This situation harms aquaculture in the face of bacterial resistance due to misuse or overuse of tetracycline in fish farming [48,49]. As a result, bacteria in water and fish pathogens might develop antibacterial resistance.

3.1. The Adverse Effects of Tetracycline on Algal and Plankton Communities

Tetracycline is harmful for algal communities, inhibiting growth of different algae in the concentration range 0.25–30 mg/L. It is not surprising that the higher the dose, the more profound are the effects. Such, 94% growth inhibition of mixed algae is observed at a concentration of 30 mg/L. Eukaryotic algae species are more vulnerable to tetracycline [50]. Freshwater green algae are sensitive both to tetracycline and its degradation products. According to Xu et al., exposure to tetracycline and its metabolites increases the permeability of algal cells and causes structural changes, including plasmolysis, starch granule deposition, deformation of the thylakoid lamellae in the chloroplasts, and enlargement of the vacuoles. These effects are more profound at higher tetracycline concentrations (>5 mg/L) [51]. The ability of tetracycline to impact the protein synthesis machinery stands behind these alterations [52].

Tetracycline also affects phytoplankton and zooplankton communities in a dose-dependent manner. These effects include reduction in abundance and species richness, which recover after exposure to tetracycline is discontinued. In addition, elevated concentrations of tetracycline decrease water clarity and lower levels of dissolved oxygen [53]. Tetracycline is capable of inducing the cyanobacterial bloom increasing the density of bacteria more than two-fold. The shift observed is in favor of *Synechococcus, Microcystis,* and *Oscillatoria* and against eukaryotic microalgae [54].

3.2. The Adverse Effects of Tetracycline on Fish Community

Apart from algae and plankton, tetracycline has many negative effects for the fish community, among which is embryotoxicity. Zebrafish (Danio rerio) have recently gained popularity as a potential animal model for research into the toxicity of various antibiotics, including tetracycline. Zhang et al. (2015) identified the toxic impact of tetracycline antibiotics on zebrafish embryos. It was stated that the drug could activate cell apoptosis by causing oxidative stress, which impedes the development of zebrafish embryos. Additionally, tetracycline induces caspase-dependent apoptosis in the early stages of zebrafish [55].

Oliveira et al. (2013) assessed the effects of tetracycline on zebrafish development and concluded that it causes delayed hatching of embryos [56]. According to Yu et al. (2020), prolonged exposure of zebrafish embryos to tetracycline at environmentally relevant concentrations causes elevated transcription of genes involved in thyroid synthesis, which might lead to thyroid dysfunction. Moreover, the authors reported that with an increase in exposure to tetracycline, zebrafish showed a decline in body length, weight, and BMI [57]. The sensitivity to tetracycline appears to vary depending on the developmental stage. Zebrafish embryos absorb more tetracycline at 3 days postfertilization than at 6 h postfertilization. Exposure to tetracycline at 0.4 mg/mL results in zebrafish death [58].

Jia et al. (2020) investigated the impact of tetracycline on aquatic culture. They conducted a study on the goldfish *Carassius auratus* (Linnaeus, 1758) treating them with tetracycline antibiotics at concentrations that are real to environmental conditions. This study discovered the negative impact of tetracycline on fish gut microbial flora. Jia identified the adverse effects of treatment with tetracycline on different *Aeromonas* species tolerance and changes in bacterial communications due to exposure to tetracycline. According to their results, tetracycline stress dramatically increased the resistance ratio in cultivated gut bacteria, and there was growth in antibiotic tolerance of *Aeromonas* species [59]. Coincidentally, there was a significant change in the structure of the gut microflora of goldfish and the abundance of antibacterial resistance genes, which can encode efflux of tetracycline antibiotics as a result of treatment with tetracycline [59].

Another dangerous effect of tetracycline on aquatic culture was found in the study of Yu et al. (2019). A study showed that tetracycline antibiotics cause antioxidative stress in fish organisms [60]. The stress response of an organism is protection caused by external stimuli in the face of variations in hormone levels, energy metabolism, motor control, and electrolyte balance [61]. For instance, in fish organisms, cortisol is one of the main significant stress indicators that can regulate the response to stress and glucose metabolism [62].

Yu et al. (2019) discovered that glucose, an energy source and intermediate of metabolism, was drastically decreased in zebrafish due to exposure to tetracycline, while significant alterations were not shown in cortisol levels. Consequently, it is assumed that fish require more energy sources to maintain the excessive level of reactive oxygen species (ROS) production by tetracycline antibiotics [60]. Treatment with tetracycline dramatically decreases glucose and NrF2 mRNA and protein levels in zebrafish larvae. Moreover, tetracycline molecules could dock with more stable hydrogen bonds into the binding pocket of PI3K of zebrafish larvae, an important protein that activates NrF2. In conclusion, tetracycline antibiotics could notably induce oxidative stress responses in zebrafish larvae. Additionally, tetracycline inhibits the activation of NrF2 and reduces the capacity of antioxidation by inhibiting the PI3K enzyme [60].

Another long-term effect of exposure to tetracycline is alterations in fish behavior. As Almeida et al. (2019) identified that exposure of zebrafish to low concentrations of tetracycline results in increased exploratory behavior. Interestingly, tetracycline treatment induced photosensibility that changed the swimming pattern of zebrafish. These effects were partially reversible after the exposure was discontinued [63]. Petersen et al. (2021) also reported alterations in zebrafish behavior following acute exposure to tetracycline. These changes included impaired locomotor activity, memory/learning processes, and proneness to aggressive behavior [64]. Several mechanisms could be proposed to explain alterations in fish behavior following tetracycline exposure. From one side, tetracycline leads to intestinal dysbiosis and this might influence the gut brain axis of fish. From the other side, prolonged exposure to tetracycline alters the levels of triiodothyronine and thyroid-stimulating hormone which might be the sign of the hypothalamus–pituitary–thyroid axis involvement. In addition, a decrease in cortisol levels is observed after tetracycline exposure, which impacts anxiety-related behaviors [65].

Concerning the above, it could be concluded that tetracycline pollution harms the aquatic environment and culture, affecting fish embryonic development and the gut microbiome, altering fish behavior, and causing oxidative stress. Tetracycline pollution negatively affects other aquatic organisms, apart from fish. Acute and chronic exposure to tetracycline may lead to an increased prevalence of diseases related to the digestive, nervous and immune systems of fish, which might also be influenced by the development of antibiotic resistance.

3.3. Development of Antibiotic Resistance in Bacteria

It was estimated that 90% of bacteria in the aquatic environment are resistant to at least one antibiotic and 20% are multi drug resistant [66]. Bacteria develop antibiotic resistance via molecular and genetic pathways. There are four well-defined mechanisms: efflux pumps, tetracycline-inactivating enzymes, ribosomal protection proteins and spontaneous mutations in target genes. Approximately 50 tetracycline-resistance genes are known up to now, which are typically encoded in plasmids and transposons (some tetracycline genes reside on chromosomes) and are passed from one species to another [67]. Once provoked, antibiotic resistance spreads rapidly among aquatic microbial populations eventually reaching human pathogens by means of horizontal gene transfer. This results in the appearance of resistant strains that are more difficult to treat with available antibiotics and increase in the occurrence of infectious diseases, which also tend to be more severe [68].

More research is needed to demonstrate a link between molecular events and physiological as well as pathological effects of tetracycline exposure in fish and other aquatic organisms. In addition, it is important to investigate the ability of aquatic organisms to recover from tetracycline exposure. Since the contamination of aquatic environments with antibiotics is likely to grow, there is a need to search for methods that can effectively remove them.

4. Effective Methods of Tetracycline Removal from the Aquatic Environment

As discussed above, tetracycline pollution has seriously threatened human health and the environment. Ineffective wastewater systems are one of the main reasons for the increased antibiotic concentrations in aquatic sources [69]. Moreover, Ahmad et al. (2021) state that oxidation of tetracycline is difficult in the environment due to its stable compound. Tetracycline can also be unstable at low pH because of their epi- and anhydrous-product formation, but it makes them less degradable due to their low volatility [30]. Another reason for the difficulty of tetracycline removal from water sources is because of its ability to form stable compounds by binding Ca^{2+} and other ions [70,71]. However, some methods can degrade tetracycline by breaking it down into small molecules with less harmful or nonhazardous effects.

A number of approaches have been developed for the degradation of pharmaceuticals from the aquatic environment. Thus, there is a range of traditional treatment methods used for removal purposes. These include biological, chemical and physical removal, such as membrane filtration, coagulation, prechlorination, adsorption, and flocculation [72]. These methods have many benefits but also drawbacks, including maintenance requirements and cost considerations [73].

4.1. Removal of Tetracycline by Adsorption

In general, adsorption of tetracycline is a relatively inexpensive and simple method. Adsorption techniques are increasingly used to remove organic particles from contaminated streams. Currently, various adsorbents are available, such as chitosan particles, graphene oxide, kaolinite, magnesium oxide, smectite clay, rectorite, aluminum oxide, palygorskite, coal humic acid, activated carbon, and others [74]. Accumulation of a contaminant from liquids/gases to the adsorbent surface is the nature of adsorption process. The efficiency of adsorption depends on the adsorbent properties, i.e., porosity (both at micro and macro levels), pore diameter, and specific surface area. For chemical adsorption, functional groups also play an important role. Several adsorption mechanisms participate in removal of antibiotics from liquid media: electrostatic attraction, pore-filling, partition into uncarbonized fractions, hydrophobic interaction, surface precipitation and formation of hydrogen bonds [75].

Yu et al. utilized oxidized multi-walled carbon nanotubes to remove tetracycline from water and found out that chemical properties of aqueous solution (ionic strength, pH, and the presence of Cu^{2+}) play an important role in tetracycline adsorption [76]. As the application of adsorbents for tetracycline removal generates waste, photodegradation or other techniques are commonly used for pollutants removal from adsorbents. Bhangi and Ray applied kappa-carrageenan and iron oxide nanoparticle-filled poly composite gel with subsequent photocatalytic degradation to remove tetracycline from water. The solution pH, dose of the polymer, and initial concentration of tetracycline strongly influenced the efficiency of tetracycline removal. High regeneration and recyclability were among the benefits of nanocomposite adsorbent [77].

Biochars are carbon-based adsorbents that have many advantages, such as low cost, large surface area and ease of regeneration. Natural biomasses, including solid wastes, could be used for their production. Biochars appear to be ideal adsorbents, owing to enriched surface functional groups. In most instances, biochars do not require additional activation processing, although it could be performed [75]. The interest in the application of biochars for tetracycline removal increased over the past decade reflecting intense research efforts. Seaweed biochar derived from *Sargassum species* was utilized by Song et al. to adsorb tetracycline from water. The uptake of tetracycline decreased with increasing pH and the removal efficiency of biochar regenerated in different solutions could be as high as 91.2% [78]. Shrimp shell waste can also be used for biochar production, as reported by Chang et al. This environmentally friendly adsorbent removes high concentrations of tetracycline very efficiently and the maximum adsorption capacity was 229.98 mg/g for 36 h at 55 °C [79]. Chitosan and its composites appear to be another attractive biochar that can be produced from seafood wastes by chitin extraction. It can be used alone or in combination with other adsorbents, such as carbon nanotubes and graphene oxide. Da Silva Bruckmann et al. investigated the utility of magnetic chitosan ($CS \cdot Fe_3O_4$) to remove tetracycline after several adsorption/desorption cycles. The authors concluded that adsorption capacity is influenced by several factors, such as initial concentration of tetracycline, adsorbent dosage, ionic strength, and pH [80]. However, translational studies are needed to evaluate the performance of adsorption methods in practical settings.

4.2. Removal of Tetracycline by Photodegradation

One of the methods of tetracycline removal is an advanced oxidative process (AOP). This process requires the reaction between hydroxyl radicals (•HO), which have high oxidative reactivity, and organic compounds [81]. These highly reactive hydroxyl radicals can be generated by hydrogen peroxide, ozone, and metal or semimetal catalysts. AOP can produce substrates with low toxicity and then mineralize them [82]. Advanced oxidation processes can be divided into techniques such as Fenton, ozonation, and UV photolysis, depending on the catalysts used and ultrasounds [83]. One of the effective oxidizing agents for tetracycline degradation is ozone. Ozone can react with tetracycline in protonated form by adding one oxygen atom at C11a-C12 and two oxygen atoms at C2-C3 [84]. Even though ozonation is considered to be effective for tetracycline removal, several factors, such as pH and TC concentration, might impact its efficacy. The study by Ahmad et al. (2021) suggests that the pH level has a crucial influence on the ozonation process. If the pH is low, then the hydroxyl group at ring I of tetracycline cannot be dissociated, which decreases electron densities in the C2-C3 locations. As a result of reduced electron densities, the possibility of ozone reacting with the C2-C3 position will decline [30,85]. Therefore, it will negatively affect the effectiveness of the degradation process.

Although tetracycline does not degrade under visible light, it can be degraded via exposure to ultraviolet irradiation at both 254 and 185 nm wavelengths. This approach enables disinfection and removal of other pollutants, apart from tetracycline. In general, exposure to 185 nm UV resulted in better degradation of tetracycline than exposure to 254 nm UV. This could be explained by the ability of 185 nm UV to cause the photodissociation of water molecules and direct photolysis [86]. As a result, highly reactive hydroxyl radicals are formed in elevated concentrations. Moreover, the presence of dissolved oxygen increases degradation rates by an additional 16%, which is probably associated with the increased formation of oxidative radical species. The combination of UV with hydrogen peroxide or Fe^{2+} also improves the degradation of tetracycline, as well as the combination with ozone and hydrogen peroxide [87]. Fortification of UV radiation by application of peroxomonosulfate or persulfate helps to increase the rate of tetracycline degradation. This is also associated with the generation of oxidative radical species (both hydroxyl radicals and SO_4^{2-}). The resulting removal efficiency may even exceed 80% [88]. Table 1 presents the effectiveness of adsorption and photodegradation methods in the removal of tetracycline from aquatic environments.

4.3. Removal of Tetracycline by Physico-Chemical Methods

Once physical and chemical methods proved to be successful in the removal of tetracycline from water and wastewater, it is reasonable to conclude that a combination of these methods will enable higher clearance. Sonolysis is a physico-chemical process and is an efficient method for the full mineralization of wastewater. This is a relatively new advanced oxidation process. Ultrasound and associated cavitation produce both physical and chemical effects. The chemical effects of ultrasound involve the generation of high temperature and pressure, which result in the formation of various oxidizing species, such as hydrogen, hydroxide, hydroperoxide, hydrogen peroxide, etc. These are very active oxidizing species that can instantly attack the organic molecules in the majority of refractory organic contaminants and destroy them. The physical effects of ultrasound mostly include intense mixing or convection in the medium, resulting in microstreaming [89].

Table 1. Studies on the effectiveness of adsorption and photodegradation methods in removal of tetracycline.

First Author, Year of Publication, Reference	Initial Concentration of Tetracycline	Matrix	Removal Method	Reported Effectiveness
Yu et al., 2014 [76]	7.3–151.6 mg/L^{-1}	Deionized water	Adsorption (Oxidized multi-walled carbon nanotubes)	The removal rate approximated 70% (at pH range of 3.3–8.0).
Bhangi and Ray, 2022 [77]	50–300 mg/L^{-1}	Deionized water	Adsorption and photocatalytic degradation by kappa-carrageenan and iron oxide nanoparticle-filled poly composite gel	The efficiency of photo-degradation was 86.1% after 2 hours.
Song et al., 2019 [78]	500 mg/L^{-1}	Deionized water	Adsorption (biochar derived from seaweed)	The removal efficiency ranged from 89.2 to 91.2%.
Chang et al., 2020 [79]	400 mg/L^{-1}	Deionized water	Adsorption (biochar derived from shrimp shell waste)	The maximum adsorption capacity was 229.98 mg/g for 36 h at 55 °C.
Da Silva Bruckmann et al., 2022 [80]	10–200 mg/L^{-1}	Deionized water	Adsorption (magnetic chitosan, CS·Fe_3O_4)	The highest adsorption capacity reached 211.21 mg/g^{-1} (at pH 7.0).
Dalmázio et al., 2007 [84]	52.8 mg/L^{-1}	Deionized water	Ozone/air gas stream	Almost complete degradation after 120 min.
Gulnaz et al., 2016 [85]	400 mg/L^{-1}	Deionized water	Ozone/air gas stream	Complete removal after 40 min.
Luu and Lee, 2014 [87]	20 mg/L^{-1}	Artificial wastewater	Ozone/ultraviolet, Ozone/hydrogen peroxide/ultraviolet	Complete removal.
Xu et al., 2020 [88]	18.22 g/L^{-1}	Natural water (tap water, Xincheng river and Taihu lake)	Ultraviolet C, Ultraviolet C/persulfate	The removal efficiency exceeded 80%.

Hou et al. (2016) reported their experience utilizing the coupled ultrasound/Fenton-like process to degrade tetracycline over an Fe_3O_4 catalyst. According to the study findings, the application of ultrasound considerably increased the catalyst's stability. After 60 min of treatment, 93.6% of tetracycline was eliminated under ideal circumstances [90]. Wang et al. (2011) used ultrasound-amplified catalytic ozonation by a goethite catalyst in an air-lift reactor. The authors reported a 100% removal of tetracycline, which was influenced by the high concentration of gaseous ozone (13.8 mg/L), increasing gas flow rate and power density (ultrasound frequency was 20 kHz and power was 250 W) [91].

Over the past decade, photocatalytic strategies for tetracycline removal have been extensively studied in combination with ultrasound. P25 titanium dioxide nanopowder was used to induce photocatalytic degradation with simultaneous application of hydrodynamic cavitation. The highest degradation of tetracycline was 78.2%, and the reaction time was 90 min [92]. Ghoreishian et al. (2019) reported sonophotocatalytic degradation of tetracycline with the help of reduced graphene oxide/cadmium tungstate composite hierarchical structures. The authors stated a complete degradation of tetracycline (the initial concentration was 13.54 mg/L). The overall time of ultrasound-assisted reaction equaled 1 h, and the catalyst loading was 0.216 g/L [93]. Heidari et al. (2018) used a composite photocatalytic material ($Bi_2Sn_2O_7$-C_3N_4/Y) for the degradation of tetracycline. The maximum rate of tetracycline degradation was 80.4%, and the concentration of $Bi_2Sn_2O_7$-C_3N_4/Y zeolite was 1 g/L with a reaction time equal to 90 min [94].

Although the above-described methods of physico-chemical removal of tetracycline have many advantages, primarily high effectiveness, they may also yield dangerous transformation byproducts. The photolysis technique is capable of producing even more toxic intermediates than tetracycline itself [95]. In addition, some of them pose high requirements for reagents or have increased energy demands. Therefore, the development of biological methods for tetracycline removal appears to be a promising approach. Table 2 summarizes the results of different studies on the effectiveness of physico-chemical methods used for tetracycline removal from aquatic environment.

Table 2. Studies on the effectiveness of physico-chemical methods in removal of tetracycline.

First Author, Year of Publication, Reference	Initial Concentration of Tetracycline	Matrix	Removal Method	Reported Effectiveness
Hou et al., 2016 [90]	100 mg/L^{-1}	Deionized water	Ultrasound/heterogeneous Fenton process	93.6% of tetracycline was removed after 60 min.
Wang et al., 2011 [91]	100 mg/L^{-1}	Deionized water	Ultrasound/goethite/ozone	Complete removal.
Wang et al., 2017 [92]	30 mg/L^{-1}	Deionized water	Photocatalysis/hydrodynamic cavitation	78.2% removal after 90 min.
Ghoreishian et al., 2019 [93]	13.54 mg/L^{-1}	Deionized water	Sonophotocatalysis	Complete removal (after 60 min).
Heidari et al., 2018 [94]	10–30 mg/L^{-1}	Deionized water	Sonophotocatalysis	80.4% degradation after 90 min.

4.4. Removal of Tetracycline by Biological Methods

Biodegradation and biosorption are two main biological methods used to remove antibiotics from the aquatic environment. Microbial metabolism and cometabolism are both a part of biodegradation. In microbial metabolism, microorganisms use antibiotics as carbon sources and energy substrates for their growth. Meanwhile, in the case of microbial cometabolism, antibiotics can be destroyed by homologous enzymes released by the microbial population. Biosorption applies to the removal of antibiotics by electrostatic and hydrophobic interactions [96].

Enzymes are frequently used for the treatment of various contaminants. They are characterized by mild reaction conditions, rapid reaction times, high efficiency, and minimal energy consumption [97]. It was demonstrated that horseradish peroxidase can remove 50% of tetracycline within 1 h [98]. Meanwhile, *Phanerochaete chrysosporium* expresses three key ligninolytic enzymes: lignin peroxidase, manganese peroxidase, and laccase. Sun et al. (2021) utilized manganese peroxidase from *Phanerochaete chrysosporium* to biodegrade tetracycline and showed that it can transform as much as 80% of tetracycline within 3 h [99]. Yang et al. (2017) developed a review on the potency of laccases to remove tetracycline [100]. According to Becker et al. (2016), the use of immobilized laccase from *Trametes versicolor* helped to remove >70% of tetracycline within 24 h [101]. Wen and Li (2009) used crude lignin peroxidase from *Phanerochaete chrysosporium* to biodegrade tetracycline. This enzyme can remove up to 95% of tetracycline within 5 min under optimal conditions [102].

There is a series of computational studies that model the ability of different enzymes to biodegrade antibiotics, including tetracycline. Currently, bioinformatics presents an economically viable way to predict the molecule's properties prior to experimental trials. For this purpose, molecular docking and molecular dynamics analyses are applied. Cárdenas-Moreno et al. (2019) modeled the interactions between laccases from *Ganoderma weberianum* and tetracycline. The root mean square deviation of the laccase-tetracycline interaction was 1.991. As lower values indicate higher similarity, it may be concluded that laccase can effectively bind to tetracycline [103].

Several mechanisms could be proposed to explain how microorganisms can remove tetracycline via biodegradation. Microorganisms can biodegrade tetracycline by opening loop structures and cutting functional groups, such as N-methyl, carbonyl, and amino groups [104–106]. Tetracycline is degraded by a range of microorganisms, including *Bacillus* sp., *Stenotrophomonas maltophilia, Klebsiella* sp., *Sphingobacterium* sp., *Trichosporon mycotoxinivorans, and Shewanella species* [107]. *Stenotrophomonas maltophilia* has been linked to a number of potential degradative pathways, and processes such as decarbonylation, denitromethylation, and deamination have all been identified [108]. Similarly, *Klebsiella* sp.

uses hydrolysis ring-opening, oxidation, deamination, decarbonylation, and demethylation reactions in the process of tetracycline degradation [109]. At the same time, *Trichosporon mycotoxinivorans* utilizes proton-transfer pathway reactions, dehydration, and epimerization as parts of the tetracycline breakdown process [30].

A novel method of wastewater treatment known as a membrane bioreactor (MBR) combines the conventional activated sludge process with membrane separation technology. According to Tran et al. (2016), MBRs can be implemented for treating wastewater for the removal of tetracycline. It was demonstrated that acclimated sludge from an MBR can degrade up to 40 mg tetracycline with 83.3–95.5% antibiotic removal compared to the conventional process with 44.3–87.6% efficiency [106]. Xu et al. (2019) showed that MBRs can remove more than 90% of tetracycline via both biodegradation and adsorption [110]. Sheng et al. (2018) proved that MBRs have high removal efficiency for tetracycline (87.6–100%) at environmentally relevant concentrations (1 mg/L). Nevertheless, it had inadequate removal at higher tetracycline concentrations (i.e., 10 mg/L) [111]. These data illustrate that tetracycline removal by membrane bioreactors is an effective option for wastewater treatment, but only if the concentration of tetracycline is relatively low.

On the basis of all the above stated, it might be concluded that there is a need for the continuous search and development of innovative methods of tetracycline removal from various aquatic environments. This will help to overcome the issue of environmental pollution caused by tetracycline and minimize the associated negative effects. The treatment of wastewater requires special attention. Table 3 summarizes the effectiveness of biological methods used for tetracycline removal.

Table 3. Studies on the effectiveness of biological methods in removal of tetracycline.

First Author, Year of Publication, Reference	Initial Concentration of Tetracycline	Matrix	Removal Method	Reported Effectiveness
Leng et al., 2020 [98]	0.13 mg/L^{-1}	Wastewater collected from the Tudhoe Mill Sewage Treatment Plant, UK	Enzymatic treatment with horseradish peroxidase, horseradish peroxidase/redox mediator	The mean degradation was 47.57% after 30 min and 67.90% after 8 h.
Sun et al., 2021 [99]	10–50, 100 mg/L^{-1}	Pure water	Enzymatic treatment with manganese peroxidase	The degradation rate was 80% (<50 mg L^{-1}) and 60% (≥50 mg L^{-1}).
Becker et al., 2016 [101]	10 mg/L^{-1}	Deionized water	Enzymatic treatment with fungal laccase	70% removal within 24 h.
Wen et al., 2009 [102]	50 mg/L^{-1}	High purity water	Enzymatic treatment with lignin peroxidase	95% removal after 5 min.
Tran et al., 2016 [106]	Median concentration 3604 ng/L^{-1}	Wastewater from a conventional wastewater treatment plant	Conventional activated sludge, membrane bioreactor	Membrane bioreactor removed 83.3–95.5% and conventional process had 44.3–87.6% efficiency.
Xu et al., 2019 [110]	1000 µg/L^{-1}	Wastewater from a conventional wastewater treatment plant	Membrane bioreactor	90% of tetracycline was removed.
Sheng et al., 2018 [111]	1, 10, 100 µg/L^{-1}; 1, 10 mg/L^{-1}	Activated sludge from a conventional wastewater treatment plant	Nitritation membrane bioreactor	The removal rate was 87.6–100% at low concentration (≤1 mg/L) but poor at higher concentration (≥10 mg/L).

5. Conclusions

Tetracycline is one of the most common antibiotics used for human and animal therapy in agriculture and aquaculture to promote growth. Globally, aquatic environments are polluted by tetracycline due to its widespread use and high stability. This promotes antibiotic resistance and necessitates development of novice antibacterial drugs. In addition, tetracycline has many toxic effects on aquatic organisms and breaks the equilibrium, causing dysbiosis. The negative effects of tetracycline are dose-dependent and there is a need for continuous monitoring of tetracycline pollution in different aquatic systems. A range of methods for tetracycline removal has been proposed and future research needs to focus on evaluation of their effectiveness in real world practice. Antibiotic pollution of wastewaters is another major concern. Biodegradation appears to be a promising method to solve this issue, yet a lot needs to be done before it becomes a routine approach in conventional wastewater treatment plants.

Author Contributions: Conceptualization, Y.A. and Y.S.; methodology, Y.A.; investigation, M.D.; resources, M.A.; data curation, G.B.; writing—original draft preparation, Y.A.; writing—review and editing, G.B.; visualization, G.B.; supervision, Y.A.; project administration, M.A.; funding acquisition, Y.A. All authors have read and agreed to the published version of the manuscript.

Funding: This research received no external funding.

Data Availability Statement: Not applicable.

Conflicts of Interest: The authors declare no conflict of interest.

References

1. Begum, S.; Begum, T.; Rahman, N.; Khan, R.A. A review on antibiotic resistance and way of combating antimicrobial resistance. *GSC Biol. Pharm. Sci.* **2021**, *14*, 87–97. [CrossRef]
2. Wang, B.; Zhang, Y.; Zhu, D.; Li, H. Assessment of bioavailability of biochar-sorbed tetracycline to escherichia coli for activation of antibiotic resistance genes. *Environ. Sci. Technol.* **2020**, *54*, 12920–12928. [CrossRef]
3. Cowieson, A.; Kluenter, A. Contribution of exogenous enzymes to potentiate the removal of antibiotic growth promoters in poultry production. *Anim. Feed Sci. Technol.* **2019**, *250*, 81–92. [CrossRef]
4. Han, Q.F.; Zhao, S.; Zhang, X.R.; Wang, X.L.; Song, C.; Wang, S.G. Distribution, combined pollution and risk assessment of antibiotics in typical marine aquaculture farms surrounding the Yellow Sea, North China. *Environ. Int.* **2020**, *138*, 105551. [CrossRef]
5. Adel, M.; Dadar, M.; Oliveri Conti, G. Antibiotics and malachite green residues in farmed rainbow trout (*Oncorhynchus mykiss*) from the Iranian markets: A risk assessment. *Int. J. Food Prop.* **2017**, *20*, 402–408. [CrossRef]
6. Scaria, J.; Anupama, K.; Nidheesh, P. Tetracyclines in the environment: An overview on the occurrence, fate, toxicity, detection, removal methods, and sludge management. *Sci. Total Environ.* **2021**, *771*, 145291. [CrossRef]
7. Klein, E.Y.; Van Boeckel, T.P.; Martinez, E.M.; Pant, S.; Gandra, S.; Levin, S.A.; Laxminarayan, R. Global increase and geographic convergence in antibiotic consumption between 2000 and 2015. *Proc. Natl. Acad. Sci. USA* **2018**, *115*, 3463–3470. [CrossRef] [PubMed]
8. Wencewicz, T.A. Crossroads of antibiotic resistance and biosynthesis. *J. Mol. Biol.* **2019**, *431*, 3370–3399. [CrossRef] [PubMed]
9. Greenfield, B.K.; Shaked, S.; Marrs, C.F.; Nelson, P.; Raxter, I.; Xi, C.; McKone, T.E.; Jolliet, O. Modeling the emergence of antibiotic resistance in the environment: An analytical solution for the minimum selection concentration. *Antimicrob. Agents Chemother.* **2018**, *62*, e01686-17. [CrossRef] [PubMed]
10. Grossman, T.H. Tetracycline antibiotics and resistance. *Cold Spring Harb. Perspect. Med.* **2016**, *6*, a025387. [CrossRef]
11. Nguyen, F.; Starosta, A.L.; Arenz, S.; Sohmen, D.; Dönhöfer, A.; Wilson, D.N. Tetracycline antibiotics and resistance mechanisms. *Biol. Chem.* **2014**, *395*, 559–575. [CrossRef] [PubMed]
12. Brodersen, D.E.; Clemons, W.M., Jr.; Carter, A.P.; Morgan-Warren, R.J.; Wimberly, B.T.; Ramakrishnan, V. The structural basis for the action of the antibiotics tetracycline, pactamycin, and hygromycin B on the 30s ribosomal subunit. *Cell* **2000**, *103*, 1143–1154. [CrossRef] [PubMed]
13. Fuoco, D. Classification framework and chemical biology of tetracycline-structure-based drugs. *Antibiotics* **2012**, *1*, 1–13. [CrossRef] [PubMed]
14. Chang, Q.; Wang, W.; Regev-Yochay, G.; Lipsitch, M.; Hanage, W.P. Antibiotics in agriculture and the risk to human health: How worried should we be? *Evol. Appl.* **2015**, *8*, 240–247. [CrossRef] [PubMed]
15. Lu, L.; Liu, J.; Li, Z.; Zou, X.; Guo, J.; Liu, Z.; Yang, J.; Zhou, Y. Antibiotic resistance gene abundances associated with heavy metals and antibiotics in the sediments of Changshou Lake in the three Gorges Reservoir area, China. *Ecol. Indic.* **2020**, *113*, 106275. [CrossRef]
16. Granados-Chinchilla, F.; Rodríguez, C. Tetracyclines in food and feedingstuffs: From regulation to analytical methods, bacterial resistance, and environmental and health implications. *J. Anal. Methods Chem.* **2017**, *2017*, 1–25. [CrossRef]
17. Leng, Y.; Xiao, H.; Li, Z.; Wang, J. Tetracyclines, sulfonamides and quinolones and their corresponding resistance genes in coastal areas of Beibu Gulf, China. *Sci. Total Environ.* **2020**, *714*, 136899. [CrossRef]
18. Monahan, C.; Harris, S.; Morris, D.; Cummins, E. A comparative risk ranking of antibiotic pollution from human and veterinary antibiotic usage–An Irish case study. *Sci. Total Environ.* **2022**, *826*, 154008. [CrossRef]

19. Dong, H.; Yuan, X.; Wang, W.; Qiang, Z. Occurrence and removal of antibiotics in ecological and conventional wastewater treatment processes: A field study. *J. Environ. Manag.* **2016**, *178*, 11–19. [CrossRef]
20. Kafaei, R.; Papari, F.; Seyedabadi, M.; Sahebi, S.; Tahmasebi, R.; Ahmadi, M.; Sorial, G.A.; Asgari, G.; Ramavandi, B. Occurrence, distribution, and potential sources of antibiotics pollution in the water-sediment of the northern coastline of the Persian Gulf, Iran. *Sci. Total Environ.* **2018**, *627*, 703–712. [CrossRef]
21. Javid, A.; Mesdaghinia, A.; Nasseri, S.; Mahvi, A.H.; Alimohammadi, M.; Gharibi, H. Assessment of tetracycline contamination in surface and groundwater resources proximal to animal farming houses in Tehran, Iran. *J. Environ. Health Sci. Eng.* **2016**, *14*, 4. [CrossRef]
22. Hong, P.Y.; Yannarell, A.; Mackie, R.I. The contribution of antibiotic residues and antibiotic resistance genes from livestock operations to antibiotic resistance in the environment and food chain. In *Zoonotic Pathogens in The Food Chain;* CABI: Wallingford, UK, 2011; pp. 119–139. [CrossRef]
23. Chen, Y.; Hu, C.; Deng, D.; Li, Y.; Luo, L. Factors affecting sorption behaviors of tetracycline to soils: Importance of soil organic carbon, pH and Cd contamination. *Ecotoxicol. Environ. Saf.* **2020**, *197*, 110572. [CrossRef] [PubMed]
24. Ding, C.; He, J. Effect of antibiotics in the environment on microbial populations. *Appl. Microbiol. Biotechnol.* **2010**, *87*, 925–941. [CrossRef] [PubMed]
25. Chen, W.R.; Huang, C.H. Transformation kinetics and pathways of tetracycline antibiotics with manganese oxide. *Environ. Pollut.* **2011**, *159*, 1092–1100. [CrossRef]
26. Wirtz, V.J.; Dreser, A.; Gonzales, R. Trends in antibiotic utilization in eight Latin American countries, 1997–2007. *Revista Panamericana de Salud Pública* **2010**, *27*, 219–225. [CrossRef]
27. Sanderson, H.; Ingerslev, F.; Brain, R.A.; Halling-Sorensen, B.; Bestari, J.K.; Wilson, C.J.; Johnson, D.J.; Solomon, K.R. Dissipation of oxytetracycline, chlortetracycline, tetracycline and doxycycline using HPLC-UV and LC/MS/MS under aquatic semi-field microcosm conditions. *Chemosphere* **2005**, *60*, 619–629. [CrossRef] [PubMed]
28. Xu, L.; Zhang, H.; Xiong, P.; Zhu, Q.; Liao, C.; Jiang, G. Occurrence, fate, and risk assessment of typical tetracycline antibiotics in the aquatic environment: A review. *Sci. Total Environ.* **2021**, *753*, 141975. [CrossRef]
29. Lundström, S.V.; Östman, M.; Bengtsson-Palme, J.; Rutgersson, C.; Thoudal, M.; Sircar, T.; Blanck, H.; Eriksson, K.M.; Tysklind, M.; Flach, C.F. Minimal selective concentrations of tetracycline in complex aquatic bacterial biofilms. *Sci. Total Environ.* **2016**, *553*, 587–595. [CrossRef]
30. Ahmad, F.; Zhu, D.; Sun, J. Environmental fate of tetracycline antibiotics: Degradation pathway mechanisms, challenges, and perspectives. *Environ. Sci. Eur.* **2021**, *33*, 64. [CrossRef]
31. Van Boeckel, T.P.; Brower, C.; Gilbert, M.; Grenfell, B.T.; Levin, S.A.; Robinson, T.P.; Laxminarayan, R. Global trends in antimicrobial use in food animals. *Proc. Natl. Acad. Sci. USA* **2015**, *112*, 5649–5654. [CrossRef]
32. Mu, Q.; Li, J.; Sun, Y.; Mao, D.; Wang, Q.; Luo, Y. Occurrence of sulfonamide-, tetracycline-, plasmid-mediated quinolone-and macrolide-resistance genes in livestock feedlots in Northern China. *Env. Sci. Pollut. Res.* **2015**, *22*, 6932–6940. [CrossRef] [PubMed]
33. Woźniak-Biel, A.; Bugla-Płoskońska, G.; Kielsznia, A.; Korzekwa, K.; Tobiasz, A.; Korzeniowska-Kowal, A.; Wieliczko, A. High prevalence of resistance to fluoroquinolones and tetracycline *Campylobacter* spp. isolated from poultry in Poland. *Microb. Drug Resist.* **2018**, *24*, 314–322. [CrossRef] [PubMed]
34. Pena-Ortiz, M. *Linking Aquatic Biodiversity Loss to Animal Product Consumption: A Review*; MSc Biological Sciences, University of Amsterdam: Amsterdam, The Netherlands, 2021.
35. Mahamallik, P.; Saha, S.; Pal, A. Tetracycline degradation in aquatic environment by highly porous MnO_2 nanosheet assembly. *Chem. Eng. J.* **2015**, *276*, 155–165. [CrossRef]
36. Daghrir, R.; Drogui, P. Tetracycline antibiotics in the environment: A review. *Environ. Chem. Lett.* **2013**, *11*, 209–227. [CrossRef]
37. Paramonov, S.; Zelikova, D.; Sklyarova, L.; Alkhutova, I. Environmental risks of micro-contamination of the environment with tetracycline. *Pharm. Formulas* **2022**, *4*, 76–88. [CrossRef]
38. Zhang, Q.Q.; Ying, G.G.; Pan, C.G.; Liu, Y.S.; Zhao, J.L. Comprehensive evaluation of antibiotics emission and fate in the river basins of China: Source analysis, multimedia modeling, and linkage to bacterial resistance. *Environ. Sci. Technol.* **2015**, *49*, 6772–6782. [CrossRef] [PubMed]
39. Kim, K.R.; Owens, G.; Kwon, S.I.; So, K.H.; Lee, D.B.; Ok, Y.S. Occurrence and environmental fate of veterinary antibiotics in the terrestrial environment. *Water Air Soil Pollut.* **2011**, *214*, 163–174. [CrossRef]
40. Chen, A.; Chen, Y.; Ding, C.; Liang, H.; Yang, B. Effects of tetracycline on simultaneous biological wastewater nitrogen and phosphorus removal. *RSC Adv.* **2015**, *5*, 59326–59334. [CrossRef]
41. Zhao, Y.; Gu, X.; Gao, S.; Geng, J.; Wang, X. Adsorption of tetracycline (TC) onto montmorillonite: Cations and humic acid effects. *Geoderma* **2012**, *183*, 12–18. [CrossRef]
42. Azanu, D.; Styrishave, B.; Darko, G.; Weisser, J.J.; Abaidoo, R.C. Occurrence and risk assessment of antibiotics in water and lettuce in Ghana. *Sci. Total Environ.* **2018**, *622*, 293–305. [CrossRef]
43. Zhang, R.; Tang, J.; Li, J.; Cheng, Z.; Chaemfa, C.; Liu, D.; Zhang, G. Occurrence and risks of antibiotics in the coastal aquatic environment of the Yellow Sea, North China. *Sci. Total Environ.* **2013**, *450*, 197–204. [CrossRef]
44. Tang, J.; Wang, S.; Fan, J.; Long, S.; Wang, L.; Tang, C.; Yang, Y. Predicting distribution coefficients for antibiotics in a river water-sediment using quantitative models based on their spatiotemporal variations. *Sci. Total Environ.* **2019**, *655*, 1301–1310. [CrossRef]

45. Cabello, F.C.; Godfrey, H.P.; Tomova, A.; Ivanova, L.; Dölz, H.; Millanao, A.; Buschmann, A.H. Antimicrobial use in aquaculture re-examined: Its relevance to antimicrobial resistance and to animal and human health. *Environ. Microbiol.* **2013**, *15*, 1917–1942. [CrossRef]
46. Burke, V.; Richter, D.; Greskowiak, J.; Mehrtens, A.; Schulz, L.; Massmann, G. Occurrence of antibiotics in surface and groundwater of a drinking water catchment area in Germany. *Water Environ. Res.* **2016**, *88*, 652–659. [CrossRef] [PubMed]
47. Hou, J.; Wang, C.; Mao, D.; Luo, Y. The occurrence and fate of tetracyclines in two pharmaceutical wastewater treatment plants of Northern China. *Environ. Sci. Pollut. Res.* **2016**, *23*, 1722–1731. [CrossRef]
48. Xiong, W.; Sun, Y.; Zhang, T.; Ding, X.; Li, Y.; Wang, M.; Zeng, Z. Antibiotics, antibiotic resistance genes, and bacterial community composition in fresh water aquaculture environment in China. *Microb. Ecol.* **2015**, *70*, 425–432. [CrossRef]
49. Cheng, W.; Li, J.; Wu, Y.; Xu, L.; Su, C.; Qian, Y.; Chen, H. Behavior of antibiotics and antibiotic resistance genes in eco-agricultural system: A case study. *J. Hazard. Mater.* **2016**, *304*, 18–25. [CrossRef]
50. Taşkan, E. Effect of tetracycline antibiotics on performance and microbial community of algal photo-bioreactor. *Appl. Biochem. Biotechnol.* **2016**, *179*, 947–958. [CrossRef]
51. Xu, D.; Xiao, Y.; Pan, H.; Mei, Y. Toxic effects of tetracycline and its degradation products on freshwater green algae. *Ecotoxicol. Environ. Saf.* **2019**, *174*, 43–47. [CrossRef] [PubMed]
52. Bashir, K.M.I.; Cho, M.G. The effect of kanamycin and tetracycline on growth and photosynthetic activity of two chlorophyte algae. *BioMed Res. Int.* **2016**, *2016*, 5656304. [CrossRef] [PubMed]
53. Wilson, C.J.; Brain, R.A.; Sanderson, H.; Johnson, D.J.; Bestari, K.T.; Sibley, P.K.; Solomon, K.R. Structural and functional responses of plankton to a mixture of four tetracyclines in aquatic microcosms. *Environ. Sci. Technol.* **2004**, *38*, 6430–6439. [CrossRef] [PubMed]
54. Xu, S.; Jiang, Y.; Liu, Y.; Zhang, J. Antibiotic-accelerated cyanobacterial growth and aquatic community succession towards the formation of cyanobacterial bloom in eutrophic lake water. *Environ. Pollut.* **2021**, *290*, 118057. [CrossRef] [PubMed]
55. Zhang, Q.; Cheng, J.; Xin, Q. Effects of tetracycline on developmental toxicity and molecular responses in zebrafish (*Danio rerio*) embryos. *Ecotoxicology* **2015**, *24*, 707–719. [CrossRef] [PubMed]
56. Oliveira, R.; McDonough, S.; Ladewig, J.C.; Soares, A.M.; Nogueira, A.J.; Domingues, I. Effects of oxytetracycline and amoxicillin on development and biomarkers activities of zebrafish (*Danio rerio*). *Environ. Toxicol. Pharmacol.* **2013**, *36*, 903–912. [CrossRef]
57. Yu, K.; Li, X.; Qiu, Y.; Zeng, X.; Yu, X.; Wang, W.; Yi, X.; Huang, L. Low-dose effects on thyroid disruption in zebrafish by long-term exposure to oxytetracycline. *Aquat. Toxicol.* **2020**, *227*, 105608. [CrossRef]
58. Zhang, F.; Qin, W.; Zhang, J.P.; Hu, C.Q. Antibiotic toxicity and absorption in zebrafish using liquid chromatography-tandem mass spectrometry. *PLoS ONE* **2015**, *10*, e0124805. [CrossRef]
59. Jia, J.; Cheng, M.; Xue, X.; Guan, Y.; Wang, Z. Characterization of tetracycline effects on microbial community, antibiotic resistance genes and antibiotic resistance of *Aeromonas* spp. in gut of goldfish *Carassius auratus* Linnaeus. *Ecotoxicol. Environ. Saf.* **2020**, *191*, 110182. [CrossRef]
60. Yu, X.; Wu, Y.; Deng, M.; Liu, Y.; Wang, S.; He, X.; Allaire-Leung, M.; Wan, J.; Zou, Y.; Yang, C. Tetracycline antibiotics as PI3K inhibitors in the Nrf2-mediated regulation of antioxidative stress in zebrafish larvae. *Chemosphere* **2019**, *226*, 696–703. [CrossRef]
61. Urbinati, E.C.; de Abreu, J.S.; da Silva Camargo, A.C.; Parra, M.A.L. Loading and transport stress of juvenile matrinxã (*Brycon cephalus*, Characidae) at various densities. *Aquaculture* **2004**, *229*, 389–400. [CrossRef]
62. Strange, R.J.; Schreck, C.B. Anesthetic and handling stress on survival and cortisol concentration in yearling chinook salmon (*Oncorhynchus tshawytscha*). *J. Fish. Board Can.* **1978**, *35*, 345–349. [CrossRef]
63. Almeida, A.R.; Domingues, I.; Henriques, I. Zebrafish and water microbiome recovery after oxytetracycline exposure. *Environ. Pollut.* **2021**, *272*, 116371. [CrossRef]
64. Petersen, B.D.; Pereira, T.C.B.; Altenhofen, S.; Nabinger, D.D.; Ferreira, P.M.D.A.; Bogo, M.R.; Bonan, C.D. Antibiotic drugs alter zebrafish behavior. *Comp. Biochem. Physiol. Part C Toxicol. Pharmacol.* **2021**, *242*, 108936. [CrossRef]
65. Gusso, D.; Altenhofen, S.; Fritsch, P.M.; Rübensam, G.; Bonan, C.D. Oxytetracycline induces anxiety-like behavior in adult zebrafish. *Toxicol. Appl. Pharmacol.* **2021**, *426*, 115616. [CrossRef]
66. Lin, J.; Nishino, K.; Roberts, M.C.; Tolmasky, M.; Aminov, R.I.; Zhang, L. Mechanisms of antibiotic resistance. *Front. Microbiol.* **2015**, *6*, 34. [CrossRef] [PubMed]
67. Schnabel, E.L.; Jones, A.L. Distribution of tetracycline resistance genes and transposons among phylloplane bacteria in Michigan apple orchards. *Appl. Environ. Microbiol.* **1999**, *65*, 4898–4907. [CrossRef] [PubMed]
68. Pepi, M.; Focardi, S. Antibiotic-resistant bacteria in aquaculture and climate change: A challenge for health in the Mediterranean Area. *Int. J. Environ. Res. Public Health* **2021**, *18*, 5723. [CrossRef] [PubMed]
69. Tran, N.H.; Gin, K.Y.H. Occurrence and removal of pharmaceuticals, hormones, personal care products, and endocrine disrupters in a full-scale water reclamation plant. *Sci. Total Environ.* **2017**, *599*, 1503–1516. [CrossRef] [PubMed]
70. Gao, P.; Ding, Y.; Li, H.; Xagoraraki, I. Occurrence of pharmaceuticals in a municipal wastewater treatment plant: Mass balance and removal processes. *Chemosphere* **2012**, *88*, 17–24. [CrossRef] [PubMed]
71. Li, B.; Zhang, T. Biodegradation and adsorption of antibiotics in the activated sludge process. *Environ. Sci. Technol.* **2010**, *44*, 3468–3473. [CrossRef] [PubMed]
72. Smol, M.; Włodarczyk-Makuła, M. The Effectiveness in the Removal of PAHs from Aqueous Solutions in Physical and Chemical Processes: A Review. *Polycycl. Aromat. Compd.* **2007**, *37*, 292–313. [CrossRef]

73. Tian, W.J.; Bai, J.; Liu, K.K.; Sun, H.M.; Zhao, Y.G. Occurrence and removal of polycyclic aromatic hydrocarbons in the wastewater treatment process. *Ecotoxicol. Environ. Saf.* **2012**, *82*, 1–7. [CrossRef]
74. Krakko, D.; Heieren, B.T.; Illes, A.; Kvamme, K.; Dóbé, S.; Záray, G. (V)UV degradation of the antibiotic tetracycline: Kinetics, transformation products and pathway. *Process Saf. Environ. Prot.* **2022**, *163*, 395–404. [CrossRef]
75. Ahmed, M.B.; Zhou, J.L.; Ngo, H.H.; Guo, W. Adsorptive removal of antibiotics from water and wastewater: Progress and challenges. *Sci. Total Environ.* **2015**, *532*, 112–126. [CrossRef] [PubMed]
76. Yu, F.; Ma, J.; Han, S. Adsorption of tetracycline from aqueous solutions onto multi-walled carbon nanotubes with different oxygen contents. *Sci. Rep.* **2014**, *4*, 5326. [CrossRef] [PubMed]
77. Bhangi, B.K.; Ray, S. Adsorption and photocatalytic degradation of tetracycline from water by kappa-carrageenan and iron oxide nanoparticle-filled poly (acrylonitrile-co-N-vinyl pyrrolidone) composite gel. *Polym. Eng. Sci.* **2022**, *2022*, 1–18. [CrossRef]
78. Song, G.; Guo, Y.; Li, G.; Zhao, W.; Yu, Y. Comparison for adsorption of tetracycline and cefradine using biochar derived from seaweed *Sargassum* sp. *Desalination Water Treat.* **2019**, *160*, 316–324. [CrossRef]
79. Chang, J.; Shen, Z.; Hu, X.; Schulman, E.; Cui, C.; Guo, Q.; Tian, H. Adsorption of tetracycline by shrimp shell waste from aqueous solutions: Adsorption isotherm, kinetics modeling, and mechanism. *ACS Omega* **2020**, *5*, 3467–3477. [CrossRef]
80. da Silva Bruckmann, F.; Schnorr, C.E.; da Rosa Salles, T.; Nunes, F.B.; Baumann, L.; Müller, E.I.; Bohn Rhoden, C.R. Highly efficient adsorption of tetracycline using chitosan-based magnetic adsorbent. *Polymers* **2022**, *14*, 4854. [CrossRef]
81. Wang, J.L.; Xu, L.J. Advanced oxidation processes for wastewater treatment: Formation of hydroxyl radical and application. *Crit. Rev. Environ. Sci. Technol.* **2012**, *42*, 251–325. [CrossRef]
82. Deng, Y.; Zhao, R. Advanced oxidation processes (AOPs) in wastewater treatment. *Curr. Pollut. Rep.* **2015**, *1*, 167–176. [CrossRef]
83. Klavarioti, M.; Mantzavinos, D.; Kassinos, D. Removal of residual pharmaceuticals from aqueous systems by advanced oxidation processes. *Environ. Int.* **2009**, *35*, 402–417. [CrossRef] [PubMed]
84. Dalmázio, I.; Almeida, M.O.; Augusti, R.; Alves, T. Monitoring the degradation of tetracycline by ozone in aqueous medium via atmospheric pressure ionization mass spectrometry. *J. Am. Soc. Mass Spectrom.* **2007**, *18*, 679–687. [CrossRef] [PubMed]
85. Gulnaz, O.; Sezer, G. Ozonolytic degradation of tetracycline antibiotic: Effect of PH. *Fresenius Environ. Bull.* **2016**, *25*, 2928–2934.
86. Krakkó, D.; Illés, Á.; Domján, A.; Demeter, A.; Dóbé, S.; Záray, G. UV and (V) UV irradiation of sitagliptin in ultrapure water and WWTP effluent: Kinetics, transformation products and degradation pathway. *Chemosphere* **2022**, *288*, 132393. [CrossRef] [PubMed]
87. Luu, H.T.; Lee, K. Degradation and changes in toxicity and biodegradability of tetracycline during ozone/ultraviolet-based advanced oxidation. *Water Sci. Technol.* **2014**, *70*, 1229–1235. [CrossRef] [PubMed]
88. Xu, M.; Deng, J.; Cai, A.; Ma, X.; Li, J.; Li, Q.; Li, X. Comparison of UVC and UVC/persulfate processes for tetracycline removal in water. *Chem. Eng. J.* **2020**, *384*, 123320. [CrossRef]
89. de Andrade, F.V.; Augusti, R.; de Lima, G.M. Ultrasound for the remediation of contaminated waters with persistent organic pollutants: A short review. *Ultrason. Sonochem.* **2021**, *78*, 105719. [CrossRef]
90. Hou, L.; Wang, L.; Royer, S.; Zhang, H. Ultrasound-assisted heterogeneous Fenton-like degradation of tetracycline over a magnetite catalyst. *J. Hazard. Mater.* **2016**, *302*, 458–467. [CrossRef]
91. Wang, Y.; Zhang, H.; Chen, L. Ultrasound enhanced catalytic ozonation of tetracycline in a rectangular air-lift reactor. *Catal. Today* **2011**, *175*, 283–292. [CrossRef]
92. Wang, X.; Jia, J.; Wang, Y. Combination of photocatalysis with hydrodynamic cavitation for degradation of tetracycline. *Chem. Eng. J.* **2017**, *315*, 274–282. [CrossRef]
93. Ghoreishian, S.M.; Raju, G.S.R.; Pavitra, E.; Kwak, C.H.; Han, Y.K.; Huh, Y.S. Ultrasound-assisted heterogeneous degradation of tetracycline over flower-like rGO/CdWO4 hierarchical structures as robust solar-light-responsive photocatalysts: Optimization, kinetics, and mechanism. *Appl. Surf. Sci.* **2019**, *489*, 110–122. [CrossRef]
94. Heidari, S.; Haghighi, M.; Shabani, M. Ultrasound assisted dispersion of $Bi_2Sn_2O_7$-C_3N_4 nanophotocatalyst over various amount of zeolite Y for enhanced solar-light photocatalytic degradation of tetracycline in aqueous solution. *Ultrason. Sonochem.* **2018**, *43*, 61–72. [CrossRef] [PubMed]
95. Sun, K.; Huang, Q.; Li, S. Transformation and toxicity evaluation of tetracycline in humic acid solution by laccase coupled with 1-hydroxybenzotriazole. *J. Hazard. Mater.* **2017**, *331*, 182–188. [CrossRef]
96. Huang, S.; Yu, J.; Li, C.; Zhu, Q.; Zhang, Y.; Lichtfouse, E.; Marmier, N. The effect review of various biological, physical and chemical methods on the removal of antibiotics. *Water* **2022**, *14*, 3138. [CrossRef]
97. Duran, N.; Esposito, E. Potential applications of oxidative enzymes and phenoloxidase-like compounds in wastewater and soil treatment: A review. *Appl. Catal. B Environ.* **2000**, *28*, 83–99. [CrossRef]
98. Leng, Y.; Bao, J.; Xiao, H.; Song, D.; Du, J.; Mohapatra, S.; Wang, J. Transformation mechanisms of tetracycline by horseradish peroxidase with/without redox mediator ABTS for variable water chemistry. *Chemosphere* **2020**, *258*, 1–10. [CrossRef]
99. Sun, X.; Leng, Y.; Wan, D.; Chang, F.; Huang, Y.; Li, Z.; Wang, J. Transformation of tetracycline by manganese peroxidase from *phanerochaete chrysosporium*. *Molecules* **2021**, *26*, 6803. [CrossRef]
100. Yang, J.; Li, W.; Ng, T.B.; Deng, X.; Lin, J.; Ye, X. Laccases: Production, expression regulation, and applications in pharmaceutical biodegradation. *Front. Microbiol.* **2017**, *8*, 832. [CrossRef]

101. Becker, D.; Della Giustina, S.V.; Rodriguez-Mozaz, S.; Schoevaart, R.; Barceló, D.; de Cazes, M.; Belleville, M.P.; Sanchez-Marcano, J.; de Gunzburg, J.; Couillerot, O.; et al. Removal of antibiotics in wastewater by enzymatic treatment with fungal laccase—Egradation of compounds does not always eliminate toxicity. *Bioresour. Technol.* **2016**, *219*, 500–509. [CrossRef]
102. Wen, X.; Jia, Y.; Li, J. Degradation of tetracycline and oxytetracycline by crude lignin peroxidase prepared from *Phanerochaete chrysosporium*—A white rot fungus. *Chemosphere* **2009**, *75*, 1003–1007. [CrossRef]
103. Cárdenas-Moreno, Y.; Espinosa, L.A.; Vieyto, J.C.; González-Durruthy, M.; del Monte-Martinez, A.; Guerra-Rivera, G.; Sánchez López, M.I. Theoretical study on binding interactions of laccase-enzyme from *Ganoderma weberianum* with multiples ligand substrates with environmental impact. *Ann. Proteom. Bioinform.* **2019**, *3*, 001–009.
104. Yin, Z.; Xia, D.; Shen, M.; Zhu, D.; Cai, H.; Wu, M.; Kang, Y. Tetracycline degradation by *Klebsiella* sp. strain TR5: Proposed degradation pathway and possible genes involved. *Chemosphere* **2020**, *253*, 126729. [CrossRef] [PubMed]
105. Leng, Y.; Bao, J.; Chang, G.; Zheng, H.; Li, X.; Du, J.; Li, X. Biotransformation of tetracycline by a novel bacterial strain *Stenotrophomonas maltophilia* DT1. *J. Hazard. Mater.* **2016**, *318*, 125–133. [CrossRef] [PubMed]
106. Tran, N.H.; Chen, H.; Reinhard, M.; Mao, F.; Gin, K.Y.H. Occurrence and removal of multiple classes of antibiotics and antimicrobial agents in biological wastewater treatment processes. *Water Res.* **2016**, *104*, 461–472. [CrossRef]
107. Shao, S.; Wu, X. Microbial degradation of tetracycline in the aquatic environment: A review. *Crit. Rev. Biotechnol.* **2020**, *40*, 1010–1018. [CrossRef]
108. Kumar, M.; Jaiswal, S.; Sodhi, K.K.; Shree, P.; Singh, D.K.; Agrawal, P.K.; Shukla, P. Antibiotics bioremediation: Perspectives on its ecotoxicity and resistance. *Environ. Int.* **2019**, *124*, 448–461. [CrossRef]
109. Zhong, S.F.; Yang, B.; Xiong, Q.; Cai, W.W.; Lan, Z.G.; Ying, G.G. Hydrolytic transformation mechanism of tetracycline antibiotics: Reaction kinetics, products identification and determination in WWTPs. *Ecotoxicol. Environ. Saf.* **2022**, *229*, 113063. [CrossRef]
110. Xu, R.; Wu, Z.; Zhou, Z.; Meng, F. Removal of sulfadiazine and tetracycline in membrane bioreactors: Linking pathway to microbial community shift. *Environ. Technol.* **2019**, *40*, 134–143. [CrossRef] [PubMed]
111. Sheng, B.; Cong, H.; Zhang, S.; Meng, F. Interactive effects between tetracycline and nitrosifying sludge microbiota in a nitritation membrane bioreactor. *Chem. Eng. J.* **2018**, *341*, 556–564. [CrossRef]

antibiotics

MDPI

Article

Molecular Typing Reveals Environmental Dispersion of Antibiotic-Resistant Enterococci under Anthropogenic Pressure

Anca Farkas [1,2,*], Cristian Coman [3], Edina Szekeres [1,3], Adela Teban-Man [3,4], Rahela Carpa [1,2] and Anca Butiuc-Keul [1,2]

1 Department of Molecular Biology and Biotechnology, Faculty of Biology and Geology, Babeș-Bolyai University, 1 M. Kogălniceanu Street, 400084 Cluj-Napoca, Romania
2 Centre for Systems Biology, Biodiversity and Bioresources, Babeș-Bolyai University, 5–7 Clinicilor Street, 400006 Cluj-Napoca, Romania
3 National Institute of Research and Development for Biological Sciences (NIRDBS), Institute of Biological Research, 48 Republicii Street, 400015 Cluj-Napoca, Romania
4 Department of Taxonomy and Ecology, Faculty of Biology and Geology, Babeș-Bolyai University, 1 M. Kogălniceanu Street, 400084 Cluj-Napoca, Romania
* Correspondence: ancuta.farkas@ubbcluj.ro

Abstract: As a consequence of global demographic challenges, both the artificial and the natural environment are increasingly impacted by contaminants of emerging concern, such as bacterial pathogens and their antibiotic resistance genes (ARGs). The aim of this study was to determine the extent to which anthropogenic contamination contributes to the spread of antibiotic resistant enterococci in aquatic compartments and to explore genetic relationships among *Enterococcus* strains. Antimicrobial susceptibility testing (ampicillin, imipenem, norfloxacin, gentamycin, vancomycin, erythromycin, tetracycline, trimethoprim-sulfamethoxazole) of 574 isolates showed different rates of phenotypic resistance in bacteria from wastewaters (91.9–94.4%), hospital effluents (73.9%), surface waters (8.2–55.3%) and groundwater (35.1–59.1%). The level of multidrug resistance reached 44.6% in enterococci from hospital effluents. In all samples, except for hospital sewage, the predominant species were *E. faecium* and *E. faecalis*. In addition, *E. avium*, *E. durans*, *E. gallinarum*, *E. aquimarinus* and *E. casseliflavus* were identified. *Enterococcus faecium* strains carried the greatest variety of ARGs (*bla*$_{TEM-1}$, *aac(6′)-Ie-aph(2″)*, *aac(6′)-Im*, *vanA*, *vanB*, *ermB*, *mefA*, *tetB*, *tetC*, *tetL*, *tetM*, *sul1*), while *E. avium* displayed the highest ARG frequency. Molecular typing using the ERIC2 primer revealed substantial genetic heterogeneity, but also clusters of enterococci from different aquatic compartments. Enterococcal migration under anthropogenic pressure leads to the dispersion of clinically relevant strains into the natural environment and water resources. In conclusion, ERIC-PCR fingerprinting in conjunction with ARG profiling is a useful tool for the molecular typing of clinical and environmental *Enterococcus* species. These results underline the need of safeguarding water quality as a strategy to limit the expansion and progression of the impending antibiotic-resistance crisis.

Keywords: antimicrobial resistance; ERIC-PCR; *Enterococcus avium*; *Enterococcus faecalis*; *Enterococcus faecium*; hospital; wastewater; freshwater

Citation: Farkas, A.; Coman, C.; Szekeres, E.; Teban-Man, A.; Carpa, R.; Butiuc-Keul, A. Molecular Typing Reveals Environmental Dispersion of Antibiotic-Resistant Enterococci under Anthropogenic Pressure. *Antibiotics* **2022**, *11*, 1213. https://doi.org/10.3390/antibiotics11091213

Academic Editor: Akebe Luther King Abia

Received: 6 August 2022
Accepted: 5 September 2022
Published: 7 September 2022

1. Introduction

Today, more than half of the world's population lives in urban areas, a proportion expected to increase to 68% by 2050, according to the United Nations (https://www.un.org/, accessed on 31 July 2022). Not only are the cities themselves expected to be highly impacted by excessive anthropogenic pressure, but also the surrounding environments. The urban–rural lifestyle in metropolitan areas is a developing phenomenon, concerning the essential human activities and services, as well as recreation and leisure. As a consequence of global demographic challenges, both the artificial and the natural environment are increasingly affected by contaminants of emerging concern. The quality of water resources is vulnerable to a wide range of microbial pollutants, such as bacterial pathogens and their antibiotic-resistance genes (ARGs).

Aquatic environments are an ideal setting for the acquisition and dissemination of antimicrobial resistance, and human exposure to antibiotic-resistant bacteria and ARGs through water may pose an additional health risk [1]. *Enterococcus* species have frequently been described as carriers of antibiotic resistance across the One-Health continuum. Hospital effluents [2], untreated sewage [3] and raw manure [4] have been identified as the main hotspots for antibiotic-resistant enterococci and sources for their environmental spread. Following contamination events, enterococci can persist for long periods of time in different environmental matrices [5,6]. *Enterococcus* bacteria are all the more dangerous as potential vectors for antimicrobial resistance when escaping wastewater treatment. They pose a constant microbiological risk in surface waters that receive treated wastewaters [3,7] and continue to spread further downstream. Antibiotic-resistant enterococci have entered the groundwater environment, being isolated from untreated drinking water springs and wells [8,9], alluvial groundwater [10] and karst aquifers [11].

Enterococci are Gram-positive bacteria belonging to the phylum *Bacillota* (synonym Firmicutes), *Bacilli* class, *Lactobacillales* order, *Enterococcaceae* family. About 58 *Enterococcus* species have been recognized so far [12]. Molecular clock estimation, together with analysis of their ecology and phenotypic diversity placed the origins of the *Enterococcus* genus 500 million years ago, around the time of animal terrestrialization. Speciation occurred along with the diversification of hosts [13], enterococci being regarded as typically commensal bacteria for a long time. Essential members of animal microbiomes, they colonize mainly the digestive and urinary tracts. In humans, enterococci are found in concentrations of approximately 10^6 to 10^7 in the intestine (up to 1% of the colon microbiota) [14]. The most frequent *Enterococcus* species in human gastrointestinal tract are *E. faecalis* and *E. faecium*, followed by *E. casseliflavus* and *E. gallinarum* [15], along with *E. durans*, *E. hirae*, *E. avium* and *E. caccae*, which are less common [16].

From an evolutionary perspective, coevolution between bacteria and animals has selected intrinsic properties in enterococci, conferring them abilities to evade host defenses, compete in the intestinal tract, persist and spread in the environment. Remarkably resilient organisms, they are able to adapt to a broad range of pH, salinity and temperatures, survive sunlight exposure, desiccation, nutrient starvation, disinfection [13,17,18], microgravity and increased cosmic radiation [19]. Therefore, enterococci are able to disseminate into the environment and survive outside the animal body, being widely used as fecal indicators in water quality monitoring. The main sources of enterococci in natural environments include sewage, agricultural and urban runoff, animal manure, wildlife waste and bather shedding. During water quality monitoring, intestinal enterococci have been found in biofilms, even in drinking water systems providing safe tap water [20]. *Enterococcus* species are able to persist in stable microcolonies for long periods of time, entering a viable nonculturable state [21]. Even with the availability of modern molecular techniques, it is still difficult to decide what populations are part of the natural or transient microbiota of the environment.

Enterococci began to emerge as leading causes of multidrug-resistant hospital-acquired infections. When pathologic changes result through direct toxin activity, or indirectly triggering inflammatory damages, certain *Enterococcus* species may become responsible for human infections [22]. According to recent data, the *Enterococcus* genus is responsible for 10.9% of nosocomial infections in the EU/EEA region [23]. The most important pathogens are *E. faecalis* and *E. faecium*, but non-faecium non-faecalis enterococci, such as *E. avium*, *E. caccae*, *E. casseliflavus*, *E. dispar*, *E. durans*, *E. gallinarum*, *E. hirae* and *E. raffinosus*, have been increasingly reported to cause human infections [24]. *Enterococcus faecium* and *E. faecalis* have evolved to become globally disseminated nosocomial pathogens. Hospital-associated *E. faecium* strains are characterized by the acquisition of adaptive genetic elements, including genes involved in antibiotic resistance. In contrast to *E. faecium*, clinical variants of *E. faecalis* are not exclusively found in hospitals but are also present in healthy individuals and animals [25]. The apparent adaptations found in hospital-associated *E. faecalis* lineages likely predate the "modern hospital" era, suggesting selection in a different niche and underscoring the generalist nature of this nosocomial pathogen [26]. Very few Romanian studies concerning antimicrobial resistance of enterococci have been published. Clinical variants of *Enterococcus* showed a high resistance profile for fluoroquinolones and penicillins [27,28], while bacterial clones from fishery lakes were highly resistant to macrolides [29]. Vancomycin resistance recently emerged in this One-Health continuum.

The aim of this study was to determine the extent to which anthropogenic contamination may contribute to the spread of antibiotic resistant enterococci in aquatic compartments and to explore genetic relationships within and between *Enterococcus* species. For this purpose, environments from low to high presumptive fecal contamination related to anthropic pressure were assessed to quantify the burden of intestinal enterococci and the levels of phenotypic and genotypic antimicrobial resistance in a collection of isolates. It was of particular interest to identify the strains and to characterize their genetic diversity under the hypothesis that similarity of DNA banding patterns may be linked to their antibiotic resistance and also to the type of water source. For this objective, the effectiveness of ERIC-PCR fingerprinting was evaluated for *Enterococcus* species and strain differentiation.

2. Results

2.1. Water Contamination by Enterococci

Water contamination by intestinal enterococci was investigated in different aquatic compartments with different degrees of anthropogenic pollution: groundwater (GW1-GW4), surface waters (SW1-SW3), wastewater influents (WWI) and effluents (WWE), and hospital effluents (HE). Enterococci were detected in all samples, except for a groundwater well, in a range from 3 ± 2 colony forming units (CFU)/100 mL in a groundwater spring located outside the city area (GW1) to (465 ± 0.2) × 10^3 CFU/100 mL in WWI. Sewage treatment contributed significantly to the reduction of microbial counts, to 99 ± 5 enterococci/100 mL in WWE. Hospital effluents harbored high concentrations of enterococci, but still below the loadings from municipal sewage. In surface waters, enterococci abundances increased along the river, from 9 ± 1 CFU/mL in SW1 to (11.7 ± 0.1) × 10^3 in SW3. Groundwater samples were differently impacted by enterococcal contamination, which was found to be up to 80 ± 6 CFU/mL in GW2, a dug well from a village upstream of the city (Table 1). A dug well from Cluj city (GW4) was sampled three times, but since no intestinal enterococci were detected, it was excluded from further investigations.

Table 1. Contamination of water by enterococci along the aquatic compartments.

Parameter	SW1	SW2	SW3	GW1	GW2	GW3	GW4	HE	WWI	WWE
Intestinal enterococci (CFU/100 mL)	9 ± 1	43 ± 5	(11.7 ± 0.1) × 10^3	3 ± 2	80 ± 6	12 ± 1	0	(18 ± 0.1) × 10^3	(465 ± 0.2) × 10^3	99 ± 5
No. of tested isolates	85	38	102	10	22	37	0	92	89	99
No. of identified isolates	3	3	7	3	4	11	0	48	33	34
E. aquimarinus	0	0	0	0	0	0	0	0	1	0
E. avium	0	0	0	0	0	0	0	26	0	0
E. casseliflavus	0	0	0	0	0	0	0	0	1	0
E. durans	0	0	0	0	0	0	0	0	1	1
E. faecalis	0	3	4	2	4	0	0	5	20	11
E. faecium	3	0	3	0	0	11	0	16	10	22
E. gallinarum	0	0	0	1	0	0	0	1	0	0

Note: CFU = colony forming units; GW = groundwater; HE = hospital effluent; SW = surface water; WWE = wastewater effluent; WWI = wastewater influent.

2.2. Resistance to Antibiotics in Enterococci

Kirby–Bauer tests were performed for 547 *Enterococcus* isolates to identify their resistance to ampicillin (AMP), imipenem (IMP), norfloxacin (NOR), gentamicin (CN), vancomycin (VAN), erythromycin (E), tetracycline (TE) and trimethoprim-sulfamethoxazole (SXT). The overall prevalence of susceptible profiles was 41.5%. In all the sampling points where intestinal enterococci were detected, there were isolates displaying phenotypic resistance, and their proportions were between 8.2% and 94.4%. Variants of enterococci resistant to all the antimicrobial agents tested in this study were isolated from HE, WWE, WWI and SW3. Resistance up to eight antibiotics per strain was observed in hospital sewage, up to seven in wastewaters, up to three in river water (SW2 and SW3) and also in shallow groundwater wells (GW2 and GW3). Isolates from spring water (GW1) were resistant to a maximum of two antimicrobial drugs, while intestinal enterococci from drinking water source (SW1) to a single antibiotic.

The antibiograms indicated that 91.3%, 91.1% and 89.7% enterococci were susceptible to gentamycin, vancomycin and ampicillin, respectively. A total of 88.2% was susceptible to imipenem, 86.6% to norfloxacin and 84.8% to erythromycin. Tetracycline and trimethoprim-sulfamethoxazole were the least effective antimicrobial agents, inhibiting only 70.2% and 55.9% of *Enterococcus* isolates, respectively.

The magnitude of phenotypic resistance of intestinal enterococci categorized based on their origin is shown in Figure 1a. The highest frequency of antimicrobial resistance was observed against trimethoprim-sulfamethoxazole, in enterococcal isolates from WWI (92%), WWE (91%) and HE (50%). Tetracycline resistance was also high in all aquatic compartments, with many isolates from HE (51%), GW2 (50%) and SW2 (34%), WWI (38%) and WWE (43%) being resistant. Resistance against erythromycin was observed in all compartments, from 42% in HE to 1% in SW1. At a maximum frequency of 27% in HE, strains resistant to ampicillin were detected in all samples, except for SW1. Isolates resistant to norfloxacin, imipenem, gentamycin and vancomycin were present most frequently in hospital sewage (38%, 32%, 32%, and 30%) and in wastewater samples, but not always in surface waters and groundwater. All *Enterococcus* isolates from GW1 and GW2 were susceptible to these four antibiotics. Besides the SXT, TE, E resistance profiles and their combinations, the following most prevalent resistance patterns were NOR-SXT and AMP-IPM-NOR-CN-VAN-E-TE-SXT. From the 82 antibiotic-resistance patterns observed in 336 *Enterococcus* isolates, 48 patterns have only appeared once. Proportions of multidrug-resistant (MDR) enterococci were 44.6% in HE, 36.4% in WWE, 33.7% in WWI, 5.3% in SW2, 4.5% in GW2 and 2% in SW3. No MDR strains were present in SW1 and GW1. The overall frequency of MDR enterococci was 7.7%.

Detection by PCR of ARGs indicated that overall, 23.9% of enterococci investigated in this study (574 isolates) carried at least one of the targeted ARGs. The proportion of isolates with genetic-encoded resistance relative to the isolates displaying phenotypic resistance (336 strains) was 40.8%. The magnitude of genotypic resistance of intestinal enterococci categorized based on their origin is shown in Figure 1b. The greatest ARG diversity was observed in *Enterococcus* spp. from HE, where 9 out of the 17 target genes were detected. None of the investigated ARGs were detected in isolates from SW1, GW2 and GW3 sites. ARG relative frequencies were 0.58 in HE, 0.21 in WWE, 0.16 in WWI, 0.03 in SW3, 0.02 in SW2 and 0.01 in GW1. The most frequently detected were *tetM*, in 0.14% of *Enterococcus* isolates, followed by *tetL* (0.13%) and *ermB* (0.1%). The genes *tetL*, *tetM* and *ermB* were present in enterococci from 6 (SW2, SW3, GW2, WWI, WWE, HI), 4 (SW3, WWI, WWE, HE) and 3 (SW2, WWE, HE) out of 9 sampling sites, respectively. In addition, $bla_{\text{TEM-1}}$, *aac(6′)-Ie-aph(2″)-Ia*, *vanA*, *vanB*, *tetB* and *tetC* were exclusively detected in HE. *Enterococcus* strains carrying the ARGs *aac(6′)-Im*, *mefA* and *sul1* as well as class 1 integron integrase *intI1* were only identified in wastewaters. The most prevalent ARG patterns were *tetL*, *ermB-tetL-tetM*, *tetM*, *tetL-tetM* and *sul1*. From the 36 ARG patterns observed, 19 had single appearances. PCR amplifications for $bla_{\text{NDM-1}}$, *ermA*, *tetA*, *sul2* and *sul3* had negative results. A moderate statistical significant correlation (R = 0.66) was found between the levels of displayed phenotypic resistance and the incidence of the investigated ARGs, suggesting that other genetic-encoded mechanisms might also be involved (Figure 2a).

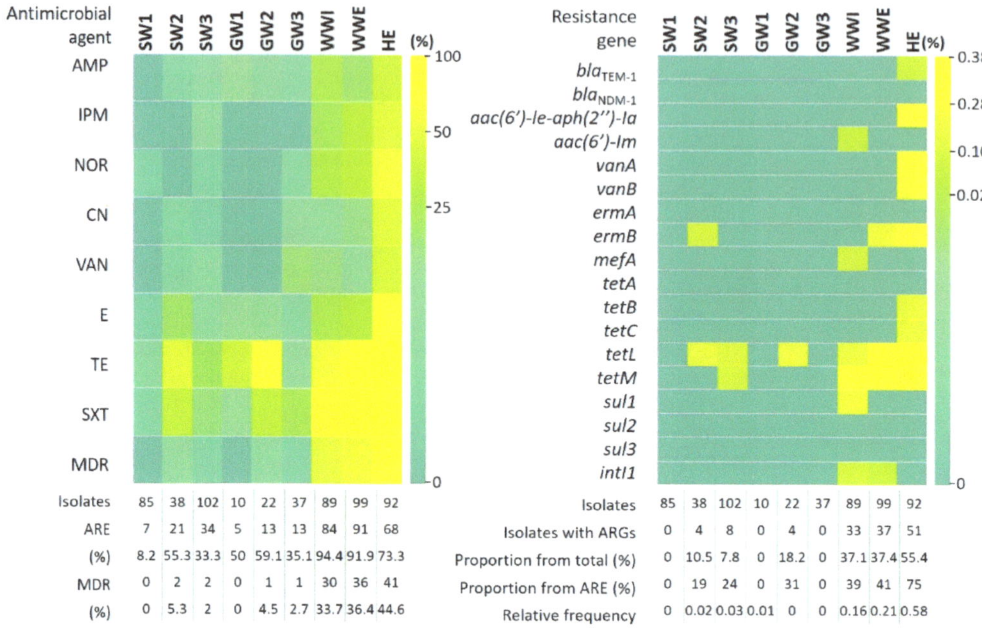

(**a**) (**b**)

Figure 1. Phenotypic (**a**) and genotypic (**b**) antibiotic resistance of *Enterococcus* spp. isolates. AMP = ampicillin; ARE = antibiotic resistant enterococci; ARGs = antibiotic resistance genes; CN = gentamicin; E = erythromycin; GW = groundwater; HE = hospital effluent; IPM = imipenem; MDR = multidrug resistance; NOR = norfloxacin; SXT = trimethoprim-sulfamethoxazole; SW = surface water; TE = tetracycline; VAN = vancomycin; WWE = wastewater effluent; WWI = wastewater influent. Quantile binning method was applied for both heat maps construction. The color code uses green for low values to yellow for high values.

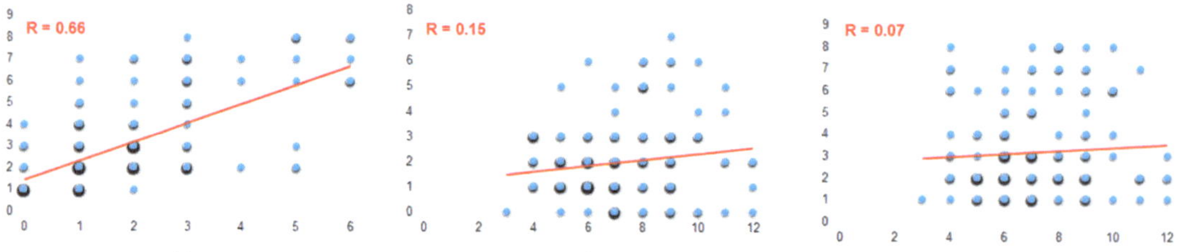

(a) (b) (c)

Figure 2. Scatter plots showing linear regression lines and correlation coefficients between the levels of phenotypic and genotypic resistance (**a**), the number of ERIC-PCR bands and phenotypic resistance (**b**), the number of ERIC-PCR bands and ARGs detected in *Enterococcus* isolates (**c**).

2.3. *Enterococcus Diversity and Association with Antibiotic Resistance Profiles*

The molecular identification of 146 resistant isolates of *Enterococcus* has led to the recovery of seven taxons in different proportions: *E. faecium* (44.5%), *E. faecalis* (33.6%), *E. avium* (17.8%), *E. durans* (1.4%), *E. gallinarum* (1.4%), *E. aquimarinus* (0.7%) and *E. casseliflavus* (0.7%). Considering the water compartments where multiple species have been recovered from, resistant *E. faecalis* was found to predominate in WWI and SW3, *E. facium* in

WWE and *E avium* in HE, respectively. From SW2, GW1 and GW2, all the resistant isolated were identified as *E. faecalis*. From SW1 and GW3, all the resistant isolates were *E. faecium*. Antibiotic-resistant *E. avium* was exclusively recovered from HE, and *E. aquimarinus* and *E. casseliflavus* from WWI, respectively (Table 1).

The genomic diversity analysis of 146 *Enterococcus* isolates was carried out using the repetitive sequence-based polymerase chain reaction (Rep-PCR) with the Enterobacterial Repetitive Intergenic Consensus (ERIC) primer ERIC2. Complex fingerprint patterns were found, consisting of 3 to 12 amplification bands. The genetic variation among isolates revealed different banding patterns, which ranged from 100 bp to 2 kb and 42% similarity. By applying the unweighted pair-group arithmetic mean method (UPGMA), dendrograms generated using Dice's similarity coefficients were comparable and useful to study the intra- and inter-species diversity of *Enterococcus* isolates.

ERIC-PCR grouped all 26 *E. avium* isolates in two clusters and resolved 12 discrete genomic patterns. A similarity of 72% was found among *E. avium* isolates. Hospital effluent had a low *E. avium* diversity, most of the strains being closely related. Within cluster A, the REP-PCR profiles of 17 isolates were highly similar. In two subgroups, three isolates (HE-2, HE-14 and HE-46) and five isolates (HE-29, HE-38, HE-53, HE-54 and HE-68), respectively, had identical ERIC-PCR profile and also shared the same antibiotic resistance pattern, suggesting clonal relatedness (Figure 3).

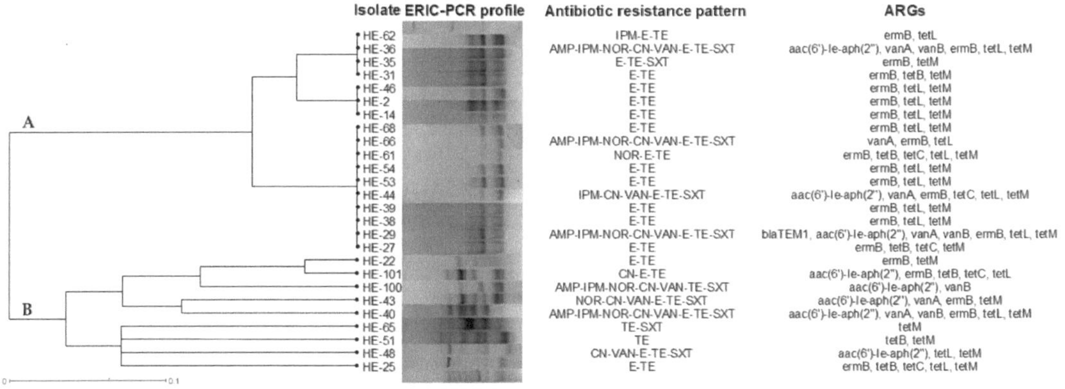

Figure 3. ERIC-PCR dendrogram and antibiotic resistance profiles of *E. avium* isolates. All isolates were from the hospital effluent.

Due to the high genetic similarity (85%), a typical ERIC-PCR fingerprint generated 16 distinct genomic patterns and grouped *E. faecalis* strains isolated from different water compartments. Among the 49 collected isolates, 45 isolates were grouped in 9 clusters. As expected, some isolates sharing the same origin clustered together, as observed for wastewater isolates in clusters D, E, F and G. However, segregation of the strains with respect to water matrices was not a general rule. The highly similar genetic patterns grouped *E. faecalis* isolates from hospital sewage, wastewater influents and effluents, from river water and groundwater together, in clusters A, B, C, H and I, despite their variability in the ARG profiles. Clonal relatedness was suggested by identical band pattern and also the ARG profile, as observed in two *E. faecalis* isolates from WWE within cluster B (WWI-12 and WWI-14), two isolates within cluster E (WWI-20 and WWI-65) and two isolates within cluster G (WWE-93 and WWE-100). In addition, within grouping I, the same ERIC-PCR and ARG profiles were observed for isolates collected from different matrices: WWI-59 and SW3-81 and also GW2-12, GW2-22, GW2-31, SW3-7, SW3-35 and SW3-53 (Figure 4).

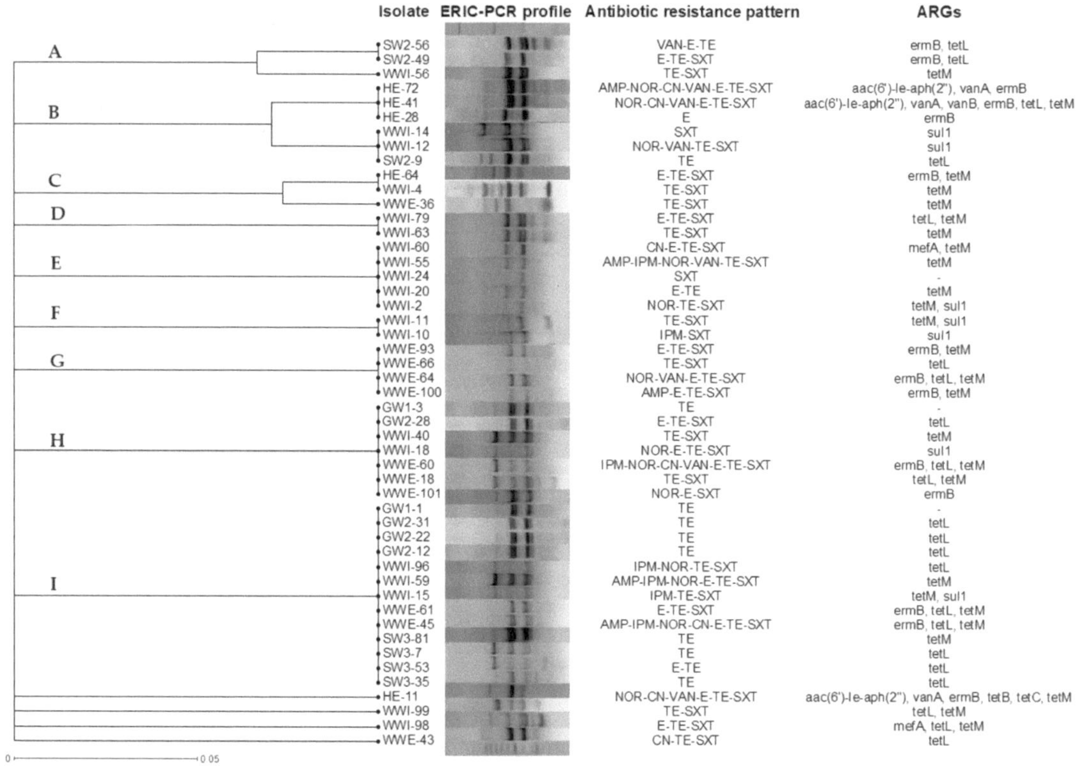

Figure 4. ERIC-PCR dendrogram and antibiotic resistance profiles of *E. faecalis* isolates. The isolates were labelled by sources: GW = groundwater; HE = hospital effluent; SW = surface water; WWI = wastewater influent; WWE = wastewater effluent.

Comparative analysis of Rep-PCR fingerprinting for the three main *Enterococcus* species revealed the most substantial genetic diversity among *E. faecium* strains. ERIC-PCR typing of 65 isolates resolved 35 discrete genomic patterns. However, bacterial isolates from different environmental compartments shared 68% genome similarity and hierarchical clustering grouped *E. faecium* strains in four main clusters. Similar to the *E. faecalis* typing results, *E. faecium* isolates sharing the same origin clustered together, but none of the ERIC-PCR patterns was exclusively specific for one aquatic regimen. The great variability of genetic patterns in grouping A was generated by strains from all aquatic compartments, with high diversity of antibiotic-resistance profiles. Clusters B and C mostly contained wastewater isolates, but also strains from groundwater. These strains displayed lower levels of antibiotic resistance, all the *E. faecium* from GW3 lacking the targeted genetic elements. Hospital effluents had a low *E. faecium* genetic diversity, most of the strains being clustered together in grouping D, together with a strain isolated from river water. Clonal relatedness suggested by identical ERIC-PCR and ARG profiles of *E. faecalis* isolates was observed within clusters A (SW1-22, SW1-35 and SW1-71), B (GW3-7, GW3-17 and GW3-37; GW3-32, GW3-33 and GW3-34; WW-1 and WWI-9) C (WWE-23 and WWE-26; WWE-12 and WWE-14; WWE-62 and WWE-63) and D (HE17 and HE-55; HE19, HE20 and HE50) (Figure 5).

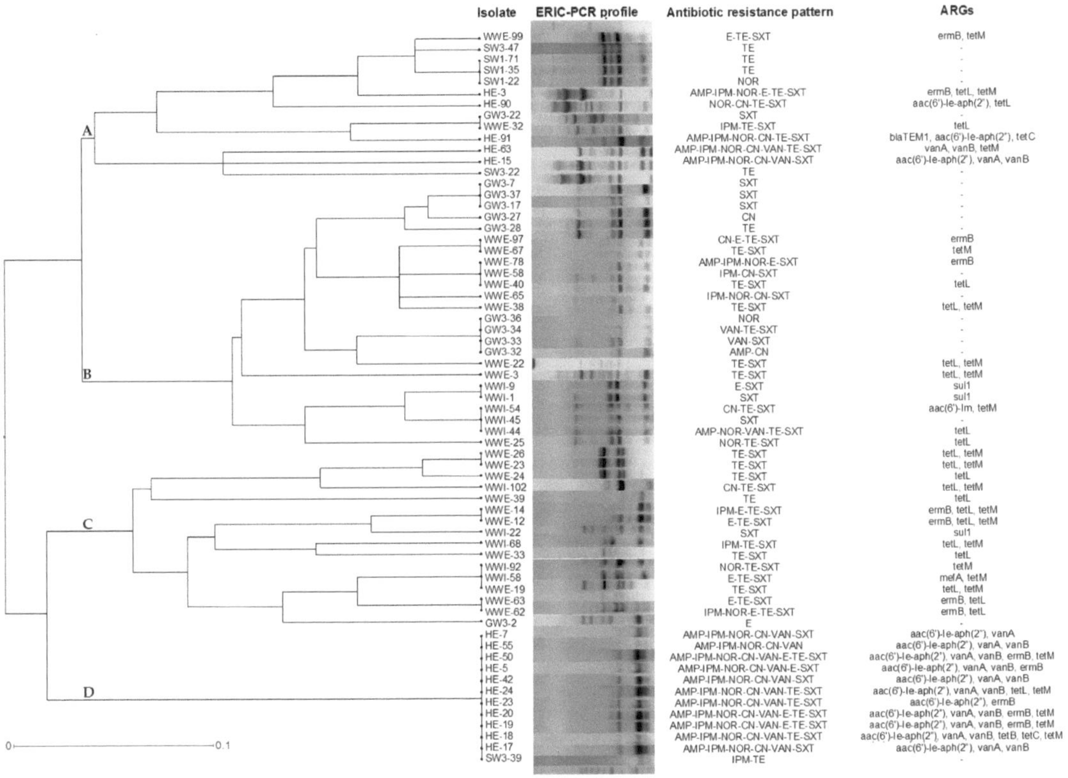

Figure 5. ERIC-PCR dendrogram and antibiotic resistance profiles of *E. faecium* isolates. The isolates were labelled by sources: GW = groundwater; HE = hospital effluent; SW = surface water; WWI = wastewater influent; WWE = wastewater effluent.

Six isolates belonging to four other species (non-predominant species) were detected and characterized during this study. They shared 33% genetic similarity and generated six ERIC-PCR patterns (Figure 6). Clonal relatedness according to genetic typing was observed for *E. durans*, but the two variants had different resistance profiles. Two *E. gallinarum* isolates differed in both their ERIC-PCR band patterns and antibiotic-resistance profiles.

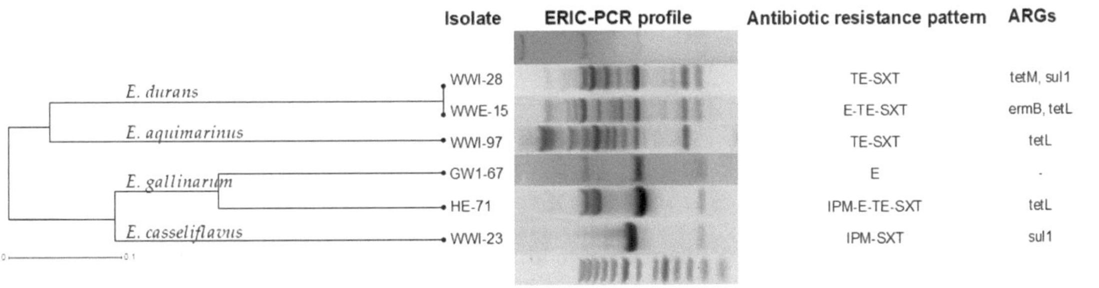

Figure 6. ERIC-PCR dendrogram and antibiotic resistance profiles of other *Enterococcus* spp. The isolates were labelled by sources: GW = groundwater; HE = hospital effluent; WWI = wastewater influent; WWE = wastewater effluent.

No statistically significant correlations were found between the number of banding patterns and the level of phenotypic or genotypic resistance (Figure 2b,c). Additional visualization tools were applied to infer the associations and differences between species. At the genus level, molecular typing revealed the clustering of *Enterococcus* isolates, both by ERIC-PCR profiles and by ARG patterns (Figure 7). Rep-PCR fingerprinting using the ERIC2 primer provided excellent discriminatory power at the species level within the genus *Enterococcus*, obvious in the UPGMA dendrogram. *Enterococcus faecium*, *E. avium* and *E. faecalis* strains clustered according to their taxonomy. Strains belonging to other species (*E. aquimarinus*, *E. durans*, *E. casseliflavus* and *E. gallinarum*) generated distinct band patterns, allowing their distinct differentiation in the UPGMA dendrogram (Figure 7a).

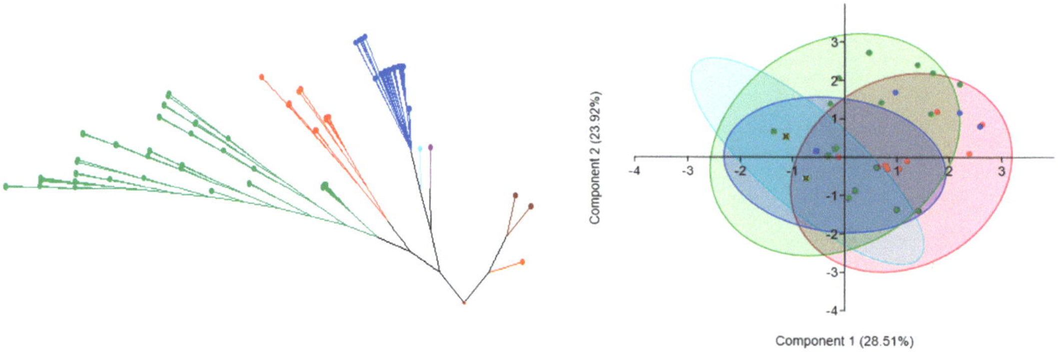

Figure 7. Molecular typing revealing clustering of *Enterococcus* spp. by: (**a**) ERIC-PCR profiles; (**b**) ARG patterns. Color codes: *E avium* (red); *E. faecalis* (blue); *E. faecium* (green); *E. aquimarinus* (aqua); *E. casseliflavus* (orange); *E. durans* (purple); *E. gallinarum* (brown). In (**b**) PCA clustering of non-predominant species appears in aqua.

Some degree of clustering according to taxonomy was observed when the principal component analysis (PCA) was employed to provide an integrative view upon the ARGs involved in variation. Genetic variation of ARGs explained by the first two principal components (52.43% of the total variation) among *Enterococcus* species revealed slightly distinct groups (Figure 7b). Besides the isolates belonging to the group of non-predominant species, *E faecalis* strains harbored the lowest diversity of ARGs, and all their encoded-genetic traits were common to *E. avium* and/or *E. faecium* and also shared with other species. *Enterococcus avium* and *E. faecium* strains benefit as well from the ARG pool specific for the family, but differences in gene frequencies resulted in their clustering.

3. Discussion

Enterococcus species are valuable fecal indicators and important predictors of anthropogenic pollution and associated risks in aquatic environments. Waters with high enterococcal loads represent an environmental and a public health hazard, since most of these bacteria carry numerous antibiotic-resistance traits. However, molecular typing clustered the strains regardless of their source or antibiotic-resistance profile.

During this study, the microbiological risk associated with contaminated waters was correlated with the magnitude of exposure to anthropogenic pressure in various aquatic matrices. The detection and enumeration of intestinal enterococci in different water compartments confirmed that they are reliable indicators of water quality and that environmental reservoirs are closely related to human activities. The highest loads of intestinal enterococci were found in raw wastewaters and in hospital sewage. The performance efficiency of the municipal treatment plant, accounting for intestinal enterococci, demonstrated an average log reduction of 1.4. Unfortunately, high enterococcal contamination was found in the river basin and in several groundwater samples. Downstream of the wastewater treatment plant, the fecal pollution of river water was reflected in a 2-log increase in *Enterococcus* counts, compared to treated effluents. This suggests that besides discharge from the wastewater treatment plant, other anthropogenic activities have substantially contributed to river pollution. Across the city, accidental sewage spills, droppings from pets, littering, illicit dumping and waste disposal have been identified as the main sources of fecal microorganisms and nutrients in urban runoff, leading to the deterioration of the Someșul Mic River and its tributaries. Moreover, unanticipated high enterococcal loads were found in surface water and groundwater upstream of the city, where fecal contamination was mainly due to surface runoff from diffuse pollution sources. In these human impacted areas, the uncontrolled discharge of wastewaters and accidental sewage spills, animal farming practices, droppings from pets and wildlife, littering, illegal dumping and waste disposal, logging and sawmilling have been identified as the main sources of fecal microorganisms and nutrients in surface runoff, leading to the deterioration of the Someșul Rece River and Tarnița Reservoir. The water quality in shallow wells was largely affected by fecal contamination due to the infiltration of surface runoff, both in the rural (GW2) and urban areas (GW3 and GW4) but was also influenced individually by specific conditions (i.e., cleaning and disinfection practices). Proper construction and routine maintenance of dug wells are important to safeguard water quality, as observed for GW4, where intestinal enterococci were not detected during this study. The outcomes of the present project regarding contamination of the river continuum are consistent with previous findings. Antibiotics, antibiotic-resistant bacteria and their ARGs have been identified as contaminants of emerging concern in hospital effluents, wastewaters, surface waters [30–33] and groundwaters [34]. International guidelines and regulations enforce water quality surveillance based on monitoring of intestinal enterococci in conjunction with *E. coli*. Despite a decades-long attempt, no other more accurate and more reliable indicators have been found. Contaminated environments may serve as reservoirs of extra-intestinal enterococci. There is no consistent evidence of enterococcal regrowth within environmental biofilms, but apparently some *Enterococcus* species or strains are able to grow in extra-enteric compartments, developing potentially naturalized environmental populations. Vegetation was recently proved to promote bacterial regrowth in a warm climate, as submerged vegetation [35] and phytoplankton [36] for *E. casseliflavus*, eelgrass for *E. casseliflavus*, *E. hirae* and *E. faecalis* [37] or dune vegetation for *E. moraviensis* [38]. Modern molecular techniques may try to distinguish natural enterococcal populations from transient microbiota in the environment. Antibiotic resistant *E. faecium* and *E. faecalis* were largely found in aquatic habitats as the dominant species. *Enterococcus faecalis* was predominant in two surface waters (SW2 and SW3), two groundwater sources (GW1 and GW2), and in municipal wastewater. *Enterococcus faecium* was predominant in the Tarnița Reservoir, the main drinking water supply for Cluj County (SW1), a groundwater well within the city (GW3) and treated wastewater. An exception of particular significance is the predominance of *E. avium* in hospital effluents. A recent study investigating non-faecium and non-faecalis hospital infections in Cluj reported that *E. avium* seems to be involved more often in infectious neurological disorders, being the only species isolated from low respiratory tract infections [39].

The *Enterococcus* spp. are intrinsically resistant to a number of antimicrobials, including cephalosporins and sulfonamides, while they are only mildly resistant to β-lactams and aminoglycosides. Clinical strains with resistance to macrolides, tetracyclines, streptogramins and glycopeptides were described previously [40]. The proportion of MDR was higher in *E. faecium* (52%) compared to *E. faecalis* (51%), but not significantly different as expected. *Enterococcus avium* isolates also displayed a high level of multidrug resistance (43%). The variant of *E. gallinarum* isolated from hospital effluent was also MDR. Strains resistant to antibiotics for human use (VAN, CN, NOR, and IPM) were found mostly in hospital effluents, while resistance to antibiotics for veterinary use (TE, and E) was also observed in surface water and groundwater, even in less-impacted environments. Municipal wastewaters harbored enterococci with resistance to all classes of antimicrobial agents, reflecting the antibiotic consumption practices in the metropolitan area. Resistance to sulphonamides was exceptionally high in urban sewage, which is a common fact for wastewater treatment plants. Differences in the antibiotic-resistance profiles are known to reflect antimicrobial use practices in each country, region, or sector of the One-Health continuum (clinical, agricultural and environmental) [40].

Due to their ability to acquire antibiotic resistance determinants, multidrug-resistant enterococci display a wide repertoire of resistance mechanisms: the modification of drug targets, inactivation of therapeutic agents and overexpression of efflux pumps. The highest level of antibiotic resistance and the greatest diversity of ARGs was found in *E. faecium*, followed by *E. avium*, *E. faecalis* and *E. durans*. *Enterococcus faecium* isolates frequently carried *tetL*, *tetM*, *aac(6′)-Ie-aph(2″)-Ia*, *vanB*, *ermB* and *vanA* genes, and less frequently *sul1*, *tetC*, *tetB*, *mefA* and *bla*$_{\text{TEM-1}}$. The ARGs detected in *E. faecalis* isolates were *tetM*, *tetL*, *ermB*, *sul1*, *aac(6′)-Ie-aph(2″)-Ia*, *vanA*, *vanB*, *tetB* and *tetC*. *Enterococcus avium* strains harbored the *ermB*, *tetM*, *tetL*, *aac(6′)-Ie-aph(2″)-Ia*, *vanA*, *tetB*, *tetC*, *vanB* and *bla*$_{\text{TEM-1}}$ genes. The genes *ermB*, *tetL*, *tetM* and *sul1* were detected in *E. durans* isolates. The lowest diversity and prevalence of ARGs was found in *E. aquimarinus* (*tetL*), *E. casseliflavus* (*sul1*) and *E. gallinarum* (*tetL*) isolates. The acquisition of genes encoding vancomycin resistance is recognized as one of the features reflecting enterococci adaptability [41]. During this study, *E. avium*, *E. faecium* and *E. faecalis* harbored both the *vanA* and *vanB* genes. The gene *vanA* was more often present in *E. avium* and *E. faecalis*, while *vanB* in *E. faecium*. *Enterococcus* species are a serious health issue worldwide, particularly due to increasing vancomycin resistance and multidrug resistance (https://resistancemap.cddep.org/AntibioticResistance.php, accessed on 31 July 2022). In the European Region, during the past 10 years, vancomycin-resistant enterococci accounted for 1.1% of all pathogens isolated from patients with hospital-acquired infections. Among patients with hospital-acquired bloodstream infections with *Enterococcus* spp., mortality attributable to vancomycin resistant variants was 33.5% [23]. Last data from European Centre for Disease Prevention and Control reported vancomycin resistance to 3.3% in *E. facecalis* and 39.3% in *E. faecium* (http://atlas.ecdc.europa.eu/public/index.aspx, accessed on 31 July 2022). Our results are consistent with official reports, the gene *vanB* being detected 10 times more frequently in *E. faecium* than in *E. faecalis* isolates. At least the *vanA*, *vanB* and *aac(6′)-Ie-aph(2″)-Ia* genes, as markers of clinical enterococci, were exclusively detected in isolates from hospital effluents. The gene *bla*$_{\text{TEM-1}}$ was detected in two multiresistant strains (*E. avium* and *E. faecium*), both from hospital sewage. This genetic feature needs further investigations, as beta-lactamases imply resistance mechanisms that are specific for Gram-negative bacteria. However, beta-lactamases were recently reported in Gram-positive bacteria [42], including the detection of *bla*$_{\text{TEM-1}}$ in *E. faecalis* [43]. The results of this screening reveal that enterococci are important vehicles for both plasmid-borne and chromosomally encoded resistance determinants. They likely function as a reservoir of drug-resistance traits and can serve as vectors for the spread of these genes to other Gram-positive pathogens [41]. The horizontal gene transfer of mobile genetic elements is the major contributor to the emergence and dissemination of multidrug resistance. Class 1 integron integrase is a molecular marker for the mobilizable chromosomal ARG platforms and for anthropogenic pollution. The *intI1* gene was detected in two *E. faecium* and one *E. faecalis* strains, all isolated from the wastewater treatment plant. The *sul1* gene was also found exclusively in wastewater isolates, but no pattern of association was found between *intI1* and *sul1*. The *sul1* gene was detected in only one out of three strains carrying *intI1*. The linkage of the *intI1* integrase and *sul1* gene is a particularity of class 1 integrons in environmental Gram-negative bacteria [44].

DNA fingerprinting by ERIC-PCR is widely applicable since ERIC primers do not exclusively target enterobacterial repetitive elements [45]. It was demonstrated that it is a reliable tool, with high discriminatory power among *Enterococcus* strains isolated from food [46–48], water samples [49], clinical specimens obtained from animals [50,51] and humans [52]. In previous studies, the genotyping assay directed ERIC1 or ERIC1 in combination with ERIC2 primers against *E. faecalis* and/or *E. faecium* genomes. For the first time, the present study provides an optimized method, using only the ERIC2 primer, which allows discrimination among seven *Enterococcus* species and offers a better overview of their diversity. The genetic typing of *Enterococcus* isolates during this study generated significant results, in agreement with previous knowledge. One particular situation worth special attention, regarding the clustering of an *E. faecium* strain from surface water (SW3-39) in the same clade with the hospital-derived variants. The segregation between commensal enterococci and hospital-adapted lineages has been partly elucidated, and it is clearer for *E. faecium* than for *E. faecalis* [25]. It is known that *E. faecium* has a defined clade that diverged about 75 years ago and is associated with human infections, being rarely encountered in healthy individuals and even less in the environment. These clinical clones are characterized by hypermutability, increase in mobile genetic elements and alterations in metabolism [53]. In contrast to *E. faecium*, clones of *E. faecalis* isolated from clinical specimens are not exclusively found in hospitals, being also present in healthy individuals and animals. Molecular epidemiology using ERIC-PCR fingerprinting showed that *E. faecium* and *E. faecalis* isolates from different aquatic matrices exhibit the same or similar genetic profiles, which warns upon contamination of water sources with clinically significant enterococci. However, diversity in their antibiotic resistance profiles excludes the clonal transmission of bacteria from hospital environment to river water and groundwater. Instead, genetic similarities between freshwater and wastewater strains confirm our hypothesis that anthropic pollution is a major source of antibiotic-resistant enterococci, contributing to their environmental spread. In addition to the enterococcal load, molecular fingerprinting indicates the magnitude of the uncontrolled discharge of untreated or insufficiently treated domestic sewage into the environment. Therefore, ERIC-PCR typing is an improved tool to assess the diversity of *Enterococcus* strains.

This study highlights the importance of water safety in the context of increasing demographic challenge. As a general trend, the population in Cluj is invariably growing, while urbanization and suburbanization affect not only the city infrastructure, but also the surrounding areas. The upstream mountains and isolated hamlets became increasingly popular, as both travel destinations and holiday homes. Recently, especially during the COVID-19 pandemic, another trend has emerged, with counter-urbanization occurring due to changing lifestyles and the opportunity of re-locating work in a home-based office. For the future, an unprecedented enhancement in anthropogenic pressure on water resources is foreseen due to other changes, such as the global warming and the risk of drought. Therefore, the implementation of adequate strategies for the protection of water resources is of paramount importance. Mitigating and adapting to the impacts of demographic change require stringent measures to enforce the regulations for the collection, treatment and discharge of wastewaters in both urban and rural areas. The identification of point sources of pollution, together with the prevention of contamination events are required in order to reduce the microbial risks and to limit the extent of the antibiotic-resistance phenomenon. Proper maintenance of domestic wastewater systems and septic tanks as well as upgrades of municipal sewerage networks and wastewater treatment plants are mandatory. In addition, routine cleaning and disinfection of groundwater wells is effective in the eradication of health hazards associated with the spread of antibiotic-resistant enterococci.

Although this study investigated a large collection of *Enterococcus* isolates and many antibiotic resistance traits, several limitations were identified, including a putative bias in the selection of bacterial isolates and in the investigated ARGs. Therefore, other genetic mechanisms, including novel resistance sequences, could also be responsible for the observed resistance phenotypes. Additional ARGs should be further investigated as more reliable predictors for antimicrobial resistance in environmental enterococci, to eventually elucidate the links between antibiotic resistance and ERIC-PCR genotyping.

4. Materials and Methods

4.1. Site Description and Sampling Strategy

With a surface of 1603 square kilometers, the Cluj metropolitan area includes Cluj-Napoca city and 19 nearby localities. Due to its dynamics, academic and economic status, and civic and cultural identity, the city constantly attracts new residents. Conducted in 2011, the last official census estimated its population at 324,000 people, while the National Institute of Statistics recorded 740,020 residents living in Cluj County on 1 January 2022 (https://cluj.insse.ro/, accessed on 31 July 2022).

Covering an area of 112 square kilometers, the study site is located in Cluj County, North Western Romania, along the Someșul Mic River basin. The sampling strategy included several types of aquatic environments, sampled in three campaigns: surface waters (SW1, SW2, SW3), groundwater (GW1, GW2, GW3, GW4), municipal wastewaters (WWI and WWE) and hospital effluents (HE). According to their estimated degree of anthropogenic pollution, from low to high, 10 sampling points were set, and a total of 30 water samples were collected. Upstream of the city, two surface waters were sampled near the foothill of Muntele Mare and Munții Gilăului mountains. Tarnița Reservoir (SW1) is a dam reservoir on the Someșul Cald River, the left headwater of Someșul Mic River. With an area of 2.15 square kilometers, a length of more than 8 km and a maximum depth of more than 70 m, it is the main source of drinking water for almost 1 million people. Someșul Rece (SW2), the right headwater of Someșul Mic River, is 49 km long and has a basin size of 330 square kilometers. Downstream of the city, surface water was sampled from Someșul Mic River (SW3), after crossing the city and receiving treated effluents from the municipal wastewater treatment plant. Four sampling points for groundwater were included: an old spring from the peri-urban area (GW1), used for drinking purposes; a shallow well upstream of the city (GW2), near the Someșul Rece River bank; and two hand-dug wells within the city (GW3 and GW4). Wastewater influents (WWI) and effluents (WWE) were sampled from the wastewater treatment plant receiving mainly municipal sewage, as well as hospital input and industrial wastewaters. The plant is designed to process around 115,000 cubic meters of wastewater per day in three-step treatment: mechanical, biological and final deep purification for nitrogen and phosphorus removal. A specialized cancer hospital with 597 beds was selected for the collection of hospital effluents (HE), before sludge treatment and disinfection.

4.2. Detection and Enumeration of Intestinal Enterococci

Water samples were collected in sterile recipients and transported in refrigerated boxes into the laboratory. Within 6 h of sampling, microbiological assays were performed for the selective cultivation of intestinal enterococci by direct inoculation or membrane filtration through 0.45 μm sterile membrane filters, according to standard methods (ISO 7899–2:2000. Water quality—Detection and enumeration of intestinal enterococci—Part 2: Membrane filtration method). Red to brown colonies developed on Slanetz Bartley agar (Oxoid, Basingstoke, UK) after 48 h at 37 °C were further confirmed as intestinal enterococci on Bile Esculin Azide Agar (Merck-Millipore, Darmstadt, Germany) by 4 h incubation at 44 °C.

4.3. Antimicrobial Susceptibility Testing

Antimicrobial susceptibility testing of 574 isolates was performed using the disk diffusion method described by reference guidelines [54]. Mueller-Hinton agar (Oxoid, Basingstoke, UK) was employed to evaluate bacterial sensitivity to eight antibiotics: ampicillin (2 μg), imipenem (10 μg), norfloxacin (10 μg), gentamicin (30 μg), vancomycin (5 μg), erythromycin (15 μg), tetracycline (30 μg) and trimethoprim-sulfamethoxazole (1.25–23.75 μg). Zone inhibition diameters were interpreted according to clinical breakpoint tables [55,56]. *Enterococcus faecalis* ATCC 2921 was used as a wild-type susceptible strain. Resistance to at least three antimicrobial families was considered multidrug resistance.

4.4. ARG Screening

After PCR confirmation with *Enterococcus* molecular markers, 338 bacterial isolates displaying phenotypic resistance were subjected to PCR screening for the detection of ARGs and class 1 integron. Cell suspensions from overnight pure cultures were standardized at 1 MacFarland density. The preparation of DNA templates included freezing, bead beating and boiling procedures for cell wall disruption and enzyme inhibition [57]. DNA amplification was performed in a 15 µL total volume, consisting of 7.5 µL of DreamTaq Green PCR Master Mix (2×) (Thermo Fisher Scientific, Waltham, MA, USA), 0.5 µM of each primer (Eurogentec, Seraing, Belgium), 5.35 µL nuclease-free water (Lonza, Basel, Switzerland), and 2 µL bacterial suspension. PCRs were performed using a TProfessional Trio (Analytik Jena, Jena, Germany) or Mastercycler Nexus (Eppendorf AG, Hamburg, Germany) thermocycler: denaturation 5 min at 94 °C and then 35 cycles of 30 s at 94 °C, 45 s at a specific annealing temperature, 45 s at 72 °C, and a final extension of 8 min at 72 °C. The specific annealing temperatures for each primer pair are given in Table 2. The amplified PCR products were separated in 1.5% *w*/*v* agarose (Cleaver Scientific Ltd., Rugby, UK) gel in 1× TBE buffer (Lonza, Basel, Switzerland) and stained with 0.5 µg/mL ethidium bromide (Thermo Fisher Scientific, Waltham, MA, USA). Data acquisition and interpretation were performed using the BDA Digital Compact System and BioDocAnalyze Software (Analytik Jena, Jena, Germany). Positive and negative controls were included in each set of amplifications. Positive controls used a collection of bacterial strains carrying the targeted genes, previously validated by sequencing.

Table 2. Primers used for PCR amplifications.

No.	Target Gene	Primer Sequence (5′–3′)	Amplicon (bp)	Annealing Temperature	NCBI Reference Sequence
1	bla_{TEM-1}	GGTCGCCGCATACACTATTC/ ATACGGGAGGGCTTACCATC	500	57 °C	AL513383.1
2	bla_{NDM-1}	GGTTTGGCGATCTGGTTTTC/ CGGAATGGCTCATCACGATC	52	55 °C	HQ256747.1
3	*aac(6′)-Im*	GGCTGACAGATGACCGTGTTCTTG/ GTAGATATTGGCATACTACTCTGC	303	53 °C	NG_052530.1
4	*aac(6′)-Ie-aph(2″)-Ia*	CCAAGAGCAATAAGGGCATA/ CACTATCATAACCACTACCG	220	51 °C	KM083808.1
5	*vanA*	GCTATTCAGCTGTACT/ CAGCGGCCATCATACGG	783	51 °C	M97297.1
6	*vanB*	CGCCATACTCTCCCCGGATAG/ AAGCCCTCTGCATCCAAGCAC	667	61 °C	KF823969.1
7	*ermA*	GAACCAGAAAAACCCTAAAGACAC/ ACAGAGTCTACACTTGGCTTAGGATG	507	57 °C	X03216.1
8	*ermB*	GAAAAGGTACTCAACCAAAT/ AGTAACGGTACTTAAATTGTTTAC	639	50 °C	AY827541.1
9	*mefA*	CATCGACGTATTGGGTGCTG/ CCGAAAGCCCCATTATTGCA	455	55 °C	AY071835.1
10	*tetA*	GCAAGCAGGACCATGATCGG/ GCCGATATCACTGATGGCGA	572	57 °C	AF534183.1
11	*tetB*	GGTTAGGGGCAAGTTTTGGG/ ATCCCACCACCAGCCAATAA	541	57 °C	NG_048168.1
12	*tetC*	TGAGATCTCGGGAAAAGCGT/ AAAGCCGCGGTAAATAGCAA	460	53 °C	NC_024960.1
13	*tetL*	TATTCAAGGGGCTGGTGCAG/ CGGCAGTACTTAGCTGGTGA	545	57 °C	AY081910.1
14	*tetM*	CCGTCTGAACTTTGCGGAAA/ CAACGGAAGCGGTGATACAG	627	57 °C	AJ585076.1
15	*sul1*	AGGCATGATCTAACCCTCGG/ GGCCCGATGAGATCAGACGTA	665	57 °C	JF969163.1

Table 2. *Cont.*

No.	Target Gene	Primer Sequence (5′–3′)	Amplicon (bp)	Annealing Temperature	NCBI Reference Sequence
16	*sul2*	GACAGTTATCAACCCGCGAC/ GAAACAGACAGAAGCACCGG	380	57 °C	AY055428.1
17	*sul3*	GTGGGCGTTGTGGAAGAAAT/ AAAAGAAGCCCATACCCGGA	370	57 °C	FJ196385.1
18	*intI1*	CCTGCACGGTTCGAATG/ TCGTTTGTTCGCCCAGC	497	55 °C	NZ_JAMYXD010000016.1
19	*16S rRNA*	AGAGTTTGATCCTGGCTCAG/ ACGGCTACCTTGTTACGACTT	1519	56 °C	AB012212.1
20	*16S Enterococcus*	GGACGMAAGTCTGACCGA/ TTAAGAAACCGCCTGCGC	221	57 °C	JQ804949.1

4.5. Molecular Identification

After the phenotypic selection of intestinal enterococci based on standard methods, molecular screening using *Enterococcus* molecular markers [58] was employed to confirm biochemical identification. The bacterial 16S ribosomal RNA gene was used for PCR amplification (Table 2) and subsequent Sanger sequencing for the identification of enterococcal isolates carrying ARGs. Raw sequencing reads were deposited in the GenBank database of National Center for Biotechnology Information (NCBI) under the accession numbers OP359225-OP359304 and OP361300-OP361306. Nucleotide sequences were processed and analyzed using bioinformatic tools available through BioEdit version 7.2, then compared to sequences stored in the GenBank nucleotide database using the blastn algorithm (http://blast.ncbi.nlm.nih.gov/Blast.cgi, accessed on 31 July 2022).

4.6. Molecular Fingerprinting of *Enterococcus* spp.

Repetitive sequence-based polymerase chain reaction (Rep-PCR) was developed using specific ERIC primers involving bacterial DNA suspensions prepared following a protocol previously optimized and demonstrated by Houf et al. [57] as the most efficient for the purpose of ERIC-PCR screening. The ERIC-PCR was carried out with a single primer, which uses the total DNA and, therefore, provides results with good reproducibility [46]. We found that ERIC2 has the greatest discriminatory power among the seven *Enterococcus* species considered in the present study. Reactions were carried out in a total volume of 20 μL containing 10 μL of DreamTaq Green PCR Master Mix (2×) (Thermo Fisher Scientific, Waltham, MA, USA), 1 μM of primer ERIC2 (5′-AAGTAAGTGACTGGGGTGAGCG-3′) (Eurogentec, Seraing, Belgium), 7.8 μL nuclease-free water (Lonza, Basel, Switzerland) and 2 μL template DNA. Amplifications were performed in a TProfessional Trio (Analytik Jena, Jena, Germany) thermocycler with a cycling program consisting of an initial denaturing step at 94 °C for 5 min, 5 cycles of denaturation at 94 °C for 5 min, annealing at 38 °C for 5 min, elongation at 72 °C for 5 min, then 30 cycles of denaturation at 94 °C for 1 min, annealing at 48 °C for 1 min and elongation at 72 °C for 5 min, and a final extension of 72 °C for 10 min. The amplified products were resolved by 1.5% gel electrophoresis at 75 V for 120 min. Data acquisition was performed using the ChemiDoc MP system (BioRad, Hercules, CA, USA) and analyzed with PyElph 1.4 software [59].

4.7. Statistical Analysis

Descriptive statistics parameters were applied to assess the mean values and standard deviations of bacterial loads. Proportions, frequencies and patterns of displayed antimicrobial resistance and ARGs were calculated. The relative frequency of ARGs took into account the number of certain gene appearances relative to the total number of ARGs. Statistical correlations between the ERIC-PCR banding patterns and the level of phenotypic and genotypic resistance were inferred using the data analysis tool pack of Microsoft Excel 2016. The heat maps were drawn with CIMminer software, using the quantile-binning method. Quantile divides the weight range of data values into intervals, each with approximately the same number of data points. This effectively spreads out the color differences between data values that are present in regions with a large number of values.

Similarity distances between ERIC-PCR profiles were calculated using the Dice coefficient, and dendrograms were constructed based on the UPGMA analysis with DarWin 6.0.021 software [60]. The PCA multivariate statistical approach was used to explore the effects of ARG variance between different *Enterococcus* species. PCA was executed for the clustering and differentiation of data sets by PAST software version 4.11 [61].

5. Conclusions

The outcomes of this study reveal that, besides their role as fecal indicators, intestinal enterococci are hosts for antibiotic resistance determinants that may serve as indicators of anthropogenic impacts on aquatic ecosystems. Rep-PCR fingerprinting using the ERIC2 primer, in conjunction with ARG profiling, is a useful tool for the molecular typing of clinical and environmental *Enterococcus* species. In the context of increasing urbanization and unsustainable human activities in the peri-urban zones, the environmental spread of *Enterococcus* species carrying ARGs is of high concern. Enterococcal release and migration under anthropic pressure leads to the dispersion of clinically relevant strains into the natural environment. These findings support the importance of future strategies for public health protection by defending the water resources. Water quality protection is not only intended to reduce the risk for waterborne outbreaks but also to limit the expansion and progression of the antibiotic resistance phenomenon.

Author Contributions: Conceptualization, A.F. and C.C.; methodology, A.F., C.C. and A.B.-K.; software, A.F. and E.S.; validation, A.F., E.S. and A.B.-K.; formal analysis, A.F. and E.S.; investigation, A.F., E.S., A.T.-M., R.C. and A.B.-K.; data curation, A.F., C.C. and A.B.-K.; writing—original draft preparation, A.F.; writing—review and editing, C.C., E.S., A.T.-M. and A.B.-K.; supervision, C.C.; project administration, C.C. and A.B.-K.; funding acquisition, A.F., C.C. and A.B.-K. All authors have read and agreed to the published version of the manuscript.

Funding: This research was funded by the EnviroAMR project, grant number 3499/20.05.2015, financed through the EEA 2009–2014 Financial Mechanism under the RO04 programme e Reduction of hazardous substances. C.C. was supported by a grant from the Ministry of Research, Innovation and Digitalization through Program 1—Development of the National R&D System, Subprogram 1.2—Institutional Performance—Projects for Excellence Financing in RDI, contract no. 2PFE/2021. E.S. was supported by the ADVANCE Collaborative Research Project No. 28/2020 (Norway Grant Call 2019). The APC for this study was funded through Seed Grants GS-UBB-FBG-Farkas Ancuța-Cristina and GS-UBB-FBG-Butiuc Anca.

Institutional Review Board Statement: Not applicable.

Informed Consent Statement: Not applicable.

Data Availability Statement: Raw sequencing reads were deposited in the GenBank database of National Center for Biotechnology Information (NCBI) under the accession numbers OP359225-OP359304 and OP361300-OP361306.

Conflicts of Interest: The authors declare no conflict of interest.

References

1. Amarasiri, M.; Sano, D.; Suzuki, S. Understanding human health risks caused by antibiotic resistant bacteria (ARB) and antibiotic resistance genes (ARG) in water environments: Current knowledge and questions to be answered. *Crit. Rev. Environ. Sci. Technol.* **2020**, *50*, 2016–2059. [CrossRef]
2. Rozman, U.; Duh, D.; Cimerman, M.; Turk, S.Š. Hospital wastewater effluent: Hot spot for antibiotic resistant bacteria. *J. Water Sanit. Hyg. Dev.* **2020**, *10*, 171–178. [CrossRef]
3. Gotkowska-Płachta, A. The prevalence of virulent and multidrug-resistant enterococci in river water and in treated and untreated municipal and hospital wastewater. *Int. J. Environ. Res. Public Health* **2021**, *18*, 563. [CrossRef] [PubMed]
4. Zalewska, M.; Błażejewska, A.; Czapko, A.; Popowska, M. Antibiotics and antibiotic resistance genes in animal manure-consequences of its application in agriculture. *Front. Microbiol.* **2021**, *12*, 610656. [CrossRef] [PubMed]

5. Novais, C.; Coque, T.M.; Ferreira, H.; Sousa, J.C.; Peixe, L. Environmental contamination with vancomycin-resistant enterococci from hospital sewage in Portugal. *Appl. Environ. Microbiol.* **2005**, *71*, 3364–3368. [CrossRef]
6. Young, S.; Nayak, B.; Sun, S.; Badgley, B.D.; Rohr, J.R.; Harwood, V.J. Vancomycin-resistant enterococci and bacterial community structure following a sewage spill into an aquatic environment. *Appl. Environ. Microbiol.* **2016**, *82*, 5653–5660. [CrossRef]
7. Hamiwe, T.; Kock, M.M.; Magwira, C.A.; Antiabong, J.F.; Ehlers, M.M. Occurrence of enterococci harbouring clinically important antibiotic resistance genes in the aquatic environment in Gauteng, South Africa. *Environ. Pollut.* **2019**, *245*, 1041–1049. [CrossRef]
8. Sapkota, A.R.; Curriero, F.C.; Gibson, K.E.; Schwab, K.J. Antibiotic-resistant enterococci and fecal indicators in surface water and groundwater impacted by a concentrated Swine feeding operation. *Environ. Health Perspect.* **2007**, *115*, 1040–1045. [CrossRef]
9. Macedo, A.S.; Freitas, A.R.; Abreu, C.; Machado, E.; Peixe, L.; Sousa, J.C.; Novais, C. Characterization of antibiotic resistant enterococci isolated from untreated waters for human consumption in Portugal. *Int. J. Food Microbiol.* **2011**, *145*, 315–319. [CrossRef]
10. Li, X.; Atwill, E.R.; Antaki, E.; Applegate, O.; Bergamaschi, B.; Bond, R.F.; Chase, J.; Ransom, K.M.; Samuels, W.; Watanabe, N.; et al. Fecal indicator and pathogenic bacteria and their antibiotic resistance in alluvial groundwater of an irrigated agricultural region with dairies. *J. Environ. Qual.* **2015**, *44*, 1435–1447. [CrossRef] [PubMed]
11. Kaiser, R.A.; Polk, J.S.; Datta, T.; Parekh, R.R.; Agga, G.E. Occurrence of antibiotic resistant bacteria in urban karst groundwater systems. *Water* **2022**, *14*, 960. [CrossRef]
12. García-Solache, M.; Rice, L.B. The *Enterococcus*: A model of adaptability to its environment. *Clin. Microbiol. Rev.* **2019**, *32*, e00058-18. [CrossRef]
13. Lebreton, F.; Manson, A.L.; Saavedra, J.T.; Straub, T.J.; Earl, A.M.; Gilmore, M.S. Tracing the enterococci from Paleozoic origins to the hospital. *Cell* **2017**, *169*, 849–861. [CrossRef]
14. Krawczyk, B.; Wityk, P.; Gałęcka, M.; Michalik, M. The many faces of *Enterococcus* spp.—Commensal, probiotic and opportunistic pathogen. *Microorganisms* **2021**, *9*, 1900. [CrossRef]
15. Qin, J.; Li, R.; Raes, J.; Arumugam, M.; Burgdorf, K.S.; Manichanh, C.; Nielsen, T.; Pons, N.; Levenez, F.; Yamada, T.; et al. A human gut microbial gene catalogue established by metagenomic sequencing. *Nature* **2010**, *464*, 59–65. [CrossRef] [PubMed]
16. Lebreton, F.; Willems, R.J.L.; Gilmore, M.S. Enterococcus diversity, origins in nature, and gut colonization. In *Enterococci: From Commensals to Leading Causes of Drug Resistant Infection*; Gilmore, M.S., Clewell, D.B., Ike, Y., Shankar, N., Eds.; Massachusetts Eye and Ear Infirmary: Boston, MA, USA, 2014; ID:NBK190420.
17. Fisher, K.; Phillips, C. The ecology, epidemiology and virulence of *Enterococcus*. *Microbiology* **2009**, *155*, 1749–1757. [CrossRef] [PubMed]
18. Byappanahalli, M.N.; Nevers, M.B.; Korajkic, A.; Staley, Z.R.; Harwood, V.J. Enterococci in the environment. *Microbiol. Mol. Biol. Rev.* **2012**, *76*, 685–706. [CrossRef]
19. Bryan, N.C.; Lebreton, F.; Gilmore, M.; Ruvkun, G.; Zuber, M.T.; Carr, C.E. Genomic and functional characterization of *Enterococcus faecalis* isolates recovered from the International Space Station and their potential for pathogenicity. *Front. Microbiol.* **2021**, *11*, 515319. [CrossRef] [PubMed]
20. Farkas, A.; Drăgan-Bularda, M.; Ciatarâş, D.; Bocoş, B.; Ţigan, Ş. Opportunistic pathogens and faecal indicators in drinking water associated biofilms in Cluj, Romania. *J. Water Health* **2012**, *10*, 471–483. [CrossRef] [PubMed]
21. del Mar Lleò, M.; Bonato, B.; Benedetti, D.; Canepari, P. Survival of enterococcal species in aquatic environments. *FEMS Microbiol. Ecol.* **2005**, *54*, 189–196. [CrossRef]
22. Selleck, E.M.; Van Tyne, D.; Gilmore, M.S. Pathogenicity of enterococci. *Microbiol. Spectr.* **2019**, *7*, 4. [CrossRef]
23. Brinkwirth, S.; Ayobami, O.; Eckmanns, T.; Markwart, R. Hospital-acquired infections caused by enterococci: A systematic review and meta-analysis, WHO European Region, 1 January 2010 to 4 February 2020. *Euro Surveill.* **2021**, *26*, 2001628. [CrossRef]
24. Said, M.S.; Tirthani, E.; Lesho, E. *Enterococcus* Infections. In: StatPearls. Available online: https://www.ncbi.nlm.nih.gov/books/NBK567759/ (accessed on 1 August 2022).
25. Guzman Prieto, A.M.; van Schaik, W.; Rogers, M.R.; Coque, T.M.; Baquero, F.; Corander, J.; Willems, R.J. Global emergence and dissemination of enterococci as nosocomial pathogens: Attack of the clones? *Front. Microbiol.* **2016**, *7*, 788. [CrossRef]
26. Pöntinen, A.K.; Top, J.; Arredondo-Alonso, S.; Tonkin-Hill, G.; Freitas, A.R.; Novais, C.; Gladstone, R.A.; Pesonen, M.; Meneses, R.; Pesonen, H.; et al. Apparent nosocomial adaptation of *Enterococcus faecalis* predates the modern hospital era. *Nat. Commun.* **2021**, *12*, 1523. [CrossRef]
27. Farkas, A.; Tarco, E.; Crăciunaş, C.; Bocoş, B.; Butiuc-Keul, A. Screening for phenotypic and genotypic resistance to antibiotics in Gram positive pathogens. *Stud. Univ. Babes-Bolyai Biol.* **2017**, *62*, 85–96. [CrossRef]
28. Arbune, M.; Gurau, G.; Niculet, E.; Iancu, A.V.; Lupasteanu, G.; Fotea, S.; Vasile, M.C.; Tatu, A.L. Prevalence of antibiotic resistance of ESKAPE pathogens over five years in an infectious diseases hospital from South-East of Romania. *Infect. Drug Resist.* **2021**, *14*, 2369–2378. [CrossRef] [PubMed]
29. Lazăr, V.; Gheorghe, I.; Curutiu, C.; Savin, I.; Marinescu, F.; Cristea, V.C.; Dobre, D.; Popa, G.L.; Chifiriuc, M.C.; Popa, M.I. Antibiotic resistance profiles in cultivable microbiota isolated from some romanian natural fishery lakes included in Natura 2000 network. *BMC Vet. Res.* **2021**, *17*, 52. [CrossRef] [PubMed]
30. Farkas, A.; Bocoş, B.; Butiuc-Keul, A. Antibiotic resistance and *intI1* carriage in waterborne *Enterobacteriaceae*. *Water Air Soil Poll.* **2016**, *227*, 251. [CrossRef]

31. Szekeres, E.; Baricz, A.; Chiriac, C.M.; Farkas, A.; Opris, O.; Soran, M.L.; Andrei, A.S.; Rudi, K.; Balcázar, J.L.; Dragos, N.; et al. Abundance of antibiotics, antibiotic resistance genes and bacterial community composition in wastewater effluents from different Romanian hospitals. *Environ. Pollut.* **2017**, *225*, 304–315. [CrossRef]
32. Teban-Man, A.; Farkas, A.; Baricz, A.; Hegedus, A.; Szekeres, E.; Pârvu, M.; Coman, C. Wastewaters, with or without hospital contribution, harbour MDR, carbapenemase-producing, but not hypervirulent *Klebsiella pneumoniae*. *Antibiotics* **2021**, *29*, 361. [CrossRef] [PubMed]
33. Butiuc-Keul, A.; Carpa, R.; Podar, D.; Szekeres, E.; Muntean, V.; Iordache, D.; Farkas, A. Antibiotic resistance in *Pseudomonas* spp. through the urban water cycle. *Curr. Microbiol.* **2021**, *78*, 1227–1237. [CrossRef] [PubMed]
34. Szekeres, E.; Chiriac, C.M.; Baricz, A.; Szőke-Nagy, T.; Lung, I.; Soran, M.L.; Rudi, K.; Dragos, N.; Coman, C. Investigating antibiotics, antibiotic resistance genes, and microbial contaminants in groundwater in relation to the proximity of urban areas. *Environ. Pollut.* **2018**, *236*, 734–744. [CrossRef]
35. Badgley, B.D.; Thomas, F.I.; Harwood, V.J. The effects of submerged aquatic vegetation on the persistence of environmental populations of *Enterococcus* spp. *Environ. Microbiol.* **2010**, *12*, 1271–1281. [CrossRef]
36. Mote, B.L.; Turner, J.W.; Lipp, E.K. Persistence and growth of the fecal indicator bacteria enterococci in detritus and natural estuarine plankton communities. *Appl. Environ. Microbiol.* **2012**, *78*, 2569–2577. [CrossRef] [PubMed]
37. Ferguson, D.M.; Weisberg, S.B.; Hagedorn, C.; De Leon, K.; Mofidi, V.; Wolfe, J.; Zimmerman, M.; Jay, J.A. *Enterococcus* growth on eelgrass (*Zostera marina*); implications for water quality. *FEMS Microbiol. Ecol.* **2016**, *92*, fiw047. [CrossRef]
38. Taučer-Kapteijn, M.; Hoogenboezem, W.; Medema, G. Environmental growth of the faecal indicator *Enterococcus moraviensis*. *Water Supply* **2016**, *16*, 971–979. [CrossRef]
39. Toc, D.A.; Pandrea, S.L.; Botan, A.; Mihaila, R.M.; Costache, C.A.; Colosi, I.A.; Junie, L.M. *Enterococcus raffinosus, Enterococcus durans* and *Enterococcus avium* isolated from a tertiary care hospital in Romania-retrospective study and brief review. *Biology* **2022**, *11*, 598. [CrossRef]
40. Zaheer, R.; Cook, S.R.; Barbieri, R.; Goji, N.; Cameron, A.; Petkau, A.; Polo, R.O.; Tymensen, L.; Stamm, C.; Song, J.; et al. Surveillance of *Enterococcus* spp. reveals distinct species and antimicrobial resistance diversity across a One-Health continuum. *Sci. Rep.* **2020**, *10*, 3937. [CrossRef] [PubMed]
41. Miller, W.R.; Munita, J.M.; Arias, C.A. Mechanisms of antibiotic resistance in enterococci. *Expert Rev. Anti Infect. Ther.* **2014**, *12*, 1221–1236. [CrossRef]
42. Toth, M.; Antunes, N.T.; Stewart, N.K.; Frase, H.; Bhattacharya, M.; Smith, C.A.; Vakulenko, S.B. Class D β-lactamases do exist in Gram-positive bacteria. *Nat. Chem. Biol.* **2016**, *12*, 9–14. [CrossRef] [PubMed]
43. Chouchani, C.; El Salabi, A.; Marrakchi, R.; Ferchichi, L.; Walsh, T.R. First report of *mef*A and *msr*A/*msr*B multidrug efflux pumps associated with $bla_{\text{TEM-1}}$ β-lactamase in *Enterococcus faecalis*. *Int. J. Infect. Dis.* **2012**, *16*, e104–e109. [CrossRef]
44. Farkas, A.; Crăciunaş, C.; Chiriac, C.; Szekeres, E.; Coman, C.; Butiuc-Keul, A. Exploring the role of coliform bacteria in class 1 integron carriage and biofilm formation during drinking water treatment. *Microb Ecol.* **2016**, *72*, 773–782. [CrossRef] [PubMed]
45. Gillings, M.; Holley, M. Repetitive element PCR fingerprinting (rep-PCR) using enterobacterial repetitive intergenic consensus (ERIC) primers is not necessarily directed at ERIC elements. *Lett. Appl. Microbiol.* **1997**, *25*, 17–21. [CrossRef] [PubMed]
46. Jurkovic, D.; Krizková, L.; Sojka, M.; Takácová, M.; Dusinský, R.; Krajcovic, J.; Vandamme, P.; Vancanneyt, M. Genetic diversity of *Enterococcus faecium* isolated from Bryndza cheese. *Int. J. Food Microbiol.* **2007**, *116*, 82–87. [CrossRef] [PubMed]
47. Martín-Platero, A.M.; Valdivia, E.; Maqueda, M.; Martínez-Bueno, M. Characterization and safety evaluation of enterococci isolated from Spanish goats' milk cheeses. *Int. J. Food Microbiol.* **2009**, *132*, 24–32. [CrossRef] [PubMed]
48. Nasiri, M.; Hanifian, S. *Enterococcus faecalis* and *Enterococcus faecium* in pasteurized milk: Prevalence, genotyping, and characterization of virulence traits. *LWT* **2022**, *153*, 112452. [CrossRef]
49. Wei, L.; Wu, Q.; Zhang, J.; Guo, W.; Chen, M.; Xue, L.; Wang, J.; Ma, L. Prevalence and genetic diversity of *Enterococcus faecalis* isolates from mineral water and spring water in China. *Front. Microbiol.* **2017**, *16*, 1109. [CrossRef]
50. Blanco, A.E.; Barz, M.; Cavero, D.; Icken, W.; Sharifi, A.R.; Voss, M.; Buxadé, C.; Preisinger, R. Characterization of *Enterococcus faecalis* isolates by chicken embryo lethality assay and ERIC-PCR. *Avian Pathol.* **2018**, *47*, 23–32. [CrossRef]
51. Stępień-Pyśniak, D.; Hauschild, T.; Dec, M.; Marek, A.; Urban-Chmiel, R.; Kosikowska, U. Phenotypic and genotypic characterization of *Enterococcus* spp. from yolk sac infections in broiler chicks with a focus on virulence factors. *Poult. Sci.* **2021**, *100*, 100985. [CrossRef]
52. Heidari, H.; Emaneini, M.; Dabiri, H.; Jabalameli, F. Virulence factors, antimicrobial resistance pattern and molecular analysis of Enterococcal strains isolated from burn patients. *Microb. Pathog.* **2016**, *90*, 93–97. [CrossRef] [PubMed]
53. Lebreton, F.; van Schaik, W.; McGuire, A.M.; Godfrey, P.; Griggs, A.; Mazumdar, V.; Corander, J.; Cheng, L.; Saif, S.; Young, S.; et al. Emergence of epidemic multidrug-resistant *Enterococcus faecium* from animal and commensal strains. *ASM J.* **2013**, *4*, e00534-13. [CrossRef] [PubMed]
54. EUCAST. *Antimicrobial Susceptibility Testing. EUCAST Disk Diffusion Method, Version 5*; European Committee on Antimicrobial Susceptibility Testing: Basel, Switzerland, 2015; pp. 1–22.
55. EUCAST. *Breakpoint Tables for Interpretation of MICs and Zone Diameters, Version 9*; European Committee on Antimicrobial Susceptibility Testing: Basel, Switzerland, 2019; pp. 29–33.
56. CLSI. *Performance Standards for Antimicrobial Susceptibility Testing; Twenty-Fifth Informational Supplement M100-S25*; Clinical and Laboratory Standards Institute: Wayne, PA, USA, 2015; pp. 72–75.

57. Houf, K.; De Zutter, L.; Van Hoof, J.; Vandamme, P. Assessment of the genetic diversity among arcobacters isolated from poultry products by using two PCR-based typing methods. *Appl. Environ. Microbiol.* **2002**, *68*, 2172–2178. [CrossRef] [PubMed]
58. Ryu, H.; Henson, M.; Elk, M.; Toledo-Hernandez, C.; Griffith, J.; Blackwood, D.; Noble, R.; Gourmelon, M.; Glassmeyer, S.; Santo Domingo, J.W. Development of quantitative PCR assays targeting the 16S rRNA genes of *Enterococcus* spp. and their application to the identification of enterococcus species in environmental samples. *Appl. Environ. Microbiol.* **2013**, *79*, 196–204. [CrossRef] [PubMed]
59. Pavel, A.B.; Vasile, C.I. PyElph-a software tool for gel images analysis and phylogenetics. *BMC Bioinform.* **2012**, *13*, 9. [CrossRef]
60. Perrier, X.; Jacquemoud-Collet, J.P. DARwin Software. 2006. Available online: https://darwin.cirad.fr/ (accessed on 1 July 2022).
61. Hammer, Ø.; Harper, D.A.T.; Ryan, P.D. PAST: Paleontological statistics software package for education and data analysis. *Palaeontol. Electron.* **2001**, *4*, 1–9.

antibiotics

MDPI

Article

Prevalence and Antimicrobial Resistance Profile of Diarrheagenic *Escherichia coli* from Fomites in Rural Households in South Africa

Phathutshedzo Rakhalaru, Lutendo Munzhedzi, Akebe Luther King Abia, Jean Pierre Kabue, Natasha Potgieter and Afsatou Ndama Traore *

Department of Biochemistry and Microbiology, Faculty of Science, Engineering and Agriculture, University of Venda, Private Bag X5050, Thohoyandou 0950, South Africa; rakhalaru96@gmail.com (P.R.); lutendomunzhedzi1@gmail.com (L.M.); lutherkinga@yahoo.fr (A.L.K.A.); kabue.ngandu@univen.ac.za (J.P.K.); natasha.potgieter@univen.ac.za (N.P.)

* Correspondence: afsatou.traore@univen.ac.za

Abstract: Diarrheagenic *Escherichia coli* (DEC) pathotypes are the leading cause of mortality and morbidity in South Asia and sub-Saharan Africa. Daily interaction between people contributes to the spreading of *Escherichia coli* (*E. coli*), and fomites are a common source of community-acquired bacterial infections. The spread of bacterial infectious diseases from inanimate objects to the surrounding environment and humans is a serious problem for public health, safety, and development. This study aimed to determine the prevalence and antibiotic resistance of diarrheagenic *E. coli* found in toilets and kitchen cloths in the Vhembe district, South Africa. One hundred and five samples were cultured to isolate *E. coli*: thirty-five samples were kitchen cloths and seventy-five samples were toilet swabs. Biochemical tests, API20E, and the VITEK®-2 automated system were used to identify *E. coli*. Pathotypes of *E. coli* were characterised using Multiplex Polymerase Chain Reaction (mPCR). Nine amplified gene fragments were sequenced using partial sequencing. A total of eight antibiotics were used for the antibiotic susceptibility testing of *E. coli* isolates using the Kirby–Bauer disc diffusion method. Among the collected samples, 47% were positive for *E. coli*. DEC prevalence was high (81%), with ETEC (51%) harboring *lt* and *st* genes being the most dominant pathotype found on both kitchen cloths and toilet surfaces. Diarrheagenic *E. coli* pathotypes were more prevalent in the kitchen cloths (79.6%) compared with the toilet surfaces. Notably, hybrid pathotypes were detected in 44.2% of the isolates, showcasing the co-existence of multiple pathotypes within a single *E. coli* strain. The antibiotic resistance testing of *E. coli* isolates from kitchen cloths and toilets showed high resistance to ampicillin (100%) and amoxicillin (100%). Only *E. coli* isolates with hybrid pathotypes were found to be resistant to more than three antibiotics. This study emphasizes the significance of fomites as potential sources of bacterial contamination in rural settings. The results highlight the importance of implementing proactive measures to improve hygiene practices and antibiotic stewardship in these communities. These measures are essential for reducing the impact of DEC infections and antibiotic resistance, ultimately safeguarding public health.

Keywords: diarrheagenic; *Escherichia coli*; antibiotic resistance; households; kitchen cloths; toilets

Citation: Rakhalaru, P.; Munzhedzi, L.; Abia, A.L.K.; Kabue, J.P.; Potgieter, N.; Traore, A.N. Prevalence and Antimicrobial Resistance Profile of Diarrheagenic *Escherichia coli* from Fomites in Rural Households in South Africa. *Antibiotics* **2023**, *12*, 1345. https://doi.org/10.3390/antibiotics12081345

Academic Editor: Jie Fu

Received: 14 July 2023
Revised: 8 August 2023
Accepted: 19 August 2023
Published: 21 August 2023

1. Introduction

Diarrheal disease remains a significant public health issue particularly in rural areas where there is limited availability of clean water and adequate sanitation facilities [1,2]. The spread of pathogens through fomites is a serious concern to human health, safety, and development. Fomites act as reservoirs and potential vectors for pathogenic bacteria, including *E.coli*, leading to the spread of infections within households [3]. Pathogenic bacteria can survive on fomites for an extended period, and the duration of their survival is influenced by factors such as temperature, humidity, and the availability of other microorganisms [4,5]. Previous studies have shown the presence of *E. coli* on various fomites, including kitchen surfaces and cloths, toilet surfaces, door handles, and bathroom surfaces. These fomites serve as source of transmission, posing a potential health risk [6,7].

E. coli is a Gram-negative bacterium that typically inhabits the lower intestines of warm-blooded animals, and certain *E. coli*, O157: H7, leads to severe gastrointestinal infections in humans [8,9]. Studies by Seidman et al. [10] and Potgieter et al. [11] have reported the contamination of toilet seats in rural households with total coliforms and *E. coli*. Research findings have also revealed that kitchen cloths exhibit bacterial contamination, with *E. coli* emerging as the most frequently detected microorganism [9,12,13]. *E. coli* is generally used as an indicator of faecal pollution and indicates the presence of other pathogenic bacteria, such as *Salmonella* and *Shigella*, which have been associated with diarrhea [14]. Apart from its role as an indicator organism, *E. coli* can be classified as diarrheagenic (intestinal) or extraintestinal pathotypes [15]. Diarrheagenic *E. coli* pathotypes are categorized into six well characterized groups harboring specific genes: enteroinvasive *E. coli* (EIEC), enteropathogenic *E. coli* (EPEC), enterotoxigenic *E. coli* (ETEC), enterohemorrhagic *E. coli* (EHEC), enteroaggregative *E. coli* (EAEC), and diffusely adherent *E. coli* [16,17]. Certain *E. coli* pathotypes can acquire virulence genes from other *E. coli* strains, resulting in what is known as a hybrid pathotype [18–20]. Diarrhea caused by pathogenic *E. coli* is a leading cause of morbidity and mortality worldwide, especially in children younger than five years [21,22].

Infections caused by *E. coli* are usually treated using antibiotics such as penicillin, gentamycin, ampicillin, amoxicillin, chloramphenicol, rifampicin, and tetracycline [23]. However, some studies have documented that *E. coli* has become resistant to some antibiotics due to their widespread and inappropriate use [24,25]. Such misuse poses a serious health problem [26]; antimicrobial resistant *E. coli* strains have been reported as the main carriers of antibiotic resistance genes to ampicillin, penicillin, tetracycline, and rifampicin [27,28]. Hybrid DEC pathotypes have been reported to exhibit multidrug resistance to beta-lactam antibiotics [20,29].

In South Africa, inadequate access to water supply, sanitation services, and hygiene is considered the eleventh most significant risk factor leading to illnesses [30]. About 73% of toilets in rural households in the Vhembe District are pit holes with no water taps close to the toilets [31], suggesting that most people might not wash their hands immediately after using the toilets. Even in situation where water is accessible, most people wash their hands solely with water without using detergents [30].

Thus, poor sanitation and hygiene are still serious problems in rural households in the Vhembe district. Therefore, this study aimed to determine the prevalence and antibiotic resistance of diarrheagenic *E. coli* contamination in household fomites, highlighting the importance of implementing effective hygiene measures to mitigate transmission risks.

2. Methods and Materials

2.1. Study Area and Period

This study was conducted in Tshamutilikwa village (−22.892981245885206, 30.600267380011015) in the Vhembe district, South Africa (Figure 1), from May to August 2021. Tshamutilikwa is a place with a population of 814 people, according to the Census conducted in 2011 (https://census2011.adrianfrith.com/place/966110) (accessed on 3 August 2023). It covers an area of 1.06 square kilometers. With a population density of 766.49 people per square kilometer, Tshamutilikwa is a relatively densely populated area. The village consists of 203 households, resulting in an average of 191.15 households per square kilometer.

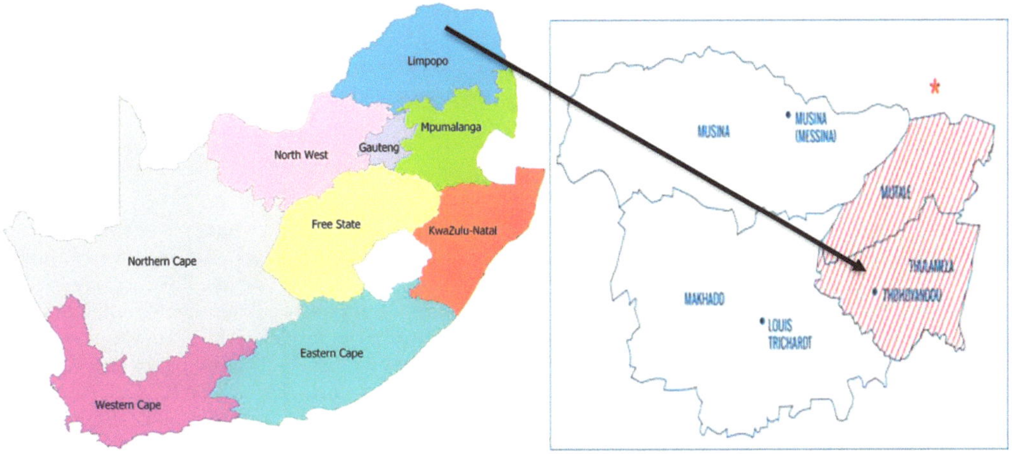

Figure 1. Map of South Africa (left) indicating sample collection site in the Vhembe District (Thulamela Municipality) where Tshamutilikwa village is located. The start indicates Vhembe District https://www.mappr.co/counties/south-africa/) (accessed on 3 August 2023).

2.2. Ethics

Ethical clearance was obtained from the University of Venda [SEA/21/MBY/02/1608]. Sampling was done after receiving permission from the household owners by signing a consent form and questionnaire to answer and sign.

2.3. Sample Collection

Kitchen cloths, toilet seats, and toilet door handle swabs were collected door-to-door from the selected households and 70 toilet (35 seats and 35 door handles) samples were collected from participating households in Tshamutilikwa. A specific prepared questionnaire was administered to household owners to obtain information on various water, sanitation, and hygiene [WASH] factors, including the source of water, usage of kitchen cloths, condition of the kitchen cloth, toilet condition, type of toilet, handwashing means after using the toilet, the incidence of diarrhea in the household, and the practice of sharing the toilet with neighbors.

Samples were collected from toilet surfaces using the peptone water sterile swab-rinse method described by Hurst et al. [32]. In addition, a total of 35 old and used kitchen cloths were collected. Participants were requested to place the kitchen cloths in sterile zipping lock bags in exchange for new kitchen cloths. Before sample analysis, a brief description of the quality of kitchen cloths based on aspects such as dirty/clean or wet/dry was recorded. The toilets were categorized as clean or dirty based on their appearance. Clean toilets had no visible dirt, while dirty toilets had visible dirt, stains, and feces on toilet seats. The samples were immediately transported in ice to the microbiology laboratory and analyzed within four hours of sampling.

2.4. Bacterial Isolation and Identification

2.4.1. Bacterial Isolation

In the laboratory, 5 cm by 5 cm (length × breadth) pieces were aseptically cut from each kitchen cloth sample and placed into a sterile flask containing 50 mL nutrient broth (Davies diagnostic (Pty) Ltd., Randburg, Gauteng, South Africa) for enrichment, vortexed for 5 min, and incubated at 37 °C overnight [33]. After incubation, 1 mL of the inoculated broth was transferred into a clean, sterile test tube containing 9 mL of sterile water. The diluted solution was mixed thoroughly by vortexing, and 0.5 mL of the diluted solution was then spread on sterile Eosin Methylene Blue (EMB) agar (Davies diagnostic (Pty) Ltd.,

Randburg, Gauteng, South Africa) plates using a sterile glass spreader and incubated for 24 h at 37 °C. Toilet seat and door handle swab samples were streaked directly on EMB agar and incubated for 24 h at 37 °C. After incubation, two distinct green metallic shiny colonies (characteristic of *E. coli*) were selected from each EMB plate and subcultured on a sterile nutrient agar plate to isolate pure colonies. All media used were prepared according to the manufacturer's specifications.

2.4.2. Bacterial Identification

The colonies obtained from sub-culturing on nutrient agar plates were analyzed using various biochemical tests such as the Kligler iron agar test [34], Urease test, Simmon citrate test [35], and the API20E (bioMérieux, Marcy I'Etoile, France). Presumptive *E. coli* isolates were further confirmed using the VITEK 2 automated system (bioMérieux, Marcy-l'Étoile, France) as described by the manufacturer. Briefly, a bacterial suspension was created by mixing *E. coli* colonies with 0.85% phosphate-buffered saline (PBS) (Thermo Fisher Scientific, Randburg, South Africa), resulting in a concentration of 1×10^8 CFU/mL Mcflarland standard. Subsequently, 2 mL of these suspensions were automatically loaded into the VITEK 2 ID system, utilizing the GNB cards specifically designed for *E. coli* identification. The cards were analyzed through kinetic fluorescence measurement, and the results were reported within 3 h.

2.5. Molecular Identification of E. coli *Isolates*

2.5.1. DNA Extraction

DNA extraction was performed as previously described by Omar et al. [36]. Briefly, 2 mL of nutrient broth with *E. coli* was aliquoted into sterile 2 mL Eppendorf tubes (Sigma-Aldrich, St Louis, MI, USA). The tubes were centrifuged at 13,000× *g* for 120 s to separate the cells from the supernatant. The DNA binding to celite was enhanced using lysis buffer mixed with 250 µL of 100% ethanol. Before washing, the celite-bound DNA was added to the spin columns. Qiagen elution buffer (Southern Cross Biotechnology®, Hilden, Germany) of 100 µL was used for DNA elution. Extracted DNA was then used as a template for PCR reactions.

2.5.2. Genotypic Identification and Classification of *E. coli* Pathotypes

Genotypic identification and classification of selected isolates into the different *E. coli* pathotypes were performed using an 11-gene multiplex PCR, as previously reported [37,38]. The primers used in this study are in (Table 1). A total volume of 20 µL reaction mixture consisted of 10 µL, 2X Qiagen® PCR multiplex mix (Qiagen®, Hilden, Germany), 1 µL 5× Q-solution, 2 µL of DNA template, 5 µL PCR grade water, and 2 µL of the primer mix containing 0.1 µM of *lt* and *mdh*, 0.5 µM of *stx1* and *st*, 0.3 µM of *eaeA* and *stx2*, and 0.2 µM of *astA*, *bfp eagg*, *ial*, and *gapdh* primers. Multiplex PCR amplification was performed in a Bio-Rad MyCycler™ Thermal cycler (Bio-Rad, Hercules, CA, USA) under the following PCR conditions: an initial activation at 95 °C for 15 min, followed by denaturation at 94 °C for 45 s, and annealing was performed at 55 °C for 45 s. Extension was done at 68 °C for 2 min (35 cycles) [38]. PCR amplifications were separated using agarose gel electrophoresis, the bacterial DNAs were loaded into pre-cast wells in the gel, and a current was applied as described by Alfinete et al. [39].

Table 1. Primers used to identify diarrheagenic *E. coli* pathotype-associated genes.

Pathogen	Primers	Sequence (5′-3′)	Size (bp)	Conc. (µM)	Reference
E. coli	*mdh* (F) *Mdh*(R)	GGT ATG GAT CGT TCC GAC CT GGC AGA ATG GTA ACA CCA GAG	300	0.1	Omar et al. [40]
EIEC	*ial* (F) *ial* (R)	GGT ATG ATG ATG AGT CCA GGA GGC CAA CAA TTA TTT CC	630	0.2	Pass et al. [41]

Table 1. *Cont.*

Pathogen	Primers	Sequence (5′-3′)	Size (bp)	Conc. (μM)	Reference
EHEC/Atypical EPEC	*eaeA* (F)	GGT ATG ATG ATG ATG AGT CCA	917	0.3	Aranda et al. [42]
	eaeA(R)	GGA GGC CAA CAA TTA TTT CC			
Typical EPEC	*bfpA* (F)	AAT GGT GCT TGC GCT TGC TGC	410		
EAEC	*eagg* (F)	AGA CTC TGG CGA AAG ACT GTA TC	194	0.2	Pass et al. [41]
	Eagg(R)	ATG GCT GTC TGT AAT AGA TGA GAA C			
EHEC	*stx1* (F)	ACA CTG GAT GAT CTC AGT GG	614	0.5	Moses et al. [43]
	stx1(R)	CTG AAT CCC CCT CCA TTA TG			
	stx2 (F)	CCA TGA CAA CGG ACA GCA GTT	779	0.3	
	Stx2(R)	CCT GTC AAC TGA GCA CTT TG			
ETEC	*lt* (F)	GGC GAC AGA TTA TAC CGT GC	330	0.1	Pass et al. [41]
	lt (R)	CGG TCT CTA TAT TCC CTG TT			
	st (F)	TTT CCC CTC TTT TAG TCA GTC AAC TG	160	0.5	
	st (R)	GGC AGG ATT ACA ACA AAG TTC ACA			
E. coli toxin	*astA (F)*	GCC ATC AAC ACA GTA TAT CC	106	0.3	Kimata et al. [44]
	astA (R)	GAG TGA CGG CTT TGT AGT C			
External Control	*gapdh* (F)	GAG TCA ACG GAT TTG GTC GT	238	0.1	Mbene et al. [45]
	gapdh (R)	TTG ATT TTG GAG GGA TCT CG			

2.6. Sequencing and Phylogenetic Analysis

Sequencing and phylogenetic analysis of *E. coli* was performed to compare the bacterial isolates obtained from the kitchen cloths and toilets within the same household and to investigate whether similar bacterial clones existed in different households, to identify any potential spread of identical clones within the community. DNA partial sequencing was performed on ABI 3500XL Genetic Analyzer POP7TM (Thermo Scientific, Waltham, MA, USA) using the same specific primers (Table 1). The reading of the DNA sequence was done and edited on FinchTV v1.4 (Geospiza Inc., Seattle, WA, USA). Nucleotide sequences of *E. coli* were compared with other reference strains on GenBank by blasting on the NCBI program (available at http://www.ncbi.nlm.nih.gov/) (accessed on 19 May 2022). For constructing the phylogenetic tree, MEGA X version 10.2.6 software was used to create phylogenetic trees by the neighbor-joining method and evaluated at 1000 bootstrap replicates for each gene [41,42].

2.7. Determination of Antibiotic Susceptibility

All the *E. coli* isolates were tested for sensitivity to different antibiotics using the Kirby–Bauer standard disc diffusion method [46,47]. For the disc diffusion assay, bacteria were grown for 24 h on Mueller–Hinton agar (Davies Diagnostics (pty) Ltd., Randburg, Gauteng, South Africa), harvested, and then suspended in 0.85% sterile PBS solution adjusted to a 0.5 McFarland turbidity standard, equivalent to 10^8 CFU/mL. The standardized bacterial suspension was streaked onto Mueller–Hinton agar plates using a sterile cotton swab and exposed to commercially available antibiotic discs (Thermo Fisher Scientific, Waltham, MA, USA). The zones of inhibition were measured using a ruler after 24 h of incubation at 37 °C. The resistance patterns of the isolates to 8 different antibiotics (Table 2) were then interpreted as either Resistant (R), Intermediate resistant (I), or Sensitive (S), following the guidelines set by the Clinical Laboratory Standards Institute (CLSI, 2020) (https://clsi.org/meetings/susceptibility-testing-subcommittees/) (accessed on 3 August 2023). The antibiotics selected (Table 2) in this study are commonly used to treat diarrheal infections caused by diarrheagenic *E. coli* pathotypes.

Table 2. List of antibiotics used, disc potencies, and zone diameter interpretative standards for *E. coli* (CLSI, 2020).

Antibiotics	Disc Code	Disc Potency (µg)	Inhibition Zone (mm)		
			Resistant	Intermediate	Sensitive
Amoxicillin-Clavulanic	AMC	30	≤19	-	≥20
Azithromycin	AMZ	30	≤13	17–19	≥20
Chloramphenicol	CN	30	≤12	13–17	≥18
Gentamicin	GM	10	≤12	13–14	≥15
Ampicillin	AMP	10	≤13	14–16	≥17
Rifampicin	C	5	≤16	17–19	≥20
Tetracycline	TE	5	≤11	12–14	≥15
Penicillin	P	10	≤14	15–20	≥21

3. Results

3.1. Study Characteristics

In all, 54.3% (19/35) of the kitchen cloths were dirty; among those, 54.6% (11/19) were dry and dirty, and 42.1% (8/19) were wet and dirty (Table 3). Of 35 toilets where swab samples were collected, 54.3% (19/35) were not clean, and two had feces on the seats.

Table 3. Demographical features of the 35 households in Tshamutilikwa village with percentage.

Variables	Category	Total Study Population (%) (n = 35)
Number of people in a household	One Two More than two	3 (8.6) 7 (20) 25 (71.4)
Source of Water	Tap Well Surface	33 (94.3) 0 2 (5.7)
Handwashing means after using the toilet	Water only Water and soap Do not wash	17 (49) 15 (43) 3 (8.6)
Type of toilet	Ventilated improved latrine Pit latrines Flush toilets	27 (77.90) 1 (2.9) 7 (20)
Toilet condition	Clean Dirty	16 (45.7) 19 (54.3)
Sharing of the toilet with neighbors	Yes No	2 (5.7) 33 (94.3)
Animal ownership	Yes No	29 (83) 6 (17)
Animals are allowed to enter the house	Yes No	1 (2.9) 34 (97.1)
Diarrhea in the household	Yes No	4 (11.4) 31 (88.6)
Condition of kitchen cloth	Clean Dirty	16 (45.7) 19 (54.3)
Kitchen cloth use	Wiping up spills Drying hands Covering food Cleaning and drying up dishes Multi-use	2 (5.7) 2 (5.7) 3 (8.6) 7 (20) 21 (60)
Washing soap	Powdered soap Bar soap Jik bleach	25 (71.4) 6 (17) 4 (11.4)

3.2. Prevalence of *E. coli* on Kitchen Cloths and Toilets

Of the 105 samples collected, 46.7% (49/105) were positive for *E. coli*. All the kitchen cloths had bacterial contamination. A total of 71.4% (25/35) of the kitchen cloths (n = 35) were contaminated with *E. coli*. Out of the 70 samples collected from the toilets, 24 (34.3%) were contaminated with *E. coli* (Table 4).

Table 4. Prevalence of *E. coli* on kitchen cloths and toilet surfaces (seats and door handle).

Samples	*E. coli*	Percentage (%)
Kitchen cloths; n = 35	25	71.4
Toilet seats; n = 35	12	34.3
Toilet door handles; n = 35	12	34.3
Total; n = 105	49	46.7

3.3. Characterization of *E. coli* Pathotypes

The *mdh* gene was used as an internal control to ensure the PCR worked for each *E. coli* isolate. A total of 43/49 (90%) isolates were positive for the *E. coli* housekeeping gene (*mdh*). All the *E. coli* isolates with *mdh* genes also tested positive for the *gapdh* gene. The m-PCR test did not show any false positives or PCR inhibition as the external control gene (*gapdh*) was detected in all samples.

Multiplex PCR detected five DEC pathotypes (EAEC, EHEC, EPEC, ETEC, and EIEC). The prevalence of commensal *E. coli* (8/43; 18.6%) was lower than that of DEC (35/43; 81%). ETEC (22/43; 51%), harboring *lt* and *st* genes, was the most dominant DEC pathotype found in kitchen cloths and on toilet surfaces.

Different hybrid pathogenic strains of *E. coli* were found, 24 (55.8%) non-hybrid pathotypes and 19 (44.2%) hybrid pathotypes. There was a high prevalence of hybrids with two pathotypes, making the percentage 18.7% (Figure 2). Most of the hybrid *E. coli* strains exhibited the presence of the Asta gene, which is known to be carried by *E. coli* toxins.

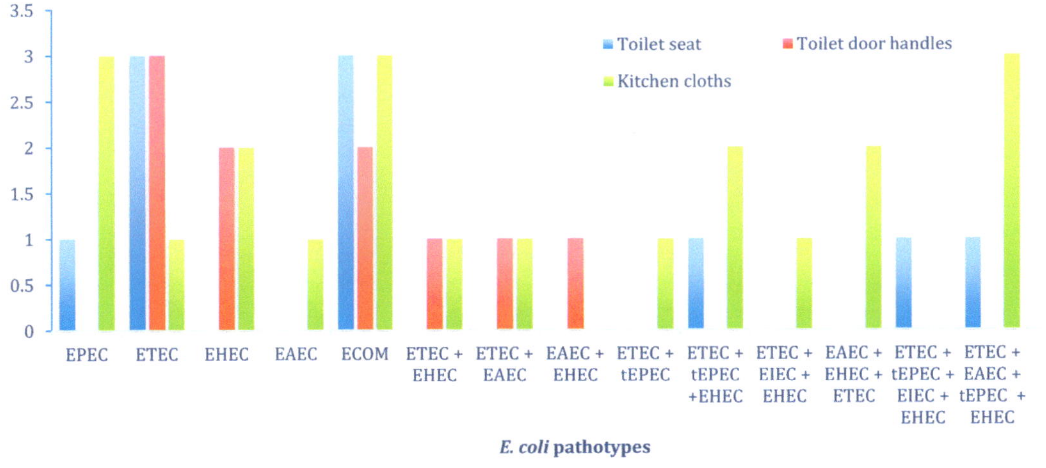

Figure 2. Prevalence of non-hybrid and hybrid *E. coli* pathotypes on kitchen cloths, toilet seats, and toilet door handles.

Based on the sample type, more diarrheagenic *E. coli* pathotypes were found in kitchen cloths (39/49, 79.6%) followed by toilet seats (20/49; 40.8%) and toilet door handles (11/49; 22.4%), respectively (Figure 2). In addition, the gel image illustrating the results of the Multiplex PCR is provided in Supplementary Figure S1.

3.4. Antibiotic Resistance Profile of *E. coli*

The *E. coli* isolates obtained from kitchen cloths exhibited varying levels of antibiotic resistance. *E. coli* isolates from the toilet surfaces and kitchen cloths displayed the highest resistance to ampicillin (24/24; 100%) and amoxicillin (24/24; 100%). (Table 5).

Table 5. Antibiotic resistance percentage of *E. coli* isolated from kitchen cloths and toilets.

Resistance to Specific Antibiotic	Kitchen Cloths (51%) n = 25	Toilet Seats (24.5%) n = 12	Toilet Door Handles (24.5%) n = 12	Total (%) n = 49
Ampicillin	25 (100)	12 (100)	12 (100)	49 (100)
Tetracycline	4 (16)	1 (8.3)	0	5 (24.3)
Amoxicillin	25 (100)	12 (100)	12 (100)	49 (100)
Chloramphenicol	5 (20)	2 (16.6)	0	7 (36.6)
Rifampicin	3 (12)	0	0	3 (12)
Azithromycin	0	0	0	0
Gentamycin	0	0	0	0
Penicillin	19 (76)	7 (58.3)	9 (75)	35 (71.42)
Ampicillin and Amoxicillin	25 (100)	12 (100)	12 (100)	49 (100)
Ampicillin, Amoxicillin, and penicillin	19 (76)	7 (58.3)	9 (75)	35 (71.4)
Multidrug resistance Amoxicillin, Ampicillin, Penicillin, Chloramphenicol, and Tetracycline	2 (8)	1 (4)	0	3 (6.1)

Some of the isolates showed resistance to more than two antibiotics; only 28.6% (14/49) of the isolates did not show resistance to three antibiotics. The multidrug resistance of *E. coli* isolates was found in 6.1% (3/49) of the isolates (Table 5). Only *E. coli* isolates with hybrid pathotypes were found to be resistant to more than three antibiotics used.

3.5. Sequence and Phylogenetic Analysis

Sequence Analysis and Phylogenetic Analysis

The study findings indicated that among the households sampled, only three households (numbers 7, 28, and 35) exhibited the consistent presence of the same pathotypes (ETEC, EHEC, and EAEC) across all three sample types: kitchen cloth, toilet seat, and toilet door handle surfaces. Specifically, household number 7 showed ETEC, 28 showed EHEC, and 35 showed EAEC detected in all sample types. Nine amplified DNA extracts were sent for partial sequencing (including three of *Stx1*, three of *lt*, and three of *Eagg*). Of the nine amplified *E. coli* isolates, only one *stx1* (1/3; 33.3%) and one *Eagg* (1/3; 33.3%) were successfully sequenced.

The two sequences obtained were blasted on GenBank for comparison with other reference *E. coli* strains. The similarities with the reference strain for the *Stx1* gene sequence ranged from 80 to 89.4%, and for the *Eagg* gene sequence ranged from 81 to 89.8% (Figures 3 and 4).

The *Stx1* sequence (accession no. 0N193544) from the present study was closely related to a reference strain isolated in water from Hungary (accession no. DQ44966.1) and shared a common ancestor with an *E. coli* strain from human feces in Bangladesh (Figure 3).

The *Eagg* sequence (accession no. 0N241000) obtained from the toilet seat in this study shared a common ancestor with an *E. coli* strain (accession no. MZ330843.1) from handwash water in the Vhembe District, South Africa (Figure 4). There were limited reference strains of *Stx1* and *Eagg* genes in Africa.

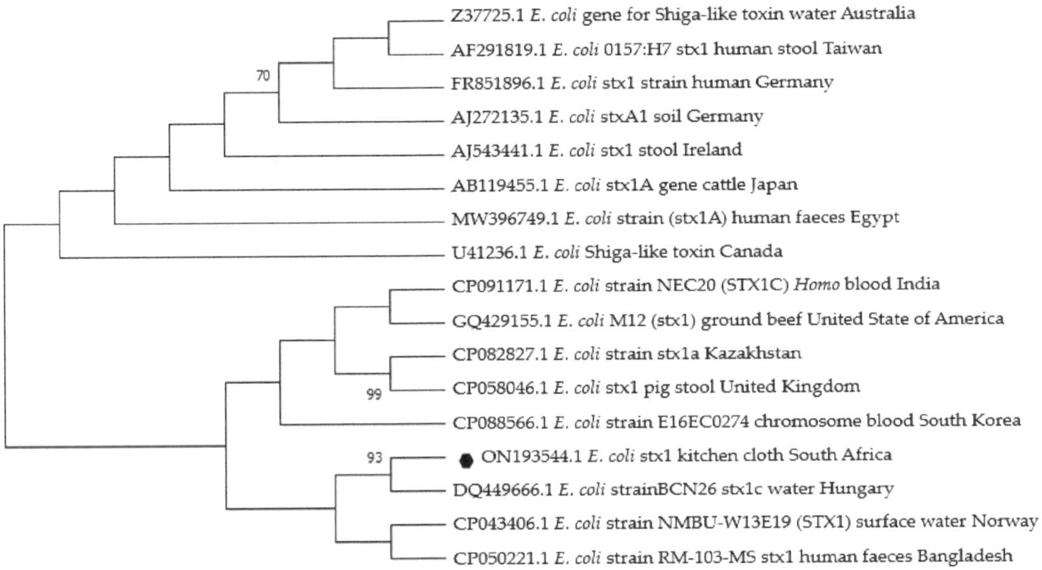

Figure 3. Phylogenetic tree based on 614 nucleotide sequences of the *E. coli* stx1 gene fragment constructed using the neighbor-joining method. The black dot indicates the sequence obtained from this study (May 2021) in the rural community of Vhembe District, South Africa. Fifteen reference *E. coli* strains with the same gene were selected randomly from GenBank. Bootstrap values greater than 70% for the branches were considered. The phylogenetic tree was constructed using Mega X version 10.2.6 software.

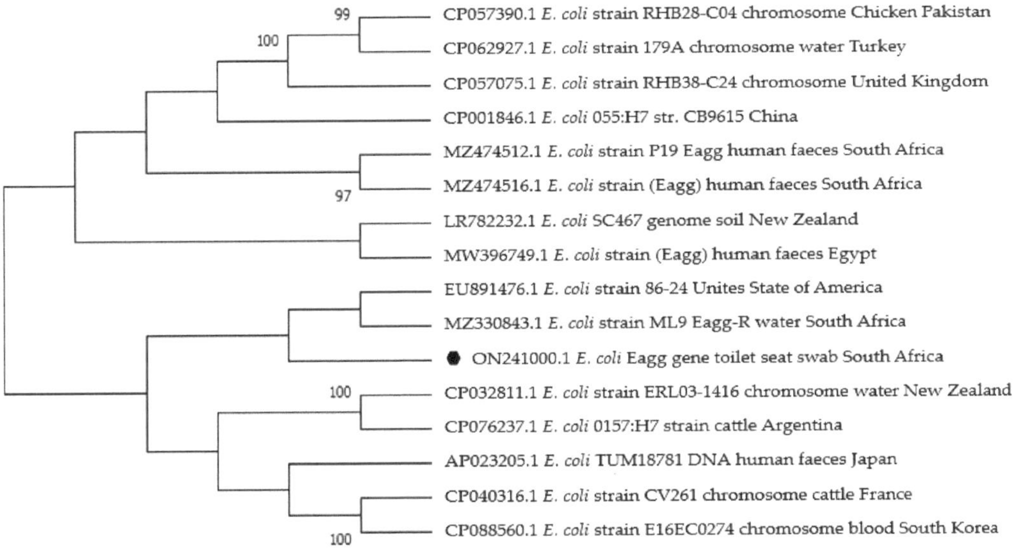

Figure 4. Phylogenetic tree based on 194 nucleotide sequence of *E. coli* eagg gene fragment constructed using the neighbor-joining method. The black dot indicates the sequence obtained from this study (May 2021) in the rural community of Vhembe District, South Africa. Fifteen *E. coli* reference strains with the same gene were selected randomly from GenBank. The phylogenetic tree was constructed using Mega X version 10.2.6 software.

4. Discussion

Poor sanitation and hygiene are still major problems in rural communities, especially in low- and middle-income countries (LMICs). They have been associated with increased diarrhea disease caused by enteric pathogens. Diarrhea is the leading cause of morbidity and mortality worldwide [42,48]. There are few reports on the prevalence and antibiotic resistance of diarrheagenic *E. coli* from household fomites in the Vhembe District. A large percentage difference was observed when comparing the bacterial rate of contamination on toilets (12/35; 34.3%) and kitchen cloths (25/35; 71.4%). This has been associated with the differences in the environmental conditions of the kitchen cloths (wet and dirty) and the toilets (dry and clean). The high frequency of *E. coli* on kitchen cloths can be attributed to the multipurpose use and the wet condition, which is suitable for the growth of bacteria [49,50]. The kitchen cloths examined in this study were highly contaminated with enterotoxigenic *E. coli*. Similar results were also reported by Chavatte et al. [12]. Furthermore, Speirs et al. [51] expressed concerns regarding the presence of enteric microorganisms in wet areas of the domestic kitchen, such as dishcloths, sink surfaces, and draining boards. These studies emphasize the potential health risks associated with dirty wet kitchen fomites that harbor bacterial contamination.

The high prevalence of DEC proves that kitchen cloths can be sources of food poisoning since ETEC, EHEC, and EPEC are pathogenic [33]. Studies have shown that the most frequently used fomites (toilets and kitchen cloths) are highly contaminated [52,53]. This study revealed a similar percentage of *E. coli* on both toilet seats and door handles. Similar findings have been previously reported [6,52,54,55]. Therefore, household toilets and kitchen cloths should be seen as important vehicles for transmitting diarrheagenic *E. coli* to humans.

Some of the presumptive *E. coli* isolates did not show the presence of the *mdh* gene, which could be due to the low DNA concentration or some PCR inhibitors and is in line with another study [40] in South Africa that reported that 15% of *E. coli* isolates were negative for the *mdh* gene. However, *E. coli* isolates that tested positive for *mdh* showed the presence of the *gapdh* gene, which was used as an external control. Using the *gapdh* gene as an external control helps ensure accurate PCR results with no false positives and no PCR inhibitors [40,56].

In this study, it was discovered that 44.2% of the *E. coli* isolate exhibited the combination of two or more genes from different pathotypes. Furthermore, hybrid pathotypes were more prevalent on kitchen cloths and toilet seats, respectively. Enterotoxigenic *E. coli* and EAEC were the most prevalent DEC in the diarrheal stool samples of young children living in the Vhembe district [22]. In addition, *E. coli* isolates with two or more virulence genes of DEC were found. Banda et al. [57] reported similar findings in the toilets and floor swabs from households in the Vhembe District, South Africa. The challenge concerning hybrid pathogens lies in their combination of virulence genes that leads to the development of severe diseases [58]. Several DEC strains with more virulence genes have been observed elsewhere in children's diarrhea stool samples [48]. Previous studies reported an increase in the number of infections due to emerging DEC hybrid pathotypes [59–61]. Identifying a substantial proportion of diarrheagenic *E. coli* hybrid pathotypes on fomites highlights the need for effective hygiene measures in rural households. These findings highlight the potential for these fomites to serve as a reservoir for harmful bacteria, increasing household members' risk of diarrheal illnesses.

A high prevalence of DEC resistance to commonly used antibiotics was found in the study area. Kitchen cloths and toilet surfaces in the rural areas of the Vhembe District were contaminated with DEC strains exhibiting high resistance to Beta-lactam antibiotics (ampicillin, amoxicillin, and penicillin). There is an increase in DEC resistance to amoxicillin and ampicillin in the current study as compared with the previous studies in Africa [60–62]. The inappropriate use of antibiotics has been identified as a contributing factor to antibiotic resistance in developing countries [10]. However, all the DEC isolates were susceptible to azithromycin and gentamycin. High *E. coli* susceptibility to gentamycin has been previously reported [63]. This study identified *E. coli* strains exhibiting resistance to multiple antibiotics. These findings agree with earlier reports on *E. coli* multidrug resistance in South Africa [64–66]. For example, Bolukaoto et al. [39], reported the multidrug resistance of DEC to two or more antibiotics (ampicillin, amoxicillin, cefotaxime, and others). This indicates a concerning situation where these commonly used antibiotics may not effectively treat infections caused by these resistant strains of DEC.

Sequences of *Stx1* and *Eagg* gene fragments identified in this study were related to reference strains associated with infections such as hemolytic uremic syndrome (HUS) and diarrhea in patients from Egypt, South Africa, China, Japan, USA, and the UK [66–72], suggesting that *Stx1* and *Eagg* strains found in this study may pose a threat to human health. The first outbreak of human *Stx1* disease in South Africa occurred in 1992, a decade after the first outbreak in the United States of America [73]. *Eagg* identified in this study from the toilet seat and *Eagg* previously isolated from handwash water in 2019 (accession no. MZ330843.1) in the Vhembe District share a similar ancestor (Figure 4). This shows inadequate hygiene and sanitation and possible routes of transmission from the toilet to humans. This reveals the continuous spread of diarrheagenic *E. coli* from 2019 to 2021 in the Vhembe District. Furthermore, Ojima et al. [65], and Sharma et al. [13] demonstrated that washing dishcloths with regular detergent or soaps was insufficient in destroying pathogenic bacteria and recommended soaking the dishcloths in sodium hypochlorite for 3 to 4 min, then washing them in hot water.

Enterotoxigenic *E. coli* and EAEC are significantly associated with hemolytic uremic syndrome (HUS), urinary tract infection, and diarrhea worldwide [66,67]. *E. coli* strains have been classified based on genetic and evolutionary relationships into four main phylogroups (A, B1, B2, and D). Some studies have reported that *E. coli* strains with *Stx1* and *Eagg* genes fall under phylogroup B2 and D, respectively [68,69]. The phylogenetic trees from this study revealed the relatedness of *Stx1* and *Eagg* from South Africa with others from different countries (Figures 3 and 4). However, there are few reference *E. coli* strains with the same genes in Africa. Therefore, *E. coli* sequences from this study play a vital role in providing valuable epidemiological data specific to Africa. By analyzing these sequences, researchers can gain insights into the prevalence, distribution, and potential transmission patterns of these particular *E. coli* strains within Africa. This information is important in understanding and addressing the region's public health implications associated with these strains.

5. Conclusions

There is a high prevalence of pathogenic and antimicrobial-resistant *E. coli* on kitchen cloths and toilet surfaces in the Vhembe District, South Africa. Kitchen cloths and toilets should be seen as important fomites for transmitting DEC. Furthermore, this study highlighted the inefficiency of regular detergents or soaps in eliminating pathogenic bacteria from kitchen cloths, emphasizing the need for proper hygiene practices such as soaking the cloths in sodium hypochlorite and washing them in hot water. The findings in this study indicate the urgency of implementing effective measures to combat antibiotic resistance and improve domestic hygiene practices in rural households to mitigate the spread of DEC.

Supplementary Materials: The following supporting information can be downloaded at: https://www.mdpi.com/article/10.3390/antibiotics12081345/s1. Figure S1. Depicts gel images A and B, showcasing the multiplex PCR results for detecting different *E. coli* genes on household kitchen cloths and toilet surfaces.

Author Contributions: Conceptualization, A.N.T. and N.P.; methodology, P.R., L.M., A.N.T. and N.P.; validation, A.N.T. and A.L.K.A.; formal analysis, P.R., J.P.K. and A.N.T.; investigation, P.R.; data curation, P.R., L.M. and J.P.K.; writing—original draft preparation, P.R.; writing—review and editing, J.P.K., A.N.T., A.L.K.A., N.P. and P.R.; supervision, A.N.T. and N.P.; project administration, P.R. and A.N.T.; funding acquisition, A.N.T. and N.P. All authors have read and agreed to the published version of the manuscript.

Funding: This research received no external funding.

Institutional Review Board Statement: This study was conducted after obtaining the approval of the Institutional Review Board (or Ethics Committee) of University of Venda (SEA/21/MBY/02/1608).

Informed Consent Statement: Informed consent was obtained from all subjects involved in this study.

Data Availability Statement: Raw sequencing reads are available in the National Center for Biotechnology Information (NCBI) GenBank database (accession numbers 0N241000 and 0N193544).

Acknowledgments: The authors would like to thank the people of Tshamutilikwa village for their support and agreement to sample in their homes. We would also like to acknowledge the support provided to this study by the Microbiology Department.

Conflicts of Interest: The authors declare no conflict of interest.

References

1. Keddy, K.H. Old and new challenges related to global burden of diarrhoea. *Lancet Infect. Dis.* **2018**, *18*, 1163–1164. [CrossRef]
2. Das, R.; Palit, P.; Haque, M.A.; Ahmed, T.; Faruque, A.G. Association between Pathogenic Variants of Diarrheagenic *Escherichia coli* and Growth in Children under 5 Years of Age in the Global Enteric Multicenter Study. *Am. J. Trop. Med. Hyg.* **2022**, *107*, 72. [CrossRef] [PubMed]
3. Stephens, B.; Azimi, P.; Thoemmes, M.S.; Heidarinejad, M.; Allen, J.G.; Gilbert, J.A. Microbial exchange via fomites and implications for human health. *Curr. Pollut. Rep.* **2019**, *5*, 198–213. [CrossRef]
4. Katzenberger, R.H.; Rösel, A.; Vonberg, R.-P. Bacterial survival on inanimate surfaces: A field study. *BMC Res. Notes* **2021**, *14*, 97. [CrossRef]
5. Van Elsas, J.D.; Semenov, A.V.; Costa, R.; Trevors, J.T. Survival of *Escherichia coli* in the environment: Fundamental and public health aspects. *ISME J.* **2011**, *5*, 173–183. [CrossRef] [PubMed]
6. Alonge, O.; Auwal, B.; Aboh, M. Bacterial contamination of toilet door handles on Baze University campus Abuja Nigeria. *Afr. J. Clin. Exp. Microbiol.* **2019**, *20*, 35–41. [CrossRef]
7. Nworie, A.; Ayeni, J.; Eze, U.; Azi, S. Bacterial contamination of door handles/knobs in selected public conveniences in Abuja metropolis, Nigeria: A public health threat. *Cont. J. Med. Res.* **2012**, *6*, 7–11.
8. Kaur, R.; Singh, D.; Kesavan, A.K.; Kaur, R. Molecular characterization and antimicrobial susceptibility of bacterial isolates present in tap water of public toilets. *Int. Health* **2020**, *12*, 472–483. [CrossRef]
9. Su, C.; Brandt, L.J. *Escherichia coli* O157: H7 infection in humans. *Ann. Intern. Med.* **1995**, *123*, 698–707. [CrossRef] [PubMed]
10. Seidman, J.; Kanungo, R.; Bourgeois, A.; Coles, C. Risk factors for antibiotic-resistant *E. coli* in children in a rural area. *Epidemiol. Infect.* **2009**, *137*, 879–888. [CrossRef]
11. Potgieter, N.; Aja-Okorie, U.; Mbedzi, R.L.; Traore-Hoffman, A.N. Bacterial contamination on household latrine surfaces: A case study in rural and Peri-urban communities in South Africa. In *Current Microbiological Research in Africa: Selected Applications for Sustainable Environmental Management*; Springer: Cham, Switzerland, 2020; pp. 175–183.
12. Chavatte, N.; Baré, J.; Lambrecht, E.; Van Damme, I.; Vaerewijck, M.; Sabbe, K.; Houf, K. Co-occurrence of free-living protozoa and foodborne pathogens on dishcloths: Implications for food safety. *Int. J. Food Microbiol.* **2014**, *191*, 89–96. [CrossRef]
13. Sharma, M.; Eastridge, J.; Mudd, C. Effective household disinfection methods of kitchen sponges. *Food Control* **2009**, *20*, 310–313. [CrossRef]
14. Ugboko, H.U.; Nwinyi, O.C.; Oranusi, S.U.; Oyewale, J.O. Childhood diarrhoeal diseases in developing countries. *Heliyon* **2020**, *6*, e03690. [CrossRef]
15. Keshav, V.; Kruger, C.A.; Mathee, A.; Naicker, N.; Swart, A.; Barnard, T.G. *E. coli* from dishcloths as an indicator of hygienic status in households. *J. Water Sanit. Hyg. Dev.* **2015**, *5*, 351–358. [CrossRef]
16. Levine, M.M. *Escherichia coli* that cause diarrhea: Enterotoxigenic, enteropathogenic, enteroinvasive, enterohemorrhagic, and enteroadherent. *J. Infect. Dis.* **1987**, *155*, 377–389. [CrossRef] [PubMed]
17. Modgil, V.; Mahindroo, J.; Narayan, C.; Kalia, M.; Yousuf, M.; Shahi, V.; Koundal, M.; Chaudhary, P.; Jain, R.; Sandha, K.S. Comparative analysis of virulence determinants, phylogroups, and antibiotic susceptibility patterns of typical versus atypical Enteroaggregative *E. coli* in India. *PLOS Neglected Trop. Dis.* **2020**, *14*, e0008769. [CrossRef] [PubMed]
18. Nyholm, O.; Halkilahti, J.; Wiklund, G.; Okeke, U.; Paulin, L.; Auvinen, P.; Haukka, K.; Siitonen, A. Comparative genomics and characterization of hybrid Shigatoxigenic and enterotoxigenic *Escherichia coli* (STEC/ETEC) strains. *PLoS ONE* **2015**, *10*, e0135936. [CrossRef]
19. Hazen, T.H.; Michalski, J.; Luo, Q.; Shetty, A.C.; Daugherty, S.C.; Fleckenstein, J.M.; Rasko, D.A. Comparative genomics and transcriptomics of *Escherichia coli* isolates carrying virulence factors of both enteropathogenic and enterotoxigenic *E. coli*. *Sci. Rep.* **2017**, *7*, 3513. [CrossRef]
20. Bolukaoto, J.Y.; Singh, A.; Alfinete, N.; Barnard, T.G. Occurrence of hybrid diarrhoeagenic *Escherichia coli* associated with multidrug resistance in environmental water, Johannesburg, South Africa. *Microorganisms* **2021**, *9*, 2163. [CrossRef]

21. Nguyen, T.V.; Le Van, P.; Le Huy, C.; Gia, K.N.; Weintraub, A. Detection and characterization of diarrheagenic *Escherichia coli* from young children in Hanoi, Vietnam. *J. Clin. Microbiol.* **2005**, *43*, 755–760. [CrossRef]
22. Ledwaba, S.; Kabue, J.; Barnard, T.; Traore, A.; Potgieter, N. Enteric pathogen co-infections in the paediatric population from rural communities in the Vhembe District, South Africa. *South Afr. J. Child Health* **2018**, *12*, 170–174. [CrossRef]
23. Beaber, J.W.; Hochhut, B.; Waldor, M.K. SOS response promotes horizontal dissemination of antibiotic resistance genes. *Nature* **2004**, *427*, 72–74. [CrossRef]
24. Ochoa, T.J.; Ruiz, J.; Molina, M.; Del Valle, L.J.; Vargas, M.; Gil, A.I.; Ecker, L.; Barletta, F.; Hall, E.R.; Cleary, T.G. High frequency of antimicrobial resistance of diarrheagenic *E. coli* in Peruvian infants. *Am. J. Trop. Med. Hyg.* **2009**, *81*, 296. [CrossRef]
25. Shigemura, K.; Yamashita, M.; Tanaka, K.; Arakawa, S.; Fujisawa, M.; Adachi, M. Chronological change of antibiotic use and antibiotic resistance in *Escherichia coli* causing urinary tract infections. *J. Infect. Chemother.* **2011**, *17*, 646–651. [CrossRef]
26. Kapil, A. The challenge of antibiotic resistance: Need to contemplate. *Indian J. Med. Res.* **2005**, *121*, 83.
27. Ventola, C.L. The antibiotic resistance crisis: Part 1: Causes and threats. *Pharm. Ther.* **2015**, *40*, 277.
28. Scaletsky, I.C.; Souza, T.B.; Aranda, K.R.; Okeke, I.N. Genetic elements associated with antimicrobial resistance in enteropathogenic *Escherichia coli* (EPEC) from Brazil. *BMC Microbiol.* **2010**, *10*, 25. [CrossRef] [PubMed]
29. Furlan, J.P.R.; Ramos, M.S.; Dos Santos, L.D.R.; da Silva Rosa, R.; Stehling, E.G. Multidrug-resistant Shiga toxin-producing *Escherichia coli* and hybrid pathogenic strains of bovine origin. *Vet. Res. Commun.* **2023**, 1–7. [CrossRef] [PubMed]
30. Wilkinson, M.; du Tout, A.; Mashimbye, D.; Cooligen, S. *Assessment of Handwashing and Hand Hygiene Behaviour*; Water Research Commission: Pretoria, South Africa, 2012.
31. Vhembe. Vhembe District Municipality 2021/22 IDP Review; Vhembe District. 2022; pp. 88–89. Available online: http://www.vhembe.gov.za/media/content/documents/2021/2025/o_2021f2087kkc2021almpu2072g2022j202112027s2023vh2022k.pdf?filename=2021%202022%202020IDP%202020REVIEW.pdf (accessed on 3 August 2023).
32. Hurst, C.J.; Crawford, R.L.; Garland, J.L.; Lipson, D.A. *Manual of Environmental Microbiology*; American Society for Microbiology Press: Washington, DC, USA, 2007.
33. Nkiwane, L.; Chigo, T. Microbial Analysis of Woven Cotton Kitchen Towels. *Zimb. J. Sci. Technol.* **2014**, *9*, 47–58.
34. Lehman, D. *Triple Sugar Iron Agar Protocols*; American Society for Microbiology: Washington, DC, USA, 2005; pp. 1–7.
35. Alam, M.; Nahar, S.; Chowdhury, M.; Hasan, M.; Islam, M.; Sikdar, B. Biochemical characterization of bacteria responsible for bacterial black pit disease of lime (Citrus aurantifolia) and their control system. *Eur. J. Biotechnol. Biosci.* **2019**, *7*, 16–22.
36. Omar, K.; Potgieter, N.; Barnard, T. Development of a rapid screening method for the detection of pathogenic *Escherichia coli* using a combination of Colilert® Quanti-Trays/2000 and PCR. *Water Sci. Technol. Water Supply* **2010**, *10*, 7–13. [CrossRef]
37. Barnard, T.; Robertson, C.; Jagals, P.; Potgieter, N. A rapid and low-cost DNA extraction method for isolating *Escherichia coli* DNA from animal stools. *Afr. J. Biotechnol.* **2011**, *10*, 1485–1490.
38. Boom, R.; Sol, C.; Salimans, M.; Jansen, C.; Wertheim-van Dillen, P.; Van der Noordaa, J. Rapid and simple method for purification of nucleic acids. *J. Clin. Microbiol.* **1990**, *28*, 495–503. [CrossRef] [PubMed]
39. Alfinete, N.W.; Bolukaoto, J.Y.; Heine, L.; Potgieter, N.; Barnard, T.G. Virulence and phylogenetic analysis of enteric pathogenic *Escherichia coli* isolated from children with diarrhoea in South Africa. *Int. J. Infect. Dis.* **2022**, *114*, 226–232. [CrossRef]
40. Omar, K.; Barnard, T. Detection of diarrhoeagenic *Escherichia coli* in clinical and environmental water sources in South Africa using single-step 11-gene m-PCR. *World J. Microbiol. Biotechnol.* **2014**, *30*, 2663–2671. [CrossRef]
41. Pass, M.; Odedra, R.; Batt, R. Multiplex PCRs for identification of *Escherichia coli* virulence genes. *J. Clin. Microbiol.* **2000**, *38*, 2001–2004. [CrossRef] [PubMed]
42. Aranda, K.R.S.; Fagundes-Neto, U.; Scaletsky, I.C.A. Evaluation of multiplex PCRs for diagnosis of infection with diarrheagenic *Escherichia coli* and *Shigella* spp. *J. Clin. Microbiol.* **2004**, *42*, 5849–5853. [CrossRef]
43. Moses, A.; Garbati, M.; Egwu, A.; Ameh, E. Detection of *E. coli* 0157 and 026 serogroups in human immunodeficiency virus-infected patients with clinical manifestation of diarrhoea in Maiduguri, Nigeria. *Res. J. Med. Med. Sci.* **2006**, *1*, 140–145.
44. Kimata, K.; Shima, T.; Shimizu, M.; Tanaka, D.; Isobe, J.; Gyobu, Y.; Watahiki, M.; Nagai, Y. Rapid categorization of pathogenic *Escherichia coli* by multiplex PCR. *Microbiol. Immunol.* **2005**, *49*, 485–492. [CrossRef]
45. Mbene, A.B.; Houreld, N.N.; Abrahamse, H. DNA damage after phototherapy in wounded fibroblast cells irradiated with 16 J/cm2. *J. Photochem. Photobiol. B: Biol.* **2009**, *94*, 131–137. [CrossRef]
46. Bauer, A.; Kirby, W.; Sherris, J.C.; Turck, M. Antibiotic susceptibility testing by a standardized single disk method. *Am. J. Clin. Pathol.* **1966**, *45*, 493–496. [CrossRef]
47. Hudzicki, J. Kirby-Bauer disk diffusion susceptibility test protocol. *Am. Soc. Microbiol.* **2009**, *15*, 55–63.
48. Natarajan, M.; Kumar, D.; Mandal, J.; Biswal, N.; Stephen, S. A study of virulence and antimicrobial resistance pattern in diarrhoeagenic *Escherichia coli* isolated from diarrhoeal stool specimens from children and adults in a tertiary hospital, Puducherry, India. *J. Health Popul. Nutr.* **2018**, *37*, 17. [CrossRef]
49. Sibiya, J.E.; Gumbo, J.R. Knowledge, attitude and practices (KAP) survey on water, sanitation and hygiene in selected schools in Vhembe District, Limpopo, South Africa. *Int. J. Environ. Res. Public Health* **2013**, *10*, 2282–2295. [CrossRef] [PubMed]
50. Borchgrevink, C.P.; Cha, J.; Kim, S. Hand washing practices in a college town environment. *J. Environ. Health* **2013**, *75*, 18–25.
51. Speirs, J.; Anderton, A.; Anderson, J. A study of the microbial content of the domestic kitchen. *Int. J. Environ. Health Res.* **1995**, *5*, 109–122. [CrossRef]

52. Barker, J.; Bloomfield, S. Survival of Salmonella in bathrooms and toilets in domestic homes following salmonellosis. *J. Appl. Microbiol.* **2000**, *89*, 137–144. [CrossRef]
53. McGinnis, S.; Marini, D.; Amatya, P.; Murphy, H.M. Bacterial contamination on latrine surfaces in community and household latrines in Kathmandu, Nepal. *Int. J. Environ. Res. Public Health* **2019**, *16*, 257. [CrossRef] [PubMed]
54. Ngonda, F. Assessment of bacterial contamination of toilets and bathroom doors handle/knobs at Daeyang Luke hospital. *Pharm. Biol. Eval.* **2017**, *4*, 193–197. [CrossRef]
55. Maori, L.; Agbor, V.O.; Ahmed, W.A. The prevalence of bacterial organisms on toilet door handles in Secondary Schools in Bokkos LGA, Jos, Plateau Sate, Nigeria. *IOSR J. Pharm. Biol. Sci.* **2013**, *8*, 85–91.
56. van Pelt-Verkuil, E.; van Belkum, A.; Hays, J.P. Ensuring PCR quality–laboratory organisation, PCR optimization and controls. In *Principles and Technical Aspects of PCR Amplification*; Springer: Dordrecht, The Netherlands, 2008; pp. 183–212.
57. Banda, N.T. Characterization of *E. coli* Strains from Rural Communities in the Vhembe District (Limpopo South Africa). Ph.D. Thesis, University of Venda, Tohoyandu, South Africa, 2019.
58. Lindstedt, B.-A.; Finton, M.D.; Porcellato, D.; Brandal, L.T. High frequency of hybrid *Escherichia coli* strains with combined Intestinal Pathogenic *Escherichia coli* (IPEC) and Extraintestinal Pathogenic *Escherichia coli* (ExPEC) virulence factors isolated from human faecal samples. *BMC Infect. Dis.* **2018**, *18*, 544. [CrossRef]
59. Borgatta, B.; Kmet-Lunaček, N.; Rello, J. *E. coli* O104: H4 outbreak and haemolytic–uraemic syndrome. *Med. Intensiv. (Engl. Ed.)* **2012**, *36*, 576–583. [CrossRef]
60. Mare, I.; Coetzee, J. The incidence of transmissible drug resistance factors among strains of *Escherichia coli* in the Pretoria area. *S. Afr. Med. J.* **1966**, *40*, 980–981. [PubMed]
61. Chiyangi, H.; Muma, J.B.; Malama, S.; Manyahi, J.; Abade, A.; Kwenda, G.; Matee, M.I. Identification and antimicrobial resistance patterns of bacterial enteropathogens from children aged 0–59 months at the University Teaching Hospital, Lusaka, Zambia: A prospective cross sectional study. *BMC Infect. Dis.* **2017**, *17*, 117. [CrossRef] [PubMed]
62. Balogun, S.; Ojo, O.; Bayode, O.; Kareem, S. High level detection of extended spectrum beta-lactamase gene encoding Enterobacteriaceae in public toilets in Abeokuta, Nigeria. *Ceylon J. Sci.* **2020**, *49*, 165–172. [CrossRef]
63. Mirsoleymani, S.R.; Salimi, M.; Shareghi Brojeni, M.; Ranjbar, M.; Mehtarpoor, M. Bacterial pathogens and antimicrobial resistance patterns in pediatric urinary tract infections: A four-year surveillance study (2009–2012). *Int. J. Pediatr.* **2014**, *2014*, 126142. [CrossRef]
64. Lamprecht, C.; Romanis, M.; Huisamen, N.; Carinus, A.; Schoeman, N.; Sigge, G.O.; Britz, T.J. *Escherichia coli* with virulence factors and multidrug resistance in the Plankenburg River. *S. Afr. J. Sci.* **2014**, *110*, 01–06. [CrossRef]
65. Ojima, M.; Toshima, Y.; Koya, E.; Ara, K.; Tokuda, H.; Kawai, S.; Kasuga, F.; Ueda, N. Hygiene measures considering actual distributions of microorganisms in Japanese households. *J. Appl. Microbiol.* **2002**, *93*, 800–809. [CrossRef]
66. Bielaszewska, M.; Karch, H. Non-O157: H7 Shiga toxin (verocytotoxin)-producing *Escherichia coli* strains: Epidemiological significance and microbiological diagnosis. *World J. Microbiol. Biotechnol.* **2000**, *16*, 711–718. [CrossRef]
67. Friedrich, A.; Bielaszewska, M.; Karch, H. Diagnosis of Shiga Toxin-Producing *Escherichia coli* Infections/Die Diagnostik von Shiga Toxin-produzierenden *Escherichia coli*-Infektionen. *LaboratoriumsMedizin* **2002**, *26*, 183–190. [CrossRef]
68. Wieler, L.H.; Semmler, T.; Eichhorn, I.; Antao, E.M.; Kinnemann, B.; Geue, L.; Karch, H.; Guenther, S.; Bethe, A. No evidence of the Shiga toxin-producing *E. coli* O104: H4 outbreak strain or enteroaggregative *E. coli* (EAEC) found in cattle faeces in northern Germany, the hotspot of the 2011 HUS outbreak area. *Gut Pathog.* **2011**, *3*, 17. [CrossRef] [PubMed]
69. Escobar-Páramo, P.; Clermont, O.; Blanc-Potard, A.-B.; Bui, H.; Le Bouguénec, C.; Denamur, E. A specific genetic background is required for acquisition and expression of virulence factors in *Escherichia coli*. *Mol. Biol. Evol.* **2004**, *21*, 1085–1094. [CrossRef] [PubMed]
70. Riley, L.W.; Remis, R.S.; Helgerson, S.D.; McGee, H.B.; Wells, J.G.; Davis, B.R.; Hebert, R.J.; Olcott, E.S.; Johnson, L.M.; Hargrett, N.T. Hemorrhagic colitis associated with a rare *Escherichia coli* serotype. *N. Engl. J. Med.* **1983**, *308*, 681–685. [CrossRef] [PubMed]
71. Aijuka, M.; Santiago, A.E.; Girón, J.A.; Nataro, J.P.; Buys, E.M. Enteroaggregative *Escherichia coli* is the predominant diarrheagenic *E. coli* pathotype among irrigation water and food sources in South Africa. *Int. J. Food Microbiol.* **2018**, *278*, 44–51. [CrossRef]
72. Van Der Hooft, J.J.; Goldstone, R.J.; Harris, S.; Burgess, K.E.; Smith, D.G. Substantial extracellular metabolic differences found between phylogenetically closely related probiotic and pathogenic strains of *Escherichia coli*. *Front. Microbiol.* **2019**, *19*, 252. [CrossRef]
73. Isaäcson, M.; Canter, P.H.; Effler, P.; Arntzen, L.; Bomans, P.; Heenan, R. Haemorrhagic colitis epidemic in Africa. *Lancet* **1993**, *341*, 961. [CrossRef]

antibiotics

MDPI

Article

Acinetobacter baylyi Strain BD413 Can Acquire an Antibiotic Resistance Gene by Natural Transformation on Lettuce Phylloplane and Enter the Endosphere

Valentina Riva, Giovanni Patania, Francesco Riva, Lorenzo Vergani, Elena Crotti and Francesca Mapelli *

Department of Food, Environmental and Nutritional Sciences (DeFENS), University of Milan, 20133 Milan, Italy
* Correspondence: francesca.mapelli@unimi.it; Tel.: +39-02-50319115; Fax: +39-02-50319238

Abstract: Antibiotic resistance spread must be considered in a holistic framework which comprises the agri-food ecosystems, where plants can be considered a bridge connecting water and soil habitats with the human microbiome. However, the study of horizontal gene transfer events within the plant microbiome is still overlooked. Here, the environmental strain *Acinetobacter baylyi* BD413 was used to study the acquisition of extracellular DNA (exDNA) carrying an antibiotic resistance gene (ARG) on lettuce phylloplane, performing experiments at conditions (i.e., plasmid quantities) mimicking those that can be found in a water reuse scenario. Moreover, we assessed how the presence of a surfactant, a co-formulant widely used in agriculture, affected exDNA entry in bacteria and plant tissues, besides the penetration and survival of bacteria into the leaf endosphere. Natural transformation frequency in planta was comparable to that occurring under optimal conditions (i.e., temperature, nutrient provision, and absence of microbial competitors), representing an entrance pathway of ARGs into an epiphytic bacterium able to penetrate the endosphere of a leafy vegetable. The presence of the surfactant determined a higher presence of culturable transformant cells in the leaf tissues but did not significantly increase exDNA entry in *A. baylyi* BD413 cells and lettuce leaves. More research on HGT (Horizontal Gene Transfer) mechanisms in planta should be performed to obtain experimental data on produce safety in terms of antibiotic resistance.

Keywords: horizontal gene transfer; phyllosphere; plant microbiome; one-health; emerging organic contaminants; surfactants; water reuse

check for updates

Citation: Riva, V.; Patania, G.; Riva, F.; Vergani, L.; Crotti, E.; Mapelli, F. *Acinetobacter baylyi* Strain BD413 Can Acquire an Antibiotic Resistance Gene by Natural Transformation on Lettuce Phylloplane and Enter the Endosphere. *Antibiotics* **2022**, *11*, 1231. https://doi.org/10.3390/antibiotics11091231

Academic Editor: Akebe Luther King Abia

Received: 29 July 2022
Accepted: 6 September 2022
Published: 10 September 2022

1. Introduction

The rise of antibiotic resistance is posing risk on a global scale for human health. Its spread has been related to the selection pressure imposed by the use of antibiotics for clinical purposes and their presence in the environment [1], where they are considered emerging organic contaminants. Contamination with sub-lethal concentrations of antibiotics can contribute to the emergence of Antibiotic Resistance Genes (ARGs) through Horizontal Gene Transfer (HGT) mechanisms into bacterial populations [2]. Accordingly, environmental bacteria displaying multi-drug resistance phenotypes against different classes of antibiotics have been found in animal, soil, and aquatic habitats [3]. Agricultural soils were indicated among the primary sources of antibiotic-resistant bacteria (ARB) threatening human health due to ARGs diffusion via manure or sewage sludge applications and the use of reclaimed wastewater for irrigation [4,5]. The plant microbiome is a nexus for the 'One-Health' approach, acting as a bridge connecting soil and water microbiomes to the human one through the food chain. In fact, the consumption of food products such as raw leafy vegetables is recognized among the possible main pathways for resistome diffusion [6,7]. Bacteria that usually inhabit the phyllosphere (i.e., the surfaces of the aerial parts of a plant, mainly represented by leaves) are overall considered harmless, but they might represent transient hosts with the capability to transfer ARGs to human pathogenic bacteria by HGT [8]. ARGs can accumulate on leaves from different pathways including air and soil particles [9] and are widely detected also on produces [10]. Nonetheless, evidence of HGT events within the microbiome that colonize edible plant portions generally consumed raw is still overlooked. Among HGT mechanisms, the role of natural transformation (i.e., the direct uptake and incorporation of extracellular DNA from a bacterium) is poorly studied in the context of environmental antibiotic resistance although recent evidence speaks in favor of greater importance than previously assumed [11,12]. *A. baylyi* BD413 strain, an environmental model bacterium [13] previously used for natural transformation studies [14,15], can be a useful tool to fill in this gap of knowledge. The genus *Acinetobacter* includes several human opportunistic pathogens, such as *Acinetobacter baumannii*, recognized as major causal agents of nosocomial infections and known for the propensity to develop resistance to the main groups of antibiotics [16,17]. On the other hand, different species of the *Acinetobacter* genus are typical members of the cultivable plant endophytic microbiome [7,18] and were isolated from fresh fruits and leafy vegetables, such as lettuce [19]. Recently, the opportunity to manage the microbiota composition of lettuce and other fresh produces has been proposed as a strategy to limit the invasion of potential human pathogens and to limit outbreaks related to the consumption of contaminated food [20,21]. *A. baylyi* species is able to horizontally transfer antibiotic resistance genes to *Escherichia coli* through the secretion of vesicles [17] and HGT between these two species has been recently demonstrated on lettuce leaf discs [22]. Moreover, the frequency of HGT events involving *A. baylyi* can be influenced by different environmental and chemical stresses [4,17,23].

This study was aimed at characterizing the possible acquisition of extracellular DNA (exDNA) on lettuce phylloplane by *A. baylyi* BD413 performing in planta experiments, to clarify the role of natural transformation as entrance pathway of ARGs into the epiphytic and/or endophytic bacterial community associated to leafy vegetables. Furthermore, based on the knowledge that surfactants can alter the permeability of biological membranes [24] and can increase the entrance of bacteria into leaf tissues [25], we tested the hypothesis that heptamethyltrisiloxane, a co-formulant widely used in agriculture, enhances *A. baylyi* BD413 membrane permeability, exDNA acquisition by bacteria and plant tissues, and bacterial leaf endosphere penetration.

2. Results

2.1. *A. baylyi BD413 Permanence as Viable and Culturable Cells into Lettuce Leaves*

The capacity of the *A. baylyi* BD413 strain to survive in a viable and cultivable state on the lettuce phylloplane (i.e., the surface of leaves) was assessed after administration by spray, to simulate sprinkler irrigation. *A. baylyi* BD413 cell suspension was prepared at a concentration of 10^8 cell/mL in physiological solution in a spray bottle. We initially evaluated the concentration of the viable and culturable bacterial cells actually released by spray (Table S1). This data was used to calculate the ratio between the CFUs/mL reisolated from the phylloplane/leaf endosphere after bacterization (i.e., survived culturable cells) and the CFUs/mL released by spray (i.e., administered cells). The experiment demonstrated that *A. baylyi* BD413 was able to adhere and survive on the leaf surface of lettuce plants (Figures 1 and S1) both 1 h and 24 h after bacterization (Table 1).

Table 1. The ratio between survived and administered cells of the strains *A. baylyi* BD413, *E. coli* DH5α, and *K. cowanii* VR04.

Strain	1 h	24 h
A. baylyi BD413	$9.39 \times 10^{-4} \pm 4.24 \times 10^{-4}$	$1.54 \times 10^{-4} \pm 5.11 \times 10^{-5}$
A. baylyi BD413-endo	-	$1.25 \times 10^{-6} \pm 3.29 \times 10^{-7}$
E. coli DH5α	$5.24 \times 10^{-3} \pm 3.87 \times 10^{-3}$	$4.34 \times 10^{-5} \pm 6.81 \times 10^{-5}$
K. cowanii VR04	$2.39 \times 10^{-2} \pm 1.19 \times 10^{-3}$	$3.01 \times 10^{-3} \pm 2.14 \times 10^{-3}$

The table reports the results obtained for each strain 1 h and 24 h after administration on the leaf surface. Furthermore, the ratio between the *A. baylyi* BD413 cells that penetrate and survived into the endosphere and those initially administered on the leaf surface has been calculated.

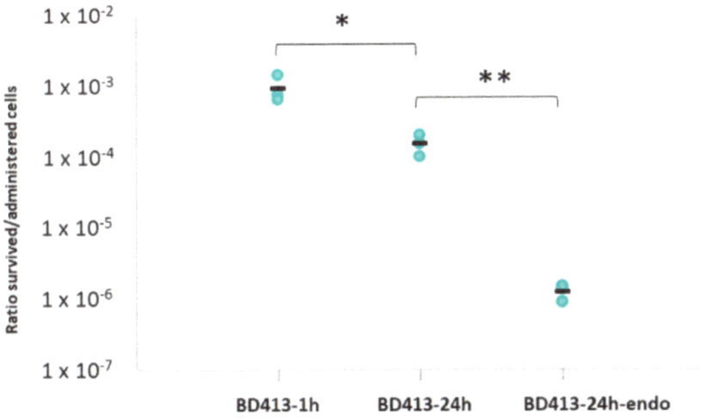

Figure 1. Permanence of *A. baylyi* BD413 as viable and culturable cells on lettuce phylloplane and into leaf tissues. The ratio between *A. baylyi* BD413 survived culturable cells and administered cells on lettuce phylloplane was assessed 1 h (BD413-1 h) and 24 h after spray administration (BD413-24 h). In addition, the survival into the leaf endosphere was assessed 24 h after bacterization (BD413-24 h-endo). The black line indicates the average value of three biological replicates. Stars indicate significant differences according to Student's *t*-test (* = p value < 0.05; ** = p value < 0.001).

However, after 24 h, the ratio between survived and administered *A. baylyi* BD413 cells showed a significantly lower value (Student's *t*-test, $p = 0.0335$) than the one obtained 1 h after administration. *A. baylyi* BD413 cells were reisolated also from the leaf endosphere 24 h after bacterization (Table 1). The ratio between the survived cells reisolated from the leaf tissues and those initially administered on the leaf surface was significantly lower (Figure 1) compared to that measured on the phylloplane at the same time point (Student's *t*-test, $p = 0.0066$).

The ability of *A. baylyi* BD413 to survive on the lettuce phylloplane was compared with those of the laboratory strain *E. coli* DH5α and the lettuce strain *K. cowanii* VR04 (Figure S2) as a benchmark to clarify its possible adaptation to this ecological niche. The CFUs/mL released by spray on lettuce leaves were measured for *E. coli* DH5α and *K. cowanii* VR04 (Table S1) to determine also for these strains the ratio between the survived and the administered cells on the leaf surface. According to ANOVA tests (Table S2), at both the experimental times the survival of *A. baylyi* BD413 into a viable and culturable state was not significantly different in comparison to *E. coli* DH5α values (Table 1). The survival of *K. cowanii* VR04 on phylloplane (Table 1) was significantly higher compared to *A. baylyi* BD413 1 h after the strain administration, while it decreased after 24 h to a value (Table 1) not significantly different from that recorded for *A. baylyi* BD413 (Figure S1, Table S2). For all survival experiments, bacterial colonies were reisolated and identified by ITS fingerprinting as *A. baylyi* BD413 (Figure S1a–c), *E. coli* DH5α (Figure S1d), and *K. cowanii* VR04 (Figure S1e).

2.2. Natural Transformation on Nitrocellulose Membrane Filters

To set up the best condition for the in vivo natural transformation assay, plasmid DNA acquisition by *A. baylyi* BD413 was initially tested on nitrocellulose membrane filters using different quantities of pZR80(gfp), comprised between 1 and 50 ng based on literature data available about exDNA concentration in wastewaters [26]. Using 1, 2, and 5 ng of plasmid DNA per transformation assay, we measured not significantly different transformation frequency values (Figure 2, Table S3). A significantly higher (ANOVA, Tukey-Kramer post-hoc test; $p < 0.0001$) transformation frequency was obtained using 10 ng of pZR80(gfp) (Figure 2, Table S3). This value further and significantly increased (Figure 2, Table S3) when performing the experiment with 20 ng and 50 ng of plasmid.

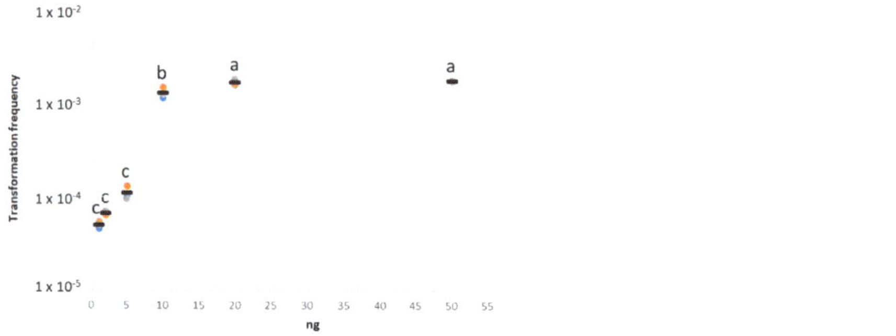

Figure 2. Selection of extracellular DNA quantities for in vivo *A. baylyi* BD413 natural transformation assays. Transformation frequency of *A. baylyi* BD413 was calculated by performing an in vitro natural transformation experiment on nitrocellulose membrane filters using a range of quantities of plasmid pZR80(gfp), chosen according to the literature information about exDNA concentration in wastewaters. The black line indicates the average value of three technical replicates. Different letters (a, b, c) indicate significant differences between the values of transformation frequency measured using DNA quantities ranging from 1 to 50 ng, according to the Tukey-Kramer post-hoc test (ANOVA, p-value < 0.0001).

Based on these results we selected the lowest quantities of plasmid DNA suitable for subsequent in vivo tests, namely 1 ng and 10 ng, which represents a compromise between the environmental conditions and the detection of natural transformation events [26]. Once the plasmid quantities have been selected, the *A. baylyi* BD413 natural transformation experiment on nitrocellulose membrane filters was repeated using four biological replicates (i.e., four different cultures of *A. baylyi* BD413) to obtain results statistically comparable with those subsequently generated on lettuce leaves. In the latter assay, the *A. baylyi* BD413 transformation frequency showed a value of $2.12 \times 10^{-3} \pm 1.43 \times 10^{-4}$ using 10 ng of plasmid (Figure 3b), while this value decreased to $2.80 \times 10^{-4} \pm 5.65 \times 10^{-5}$ performing the in vitro experiment with 1 ng of DNA (Figure 3b).

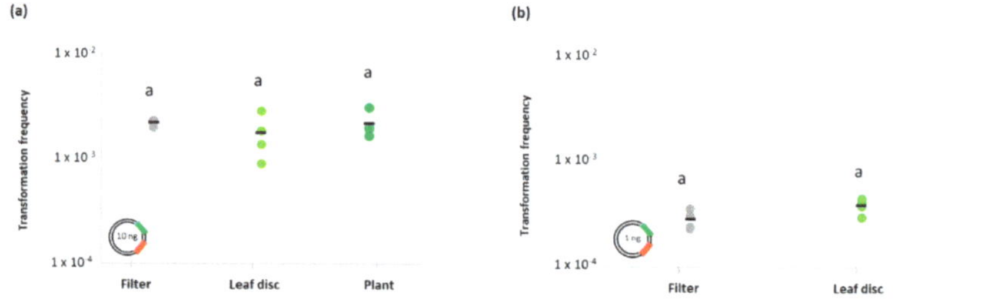

Figure 3. Natural transformation of A. baylyi BD413 under different experimental setups. Transformation frequency of *A. baylyi* BD413 was calculated using 10 ng (**a**) and 1 ng (**b**) of plasmid pZR80(gfp) on nitrocellulose membrane filters, leaf discs, and in planta. For all conditions, the black line indicates the average value of four biological replicates. The same letter (a) indicates no significant differences according to (**a**) ANOVA test (p-value > 0.05) or (**b**) Student's t-test (p-value > 0.05).

2.3. *Natural Transformation on Lettuce Leaves*

The capability of *A. baylyi* BD413 to acquire exDNA on lettuce leaf surface has been tested using both leaf discs and in planta. Using 10 ng of pZR80(gfp) plasmid, a transformation frequency of $1.70 \times 10^{-3} \pm 7.98 \times 10^{-4}$ was measured as the average value of four biological replicates (i.e., four leaf discs) (Figure 3a). Using the same amount of plasmid, the analysis was then conducted in planta on four biological replicates (i.e., four leaves of the same lettuce plant) and an average transformation frequency of $2.09 \times 10^{-3} \pm 5.94 \times 10^{-4}$

was observed (Figure 3a). The same test was repeated during a second independent experiment using a different lettuce plant, measuring not statistically different values of average transformation frequencies ($9.66 \times 10^{-3} \pm 1.59 \times 10^{-2}$, Student's *t*-test, $p = 0.3774$). Using this quantity of plasmid, the values of *A. baylyi* BD413 transformation frequencies detected on lettuce leaf discs and lettuce plant were not significantly different compared to that observed in vitro (ANOVA, $p = 0.5411$; Figure 3a).

The natural transformation assays on the leaf surface were repeated using a lower quantity of exDNA, namely 1 ng of the pZR80(gfp) plasmid, and comparing the results with those obtained in vitro. According to statistical analysis, the transformation frequencies of *A. baylyi* BD413 obtained on lettuce leaf discs ($3.81 \times 10^{-4} \pm 6.20 \times 10^{-5}$) and on nitrocellulose membrane filters ($2.80 \times 10^{-4} \pm 5.65 \times 10^{-5}$) did not show significant differences (Student's *t*-test, $p = 0.0527$) even using 1 ng of exDNA (Figure 3b). When the experiment was conducted in planta with the same quantity of plasmid, the transformation events approximate the detection limit. While total CFUs were still countable (on the serial dilution 10^{-3}), CFUs derived from transformant cells were not detectable using 1 ng of exDNA, even plating the undiluted samples, for three out of the four biological replicates. Transformant cells are a fraction of the total *A. baylyi* BD413 culturable cells, hence this data agrees with the overall decrease of two orders of magnitude presented by *A. baylyi* BD413 total CFUs values in planta compared to those obtained from the leaf disc test. Moreover, we cannot exclude that this result was directly due to the lower DNA quantity used, which could undergo a quicker degradation in planta under greenhouse conditions. We could detect transformants *A. baylyi* BD413 colonies only for one of the biological replicates (transformation frequency = $2.94 \times 10^{-5} \pm 1.47 \times 10^{-5}$, expressed as the average value of three technical replicates), a result that hampers the statistical comparison of in planta results with those observed in vitro and on leaf discs (Figure 3b).

Negative control samples (i.e., leaf discs inoculated with *A. baylyi* BD413 without plasmid) were included in all natural transformation assays, and no transformant colonies were detected on LB agar supplemented with 100 µg/mL kanamycin, confirming the reliability of the presented results. Moreover, ITS-PCR confirmed the identity of the reisolated colonies (Figure S3a,c,e), and gfp-PCR confirmed the plasmid acquisition by *A. baylyi* BD413 transformants (Figure S3b,d,f), while the gfp expression was assessed by epifluorescence microscopy (Figure S3g). The detected natural transformation events occurred on the leaf surface, and not in liquid before leaf inoculation, as demonstrated by the absence of kanamycin-resistant colonies at the end of a control experiment performed incubating in physiological solution an *A. baylyi* BD413 bacterial suspension with plasmid pZR80(gfp), at room temperature for 30 min.

2.4. *Effect of Surfactant Molecule on the Ability of* A. baylyi *BD413 to Acquire exDNA and Enter the Leaf Endosphere*

Once verified that heptamethyltrisiloxane (HPTSO, 0.021% v/v) does not cause inhibitory effects on *A. baylyi* BD413 growth, its possible influence on bacterial transformation frequency on leaf surface was tested on leaf disc and in planta using 10 ng of plasmid pZR80(gfp). When HPTSO was administered on leaf surface together with *A. baylyi* BD413, the transformation frequencies on leaf disc and in planta were $3.6 \times 10^{-3} \pm 2.5 \times 10^{-3}$ and $1.47 \times 10^{-3} \pm 3.95 \times 10^{-4}$, respectively (Figure 4a,b). Thus, in both the experimental setups, the ability of *A. baylyi* BD413 to acquire exDNA did not result significantly different in the presence and absence of HPTSO (Student's *t*-test, p-value > 0.05).

The experiment was repeated in planta to reisolate total and transformant colonies of *A. baylyi* BD413 from the leaf endosphere and measure their ratio in the presence and absence of HPTSO (Figure 4c), obtaining values that were not significantly different ($3.71 \times 10^{-3} \pm 1.33 \times 10^{-3}$ and $2.71 \times 10^{-3} \pm 1.11 \times 10^{-3}$, respectively, Student's *t*-test, $p = 0.2919$). Identity and plasmid acquisition by the putative *A. baylyi* BD413 transformants isolated from leaf tissues were confirmed by ITS-PCR and gfp-PCR (Figure S4). The effect of the tested surfactant on the permeability of *A. baylyi* BD413 cell membrane was assessed by measuring the changes in both the internal and the total cell membrane permeability in presence of HPTSO. The bacterial cell permeability was not influenced by the presence of the surfactant in the growth medium at the considered time points (Figure S5), coherently with the lack of increased natural competence (Figure 4a,b).

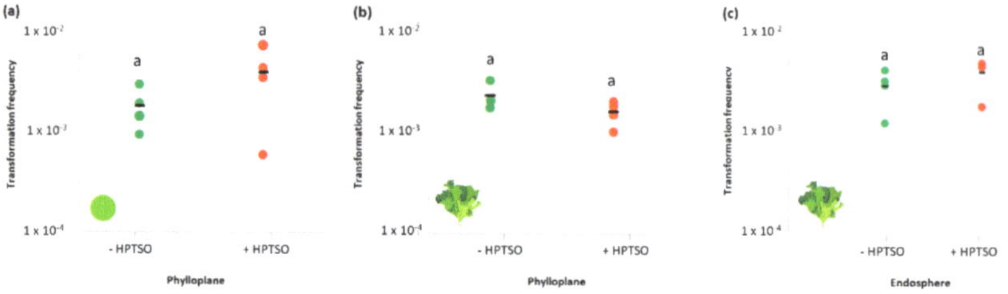

Figure 4. Influence of the heptamethyltrisiloxane surfactant on the natural transformation of *A. baylyi* BD413. Transformation frequency of *A. baylyi* BD413 with 10 ng of plasmid pZR80(gfp) on leaf disc (**a**) and in planta (**b**) in the presence (+HPTSO) or absence (-HPTSO) of the surfactant molecule heptamethyltrisiloxane. Panel (**c**) indicates the ratio between transformant and total *A. baylyi* BD413 colonies reisolated from the leaf endosphere. The black line indicates the average value of four biological replicates. The same letter (a) indicates no significant differences between the values detected in the presence or absence of HPTSO (Student's *t*-test, *p*-value > 0.05).

Considering that the application of surfactant molecules may enhance the internalization of bacteria into lettuce leaves, by performing the natural transformation experiment in planta we also aimed at measuring the concentration of *A. baylyi* BD413 total and transformant colonies in the lettuce leaf tissues. As hypothesized, the concentrations of total and transformant *A. baylyi* BD413 colonies in the lettuce endosphere showed higher values in leaves treated with HPTSO (Figure 5) and such difference was statistically significant for transformant colonies (Student's *t*-test, $p = 0.0149$). The latter result could be related to a higher uptake of exDNA by plant tissues in the presence of HPTSO resulting in the occurrence of transformation events directly in the endosphere. To test such a hypothesis, the concentration of pZR80(gfp) plasmid in the lettuce leaves was measured both in the presence and absence of the surfactant, providing the exDNA at the same quantity used for the natural transformation in planta (i.e., 10 ng which corresponded to 1.5×10^9 copies of pZR80(gfp) plasmid). The qPCR results showed that the gfp copy number per gram of leaf was higher when the exDNA was provided on the leaves together with HPTSO ($1.60 \times 10^7 \pm 2.25 \times 10^7$) although the comparison with data measured in the absence of HPTSO ($3.56 \times 10^6 \pm 9.47 \times 10^5$) revealed that the difference was not statistically significant (Student's *t*-test, $p = 0.3138$; Figure S6).

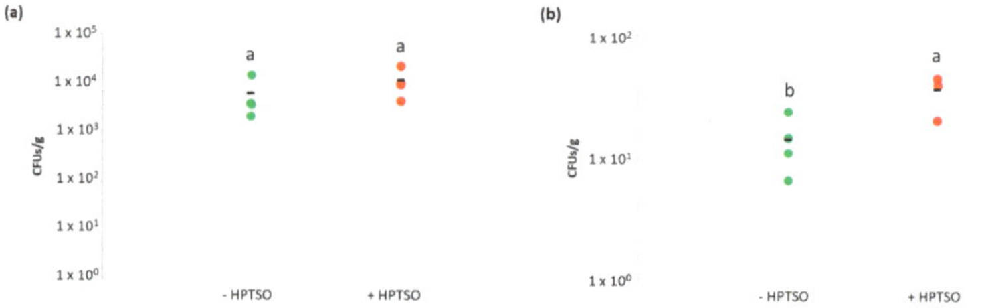

Figure 5. Entry and survival of culturable *A. baylyi* BD413 cells in lettuce endosphere. Number of total (**a**) and transformant (**b**) *A. baylyi* BD413 CFUs/g of leaf reisolated from lettuce endosphere in presence (+HPTSO) or absence (-HPTSO) of the surfactant molecule heptamethyltrisiloxane. The black line indicates the average value of four biological replicates. In each panel, different letters (a, b) indicate significant differences of the CFUs/g of *A. baylyi* BD413 detected in the presence/absence of HPTSO, according to Student's *t*-test (*p*-value > 0.05).

3. Discussion

A recent work [22] demonstrated that *A. baylyi* can transfer plasmid DNA carrying ARGs to *E. coli* clinical isolates on leaf discs and that the *E. coli* transformant cells can subsequently colonize the mouse gut and transfer the antibiotic resistance determinants to *Klebsiella pneumoniae* in vivo. In this context, the present study investigated one of the possible upstream steps, namely the acquisition of exDNA by *A. baylyi* BD413 in planta by natural transformation, using lettuce as a model leafy vegetable. Literature data indicate in fact that *Acinetobacter* spp. are abundant members of water, soil, phyllosphere, and endosphere microbiome [18,27,28], and the species *A. baylyi*, among others affiliated to this genus, was isolated from commercial lettuce [19]. During this study, we verified the ability of *A. baylyi* strain BD413 to survive on the lettuce leaf surface and enter the internal tissues when administered in a physiological solution simulating spray irrigation. The administration method was chosen considering that sprinklers are irrigation systems widely used for both field and greenhouse leafy vegetable farming. The capacity of *A. baylyi* BD413 to remain viable and culturable after spray administration was considered a prerequisite to allowing its use as a model bacterium for HGT experiments in planta. The results of the permanence assay showed that *A. baylyi* BD413 can survive on the phylloplane 1 day after administration at concentrations that were comparable to that of the lettuce strain *K. cowanii* VR04, confirming the adaptation of the genus *Acinetobacter* to the phyllosphere ecosystem [28]. This is in agreement with the previously reported capacity of *A. baylyi* to grow as an epiphytic bacterium on lettuce leaves, due to the possible use of leaf exudates as a carbon source [15].

In this study, for in vivo natural transformation, we selected two exDNA quantities (i.e., 1 and 10 ng) that mimic the environmental concentration detected in wastewater [26]. Indeed, water reuse for irrigation purposes is considered a priority, in relation to the occurrence of water shortage periods that affect crop productivity on a global scale [29]. In this framework, the recent EU legislation on water reuse aims at regulating the concentration of several emerging contaminants, including antibiotic resistance determinants in treated wastewater used for irrigation. However, the data available on antibiotic resistance in wastewater treatment plants, their effluents, and the agri-food systems, generally refer to the abundance and/or distribution of ARGs and ARB [30]. On the contrary, the mechanisms of ARG diffusion and the anthropogenic input that might increase their frequency are rarely analyzed.

Here, we demonstrated that the natural transformation of *A. baylyi* BD413 occurs on the lettuce phylloplane at the same frequency that is encountered in the laboratory applying optimal conditions in terms of temperature, nutrient provision, and absence of microbial competitors. Notably, this result was obtained not only on leaf disc but also during in planta experiment. These data corroborate previous evidence that nutrient limitation does not act in *A. baylyi* as a factor enhancing natural competence, differently from what is reported for other bacteria such as *Haemophilus influenzae* [27]. To the best of our knowledge, no previous data are available on the natural transformation frequency of environmental bacteria in planta on lettuce phylloplane. Hence, this study can add an important piece of knowledge for the risk assessment of ARGs diffusion by HGT and their entrance into the food supply chain. The frequency of HGT events in the environment could be influenced by several factors. For instance, bacterial exposure to water disinfection products used in wastewater treatment plants, such as bromoacetic acid and sodium hypochlorite, was demonstrated to enhance the process of transformation in naturally competent bacteria, promoting ARGs spread [23,31]. In this study, the possible influence of a surfactant molecule (i.e., heptamethyltrisiloxane) on *A. baylyi* BD413 natural transformation frequency was investigated. Since surfactants allow a more uniform spread of the agrochemicals over plant surfaces, they are widely used in agriculture as co-formulants in the commercial preparation of many pesticides and fertilizers provided through foliar application [25]. This class of molecule has been chosen as representative of environmental conditions that could be easily found in the field. In addition, biosurfactants can be produced by epiphytic bacteria as a strategy to move on the leaf surface towards areas where nutrients are more abundant [32]. Though the results of this study showed that heptamethyltrisiloxane did not significantly change the frequency of *A. baylyi* BD413 natural transformation, higher bacterial concentrations were observed in both reisolating wild-type and transformant *A. baylyi* BD413 cells from the lettuce endosphere, the latter retrieved at concentrations significantly higher in presence of the surfactant. The hypothesis that the higher concentration of transformant *A. baylyi* BD413 cells could be related to a higher uptake of exDNA by the leaf tissues allowing natural transformation directly in the leaf endosphere was not confirmed by the data. However, this process could be not excluded since a higher, still not significant, concentration of the pZR80(gfp) plasmid was measured in the presence of HPTSO. Regardless of the presence of the surfactant, the results of this study showed in fact that a high amount of the provided exDNA was detected in the leaf. Future studies could be focused on exDNA fate and potential to be acquired by the endophytic bacterial populations, considering the lack of overall data in the literature, where the role of exDNA is considered solely in the frame of plant-microbe interaction and plant immune response stimulation [33].

The use of Silwet L-77, a commercial product whose main component is the surfactant molecule tested in this study, was previously demonstrated to increase the entrance of a human pathogen, i.e., *Salmonella enterica*, in tomato leaf tissues and fruits [25]. Moreover, the foliar application of other commercial products, such as vegetable-derived bioactive compounds, can alter the microbiome composition of lettuce leaves promoting the growth of certain bacterial genera, including *Acinetobacter* [34]. The fact that *A. baylyi* BD413 can penetrate the lettuce leaf endosphere, where its viable and culturable populations were retrieved, is an important aspect in terms of food safety considering that once bacterial cells enter the leaf tissues they cannot be removed by washing and disinfection procedures. Since HGT between *A. baylyi* and members of the family *Enterobacteriaceae* was demonstrated [22], the relevance of the endophytic lifestyle of *A. baylyi* BD413 raises considering the frequent occurrence of *Enterobacteriaceae* in the edible tissues of lettuce [35], where they are three times more abundant compared to the root system [36].

4. Materials and Methods

4.1. *A. baylyi BD413 Survival Assay on Lettuce Phylloplane and into Leaf Endosphere*

Acinetobacter baylyi BD413, a strain resistant to rifampicin, was used for the bacterization of *Lactuca sativa* (var. Canasta) plants to verify its ability to survive in a viable and culturable state on lettuce phylloplane (i.e., leaf surface) and enter the leaf endosphere. *A. baylyi* BD413 was grown in Luria-Bertani (LB) medium (Sigma-Aldrich, St. Louis, MO, USA) supplemented with rifampicin (100 μg/mL, Sigma-Aldrich) for 24 h at 30 °C in an orbital shaker. The total cell number of the bacterial suspensions was evaluated at the optical microscope (Motic, BA310E) using a Thoma chamber. *A. baylyi* BD413 bacterial culture was centrifuged twice at 4000 rpm for 10 min and the cells were re-suspended in sterilized physiological solution (i.e., NaCl 0.9%) to obtain a final bacterial concentration of 10^8 cell/mL. The bacterial suspension was transferred in a spray bottle and dispensed on lettuce leaves. *A. baylyi* BD413 was sprayed (1 spray per leaf, corresponding to a volume of 100 μL) on five leaves per plant (number of bacterized plants = 6). Six plants were treated with a sterilized physiological solution and used as a negative control. To define the number of bacterial CFUs released on each plant from the spray bottle, five sprays were collected in a sterile tube, serially diluted, and plated in triplicates on LB agar medium supplemented with 100 μg/mL rifampicin.

Bacterized and control plants were kept in greenhouse at 25 °C. After 1 h, the epiphytic bacteria were recovered from negative control plants (n = 3) and bacterized plants (n = 3): the five treated leaves per plant were removed with a sterile scalpel and put in 20 mL of sterilized physiological solution for 1 h under shaking to detach bacterial cells from the leaf surface. Cell suspensions were serially diluted, plated in triplicate on LB agar medium supplemented with rifampicin (100 μg/mL) and CFUs were counted after incubation at 30 °C for 24 h. In addition, epiphytic *A. baylyi* BD413 cells were recovered, as described above, 24 h after plant bacterization from the remaining bacterized (n = 3) and negative control (n = 3) plants. From the latter plants, once the epiphytic *A. baylyi* BD413 cells were detached for isolation, lettuce leaves were surface sterilized with ethanol 70% for 30 sec and rinsed three times with sterilized distilled water for 3 min, to isolate *A. baylyi* BD413 cells from the leaf endosphere (protocol adapted from reference [37]). A 100 µL sample of water from the last rinsing step was plated on LB agar medium supplemented with 100 µg/mL rifampicin to confirm the complete removal of *A. baylyi* BD413 from the phylloplane. Finally, leaves were smashed using sterile mortar and pestle in physiological solution, serially diluted, and plated in triplicate on LB agar medium supplemented with 100 µg/mL rifampicin. The survival ability of *A. baylyi* BD413 was measured as the fraction between the CFUs/mL re-isolated from the phylloplane/leaf endosphere after bacterization and the CFUs/mL released by spray.

To confirm the identity of the isolates, bacterial colonies isolated from the phylloplane (n = 10) and from the leaf endosphere (n = 10) of each bacterized lettuce plant were streaked and the DNA was extracted from each colony through boiling cell lysis. The 16–23 S rRNA Intergenic Transcribed Spacer (ITS) region was amplified and isolate identification was assessed by ITS-PCR fingerprinting [38] comparing the ITS profiles of the isolated bacteria with that of the *A. baylyi* BD413 strain inoculated on lettuce.

The ability of the *A. baylyi* BD413 strain to survive on the lettuce phylloplane was compared with those of other bacteria. The described experimental procedure was adopted for the rifampicin-resistant mutants of the laboratory *Escherichia coli* strain DH5α and of the *Kosakonia cowanii* VR04, a bacterial strain previously isolated from lettuce leaf endosphere using the Violet Red Bile Lactose Agar medium (Sigma-Aldrich; Mapelli F., personal communication). Rifampicin-resistant mutants were prepared according to a published protocol [39].

4.2. *Natural Transformation Protocols*

4.2.1. Bacterial Culture Preparation

A. baylyi BD413 strain was grown in 20 mL of LB liquid medium overnight at 30 °C under shaking, subsequently inoculated in a ratio of 1:100 *v/v* in LB medium, and incubated at 30 °C until the cells reached the early exponential growth phase, corresponding to optical density (OD) value of 0.4–0.5 at 600 nm (UV/VIS Spectrophotometer 7305, Jenway, London, UK). The bacterial cells were then centrifuged at 4000 rpm for 10 min and re-suspended in sterilized physiological solution to obtain a final bacterial concentration of 10^9 cell/mL. Four aliquots of 100 µL of cells were prepared and the proper quantity of extracellular DNA (exDNA) was added and gently mixed. For each experiment, the fifth aliquot of cells was used as negative control (no DNA was added).

4.2.2. Extracellular DNA (exDNA) Preparation

Natural transformation experiments were conducted using the pZR80(gfp) plasmid as extracellular DNA. The plasmid harbors a kanamycin resistance gene (aphA-3) and a gene codifying for the green fluorescent protein (gfp) as an optical marker [14]. The plasmid was previously extracted from an overnight culture of the strain *E. coli* (pZR80(gfp)) using the QIAPrep Spin Miniprep Kit (Qiagen, Hilden, Germany) following the manufacturer's instructions and its concentration was assessed fluorometrically using the Qubit™ dsDNA HS Assay Kit (Thermo Fisher Scientific, Waltham, MA, USA).

4.2.3. Selection of the exDNA Quantity for In Vivo Experiments

To determine the quantity of exDNA to be used for in vivo natural transformation experiments, a preliminary in vitro test was conducted in triplicate using 1, 2, 5, 10, 20, and 50 ng of the pZR80(gfp) plasmid and nitrocellulose membrane filters (GSWP, 25 mm diameter, 0.22 mm pore size, Millipore, Burlington, MA, USA). The bacterial suspension (10^9 cell/mL) was mixed with the different plasmid quantities (in a final volume of 500 µL) and placed on a sterile nitrocellulose membrane filter, previously positioned on LB agar plates. After 24 h incubation at 30 °C, the cells were detached from the filter by resuspension in 1 mL of physiological solution, serially diluted, and plated on both LB agar and LB agar supplemented with 100 μg/mL kanamycin (Sigma-Aldrich) to count the total and the transformant CFU numbers present on the filter, respectively. Transformation frequency was calculated as the number of kanamycin-resistant transformant colonies over the total number of colonies. Randomly selected transformant colonies (n = 10) were checked by epifluorescence microscopy (Zeiss Axio Lab.A1) for the expression of the gfp gene harbored on the pZR80(gfp) plasmid.

4.2.4. Natural Transformation on Leaf Disc

The lowest DNA quantity that allows the detection of the transformation events on nitrocellulose membrane filters was chosen for in vivo experiments. The ability of *A. baylyi* BD413 to acquire exDNA was tested on the surface of lettuce (*Lactuca sativa* var. Canasta) leaf discs, collected using a round-shape cutting of 4.5 cm diameter, sterilized by dipping in ethanol 70% and placed in empty 60 mm diameter Petri dishes. A solution of 10^9 cell/mL bacterial cells and plasmid (or without plasmid DNA in the case of negative control) was prepared in a final volume of 100 μL and placed on the leaf disc surface and, after 24 h of incubation at 30 °C, leaf discs were placed in sterile tubes with 1 mL of physiological solution to detach the cells. The bacterial cell suspension was serially diluted and plated on LB agar and LB agar supplemented with 100 μg/mL kanamycin. After 24 h at 30 °C, CFUs were counted and the transformation frequency was calculated. Randomly selected transformant colonies (n = 30) were checked for (i) their identity through ITS-PCR fingerprinting using *A. baylyi* BD413 as positive control and (ii) the presence of the gfp gene harbored by the pZR80(gfp) plasmid. The gfp gene was amplified by PCR using the primers GFP540F (5′-CAAGAGTGCCATGCCCGAAGG-3′) and GFP875R (5′-GGTAAAAGGACAGGGCCATCGCC-3′) [40] and the following thermal protocol: 95°C for 4 min, followed by 35 cycles of 95 °C for 45 s, 60 °C for 1 min and 72 °C for 1 min and a final extension at 72 °C for 10 min.

4.2.5. Natural Transformation in Planta

Natural transformation of *A. baylyi* BD413 in presence of pZR80(gfp) plasmid was tested in planta using lettuce plants (*Lactuca sativa* var. Canasta) under greenhouse conditions. The experiment was conducted using four replicates, corresponding to four leaves of the same lettuce plant: the four leaves were inoculated with 10^9 cell/mL *A. baylyi* BD413 cell suspension mixed with 10 ng of the pZR80(gfp) plasmid (final volume of 100 μL). In addition, one leaf was inoculated with cell suspension (no plasmid, negative control) to assess the absence of native kanamycin-resistant bacteria on the lettuce phylloplane. Each bacterized leaf was covered using a sterile empty Petri dish to avoid environmental contamination from the greenhouse. After 24 h, the inoculated leaves were removed from the plant with a sterile scalpel and kept in the Petri dishes, where 1 mL of physiological solution was added to detach the cells from the leaf surface. After shaking, bacterial cell suspensions were serially diluted and plated on LB agar and LB agar supplemented with 100 μg/mL kanamycin to reisolate total and transformant *A. baylyi* BD413 colonies. CFUs were counted after incubation at 30 °C for 24 h and the transformation frequency was calculated. This experiment was repeated by applying the same conditions to reisolate total and transformant *A. baylyi* BD413 colonies from the leaf endosphere, after leaf surface sterilization. At the end of both experiments, the identity and the presence of the gfp gene were checked on randomly selected transformant colonies (n = 30) as described in the previous paragraph. To demonstrate that the HGT events occurred in planta and not in liquid (i.e., before the suspension of bacterial cells and plasmid were inoculated on the leaves), we incubated the bacterial suspension with pZR80(gfp) plasmid at room temperature for 30 min and plated the cells on LB agar medium supplemented with 100 μg/mL kanamycin. After incubation at 30 °C for 24 h, the presence of transformant colonies was checked on the Petri dishes.

4.3. Entry of Total and Transformant *A. baylyi* BD413 Cells into Leaf Endosphere

The ability of total and transformant cells of *A. baylyi* BD413 to enter the endosphere of lettuce leaves was measured during the in planta experiment described in the previous paragraph. After the removal of cells from the leaf surface, lettuce leaves were surface sterilized and smashed as described in the survival assay (see Section 4.1). Serial dilutions were prepared and plated on LB agar and LB agar supplemented with 100 μg/mL kanamycin. A 100 μL sample of water from the last rinsing step was plated on LB agar medium with and without 100 μg/mL kanamycin to confirm the complete removal of *A. baylyi* BD413 transformant and total cells from the phylloplane. After 24 h at 30 °C, the number of total and transformant CFUs present in the leaf endosphere were counted and expressed as CFUs/g of leaf tissue. All putative transformant colonies were checked for their identity and the presence of the gfp gene as described in Section 4.2.4.

4.4. Effect of a Surfactant Molecule on *A. baylyi* BD413 Transformation and Penetration into the Endosphere

Heptamethyltrisiloxane (HPTSO, Merck, Kenilworth, NJ, USA) was selected as a representative surfactant molecule for the experiment. HPTSO is the principal component (85%) of Silwet L-77, an organo-silicone surfactant used in agriculture for foliar applications of many agro-chemical products, including herbicides, insecticides, fungicides, plant growth regulators, and fertilizers with a concentration comprised between 0.025–0.1% [25]. In this experiment HPTSO was diluted in sterilized physiological water and used at 0.021% v/v, corresponding to its final concentration for foliar application on leafy green vegetables in the field, according to the Silwet L-77 product label. Firstly, the possible inhibitory effect of the surfactant on *A. baylyi* BD413 growth was analyzed in triplicate both in solid and liquid LB medium supplemented by 0.021% v/v HPTSO. Then, the effect of HPTSO on the transformation frequency of *A. baylyi* BD413 was tested on leaf discs and in planta mixing the surfactant molecule with *A. baylyi* BD413 and plasmid DNA prior to spotting the bacterial suspension on lettuce leaves (n = 4), and following the procedure described in the previous paragraph to reisolate total and transformant *A. baylyi* BD413 cells from the leaf surface. Moreover, the HPTSO influence on the *A. baylyi* BD413 ability to penetrate the leaf tissues was tested by reisolating total and transformant colonies from the endosphere, using LB agar and LB agar supplemented with 100 μg/mL kanamycin, respectively, and calculating their CFU number per gram of leaf tissue.

4.5. Bacterial Cell Membrane Permeability Assays

The effect of HPTSO on *A. baylyi* BD413 membrane permeability was determined through two different methods. The first one measures the permeability of the inner membrane and it is based on an aqueous hydrolysis reaction of o-nitrophenyl-β-Dgalactopyranoside (ONPG, Merck) [41]. The second method allows for the determination of the total cell membrane permeability using a crystal violet solution as previously described [42].

In detail, the inner membrane permeability assay was conducted growing *A. baylyi* BD413 in LB liquid medium added with 2% lactose at 30 °C overnight. Cells were recovered by centrifugation (4500× *g* for 10 min) and resuspended in physiological solution to a final concentration of 10^8 cell/mL, ONPG 2.5 mM, and HPTSO (0.021% v/v). Three biological replicates were prepared and the other three replicates without the addition of HPTSO were used as control. The samples were incubated at 30 °C and after 2, 7, and 24 h the sample OD at 415 nm was measured (UV/VIS Spectrophotometer 7305, Jenway) to monitor the production of o-nitrophenol over time.

For the determination of the total membrane permeability, *A. baylyi* BD413 was grown in LB liquid medium overnight and resuspended to a final concentration of 10^8 cell/mL in physiological solution after centrifuging the cell culture at 4500× *g* for 10 min. HPTSO (0.021% v/v) was added to three biological replicates while three samples without the surfactant molecule were used as control. Samples were incubated at 30 °C and, after 6- and 24-h, cells were harvested at 9300× *g* for 5 min and resuspended in a physiological solution containing 5 µg/mL crystal violet. Cell suspensions were incubated at 30 °C for 10 min and centrifuged at 13,400× *g* per 15 min. The OD of the supernatants was measured at 590 nm (UV/VIS Spectrophotometer 7305, Jenway). The OD value of the crystal violet initial solution used in the assay was considered 100%. The percentage of crystal violet uptake was calculated using the following formula: (OD value of the sample)/(OD value of the crystal violet solution) × 100 [42].

4.6. Lettuce Leaf Acquisition of Extracellular DNA

Acquisition of pZR80(gfp) plasmid by lettuce plants (*Lactuca sativa* var. Canasta) was tested. The experiment was conducted using four replicates (i.e., four leaves) per treatment, and each treatment was conducted on a separate plant. Leaf treatments were as follows: (i) addition of 10 ng of the pZR80(gfp) plasmid (final volume of 100 µL), (ii) addition of 10 ng of the pZR80(gfp) plasmid and HPTSO (0.021% *w*/*v*). Lastly, four replicates were put in contact with 100 µL of sterile water to serve as a negative control.

After 24 h, the treated leaves were removed from the plant with a sterile scalpel and kept in Petri dishes. Before DNA extraction from leaves, the fresh weight was measured, and surface sterilization was performed as reported in Section 4.1. Each leaf was separately crushed in a sterile mortar by N_2 liquid addition, the biological material was then collected using a sterile spatula and stored at −20 °C.

Subsequent DNA extraction from the 16 leaves was conducted by using DNeasy Plant Mini Kit (Qiagen), according to manufacturer instructions, adding an initial step of plants' material destruction by the TissueLyser II (Qiagen) to obtain higher yields of DNA. Qubit dsDNA HS kit (Invitrogen, Waltham, MA, USA) was used for the DNA concentration measurement of each sample. The DNA extracted from the leaf tissues was used as a template to perform a PCR to assess the presence of the pZR80(gfp) plasmid. The PCR targeted a fragment (1100 bp) of pZR80(gfp) plasmid including both the gfp and the aph-A genes, which was amplified using the primers GFP540F (5′-CAAGAGTGCCATGCCCGAAGG-3′) and aphA-3R2 (5′- ACTCTTCCGAGCAAAGGACG-3′), and the following thermal protocol: 95 °C for 4 min, followed by 35 cycles of 95 °C for 45 s, 59 °C for 1 min and 72 °C for 2 min and a final extension at 72 °C for 10 min. Quantitative PCR (qPCR) reactions of the gfp gene were conducted according to a published protocol [40], with slight modifications. The reactions were executed in polypropylene 96-well plates on a BIORAD CFX Connect™ Real-Time PCR Detection System by the amplification of the gfp sequence, using primers 540F (5′-CAAGAGTGCCATGCCCGAAGG-3′) and 875R (5′-GGTAAAAGGACAGGGCCATCGCC-3′) with the following conditions: 0.2 µM of each primer, 2x SsoAdvanced™Universal SYBR®Green Supermix (BIORAD), 1 µL DNA template, 12 µL final volume. The reaction conditions consisted of three-step cycles of 45 s at 98 °C and 30 s at 60 °C and 30 s at 72 °C, for a total of 40 cycles. Each plate included triplicate reactions per DNA sample and the appropriate set of standards. Melting curve analysis was conducted following each assay to confirm the amplification of specific PCR products and the number of gfp copies was related to the leaves' weights of each biological sample.

4.7. Statistical Analyses

The results of the *A. baylyi* BD413 survival assay on leaf surface at different time points and comparing epiphytic vs. endophytic permanence (24 h after administration) were analyzed statistically by Student's *t*-test.

The ratio between survived culturable cells and administered cells shown by *A. baylyi* BD413, *E. coli* DH5α, and *K. cowanii* VR04 were compared by ANOVA applying a post-hoc Dunnett's test considering *A. baylyi* BD413 as the control thesis. Natural transformation frequencies detected on nitrocellulose filters using different DNA quantities were analyzed by ANOVA applying a Tukey-Kramer post-hoc test. Likewise, the *A. baylyi* BD413 transformation frequencies detected on nitrocellulose filters, lettuce leaf discs, and in planta using 10 ng of plasmid pZR80(gfp) were analyzed by ANOVA. ANOVA and post-hoc tests indicated above were performed using JMP Pro 16 Software. All the other results related to natural transformation frequencies (e.g., in the presence and absence of HPTSO) were analyzed by a Student's *t*-test using the Microsoft Excel software. To evaluate the influence of surfactant treatment on DNA acquisition by plant tissues, the differences of gfp copy number/gram of leaf tissue were firstly checked with a Dunnett's test against the control non-treated plants using the package DescTools with the R software version 4.2.0 and then a Student's *t*-test was performed between the two treatments.

5. Conclusions

This study highlights that natural transformation is an HGT mechanism occurring on the edible part of lettuce in presence of exDNA quantities comparable to those possibly encountered in the agri-food system scenario. Moreover, the presented results indicate that after the acquisition of the plasmid pZR80(gfp), carrying an antibiotic resistance gene, transformant *A. baylyi* BD413 can enter the leaf tissues, and show that this ability is enhanced in the presence of heptamethyltrisiloxane, a surfactant adjuvant widely used in agriculture. The impact of agrochemicals on antibiotic resistance spread in agri-food systems is still overlooked and could be one of the aspects to consider for future research. All in all, we claim the importance to obtain more experimental data on HGT mechanisms directly in planta, since produces, together with animal-derived matrices, represent the possible entry point of ARGs and ARB into food production.

Supplementary Materials: The following supporting information can be downloaded at: https://www.mdpi.com/article/10.3390/antibiotics11091231/s1. Figure S1: Confirmation of strain identity after the reisolation from lettuce leaves; Figure S2: Survival in a viable and culturable state shown by *A. baylyi* BD413, *E. coli* DH5α and *K. cowanii* VR04 on lettuce phylloplane; Figure S3: Confirmation of identity and plasmid acquisition by the putative *A. baylyi* BD413 transformants isolated from the leaf surface; Figure S4: Confirmation of identity and plasmid acquisition by the putative *A. baylyi* BD413 transformants isolated in the leaf endosphere; Figure S5: Cell membrane permeability of *A. baylyi* BD413 under the influence of heptamethyltrisiloxane (HPTSO); Figure S6: Plasmid DNA entry in the lettuce leaf tissues; Table S1: Assessment of the viable and culturable bacterial cells actually released by spray administration on lettuce leaves; Table S2: Comparison between the cell survival in a culturable state the shown by strains *A. baylyi* BD413, *E. coli* DH5α and *K. cowanii* VR04. Table S3: *A. baylyi* BD413 transformation frequency values on nitrocellulose membrane filters.

Author Contributions: Conceptualization, F.M., V.R., F.R. and E.C.; methodology, V.R, E.C. and F.M.; formal analysis, V.R., G.P., F.R. and L.V.; investigation, V.R., G.P., F.R. and L.V.; resources, E.C.; writing—original draft preparation, V.R. and F.M.; writing—review and editing, G.P., F.R., E.C. and L.V.; visualization, V.R. and F.M.; supervision, F.M.; project administration, F.M.; funding acquisition, F.M. All authors have read and agreed to the published version of the manuscript.

Funding: This work was funded by the Cariplo Foundation project "Novel wastewater disinfection treatments to mitigate the spread of antibiotic resistance in agriculture—WARFARE" (GA n° 2018-0995) and supported by Università degli Studi di Milano—PSR 2021—GSA—Linea 6 within the project "One Health Action Hub: University Task Force for the resilience of territorial ecosystems". F.M. thanks personal support from "PSR2021: Linea 2 -project "ENVISAGE—Environmental Acinetobacter isolates as reservoir of antibiotic resistance potentially transferable to phylogenetically related species".

Data Availability Statement: The data presented in this study are available in the article and its supplementary material.

Conflicts of Interest: The authors declare no conflict of interest.

References

1. Larsson, D.G.J.; Flach, C.F. Antibiotic resistance in the environment. *Nat. Rev. Microbiol.* **2022**, *20*, 257–269. [CrossRef]
2. Westhoff, S.; van Leeuwe, T.M.; Qachach, O.; Zhang, Z.; van Wezel, G.P.; Rozen, D.E. The evolution of no-cost resistance at sub-MIC concentrations of streptomycin in Streptomyces coelicolor. *ISME J.* **2017**, *11*, 1168–1178. [CrossRef] [PubMed]
3. Wright, G.D. Antibiotic resistance in the environment: A link to the clinic? *Curr. Opin. Microbiol.* **2010**, *13*, 589–594. [CrossRef] [PubMed]

4. Wang, Y.; Lu, J.; Engelstädter, J.; Zhang, S.; Ding, P.; Mao, L.; Yuan, Z.; Bond, P.L.; Guo, J. Non-antibiotic pharmaceuticals enhance the transmission of exogenous antibiotic resistance genes through bacterial transformation. *ISME J.* **2020**, *14*, 2179–2196. [CrossRef] [PubMed]
5. Riva, V.; Riva, F.; Vergani, L.; Crotti, E.; Borin, S.; Mapelli, F. Microbial assisted phytodepuration for water reclamation: Environmental benefits and threats. *Chemosphere* **2020**, *241*, 124843. [CrossRef] [PubMed]
6. Chen, Q.-L.; Cui, H.-L.; Su, J.-Q.; Penuelas, J.; Zhu, Y.-G. Antibiotic Resistomes in Plant Microbiomes. *Trends Plant Sci.* **2019**, *24*, 530–541. [CrossRef]
7. Scaccia, N.; Vaz-Moreira, I.; Manaia, C.M. The risk of transmitting antibiotic resistance through endophytic bacteria. *Trends Plant Sci.* **2021**, *26*, 1213–1226. [CrossRef] [PubMed]
8. Remus-Emsermann, M.N.P.; Aicher, D.; Pelludat, C.; Gisler, P.; Drissner, D. Conjugation dynamics of self-transmissible and mobilisable plasmids into e. Coli o157:H7 on Arabidopsis thaliana rosettes. *Antibiotics* **2021**, *10*, 1–14.
9. Deng, B.; Li, W.; Lu, H.; Zhu, L. Film mulching reduces antibiotic resistance genes in the phyllosphere of lettuce. *J. Environ. Sci.* **2022**, *112*, 121–128. [CrossRef]
10. Blau, K.; Bettermann, A.; Jechalke, S.; Fornefeld, E.; Vanrobaeys, Y.; Stalder, T.; Top, E.M.; Smalla, K. The transferable resistome of produce. *mBio* **2018**, *9*, e01300-18. [CrossRef]
11. Von Wintersdorff, C.J.H.; Penders, J.; Van Niekerk, J.M.; Mills, N.D.; Majumder, S.; Van Alphen, L.B.; Savelkoul, P.H.M.; Wolffs, P.F.G. Dissemination of antimicrobial resistance in microbial ecosystems through horizontal gene transfer. *Front. Microbiol.* **2016**, *7*, 1–10. [CrossRef] [PubMed]
12. Zarei-Baygi, A.; Smith, A.L. Intracellular versus extracellular antibiotic resistance genes in the environment: Prevalence, horizontal transfer, and mitigation strategies. *Bioresour. Technol.* **2021**, *319*, 124181. [CrossRef] [PubMed]
13. de Berardinis, V.; Durot, M.; Weissenbach, J.; Salanoubat, M. Acinetobacter baylyi ADP1 as a model for metabolic system biology. *Curr. Opin. Microbiol.* **2009**, *12*, 568–576. [CrossRef]
14. Borin, S.; Crotti, E.; Mapelli, F.; Tamagnini, I.; Corselli, C.; Daffonchio, D. DNA is preserved and maintains transforming potential after contact with brines of the deep anoxic hypersaline lakes of the Eastern Mediterranean Sea. *Saline Syst.* **2008**, *4*, 10. [CrossRef] [PubMed]
15. Pontiroli, A.; Rizzi, A.; Simonet, P.; Daffonchio, D.; Vogel, T.M.; Monier, J.-M. Visual evidence of horizontal gene transfer between plants and bacteria in the phytosphere of transplastomic tobacco. *Appl. Environ. Microbiol.* **2009**, *75*, 3314–3322. [CrossRef]
16. Munoz-Price, L.S.; Weinstein, R.A. Acinetobacter infection. *N. Engl. J. Med.* **2008**, *358*, 1271–1281. [CrossRef]
17. Fulsundar, S.; Harms, K.; Flaten, G.E.; Johnsen, P.J.; Chopade, B.A.; Nielsen, K.M. Gene transfer potential of outer membrane vesicles of Acinetobacter baylyi and effects of stress on vesiculation. *Appl. Environ. Microbiol.* **2014**, *80*, 3469–3483. [CrossRef]
18. Riva, V.; Mapelli, F.; Bagnasco, A.; Mengoni, A.; Borin, S. A meta-analysis approach to defining the culturable core of plant endophytic bacterial communities. *Appl. Environ. Microbiol.* **2022**, *88*, 1–10. [CrossRef]
19. Carvalheira, A.; Silva, J.; Teixeira, P. Lettuce and fruits as a source of multidrug resistant *Acinetobacter* spp. *Food Microbiol.* **2017**, *64*, 119–125. [CrossRef]
20. Brennan, F.P.; Alsanius, B.W.; Allende, A.; Burgess, C.M.; Moreira, H.; Johannessen, G.S.; Castro, P.M.L.; Uyttendaele, M.; Truchado, P.; Holden, N.J. Harnessing agricultural microbiomes for human pathogen control. *ISME Commun.* **2022**, *2*, 1–6. [CrossRef]
21. Haelewaters, D.; Urbina, H.; Brown, S.; Newerth-Henson, S.; Aime, M. Isolation and molecular characterization of the romaine lettuce phylloplane mycobiome. *J. Fungi* **2021**, *7*, 277. [CrossRef]
22. Maeusli, M.; Lee, B.; Miller, S.; Reyna, Z.; Lu, P.; Yan, J.; Ulhaq, A.; Skandalis, N.; Spellberg, B.; Luna, B. Horizontal gene transfer of antibiotic resistance from Acinetobacter baylyi to Escherichia coli on lettuce and subsequent antibiotic resistance transmission to the gut microbiome. *mSphere* **2020**, *5*, 1–7. [CrossRef]
23. Mantilla-Calderon, D.; Plewa, M.J.; Michoud, G.; Fodelianakis, S.; Daffonchio, D.; Hong, P.Y. Water disinfection byproducts increase natural transformation rates of environmental DNA in Acinetobacter baylyi ADP1. *Environ. Sci. Technol.* **2019**, *53*, 6520–6528. [CrossRef]
24. Zdarta, A.; Pacholak, A.; Smułek, W.; Zgoła-Grześkowiak, A.; Ferlin, N.; Bil, A.; Kovensky, J.; Grand, E.; Kaczorek, E. Biological impact of octyl d-glucopyranoside based surfactants. *Chemosphere* **2019**, *217*, 567–575. [CrossRef]
25. Gu, G.; Hu, J.; Cevallos-Cevallos, J.M.; Richardson, S.M.; Bartz, J.A.; van Bruggen, A.H.C. Internal colonization of salmonella enterica serovar typhimurium in tomato plants. *PLoS ONE* **2011**, *6*, e27340. [CrossRef] [PubMed]
26. Calderón-Franco, D.; van Loosdrecht, M.C.M.; Abeel, T.; Weissbrodt, D.G. Free-floating extracellular DNA: Systematic profiling of mobile genetic elements and antibiotic resistance from wastewater. *Water Res.* **2021**, *189*, 116592. [CrossRef] [PubMed]
27. Seitz, P.; Blokesch, M. Cues and regulatory pathways involved in natural competence and transformation in pathogenic and environmental Gram-negative bacteria. *FEMS Microbiol. Rev.* **2013**, *37*, 336–363. [CrossRef]
28. Vorholt, J.A. Microbial life in the phyllosphere. *Nat. Rev. Microbiol.* **2012**, *10*, 828–840. [CrossRef] [PubMed]
29. Caparas, M.; Zobel, Z.; Castanho, A.D.A.; Schwalm, C.R. Increasing risks of crop failure and water scarcity in global breadbaskets by 2030. *Environ. Res. Lett.* **2021**, *16*, 104013. [CrossRef]
30. Miłobedzka, A.; Ferreira, C.; Vaz-Moreira, I.; Calderón-Franco, D.; Gorecki, A.; Purkrtova, S.; Bartacek, J.; Dziewit, L.; Singleton, C.M.; Nielsen, P.H.; et al. Monitoring antibiotic resistance genes in wastewater environments: The challenges of filling a gap in the One-Health cycle. *J. Hazard. Mater.* **2021**, *424*, 127407. [CrossRef]

31. Jin, M.; Liu, L.; Wang, D.; Yang, D.; Liu, W.L.; Yin, J.; Yang, Z.W.; Wang, H.R.; Qiu, Z.G.; Shen, Z.Q.; et al. Chlorine disinfection promotes the exchange of antibiotic resistance genes across bacterial genera by natural transformation. *ISME J.* **2020**, *14*, 1847–1856. [CrossRef] [PubMed]
32. Lindow, S.E.; Brandl, M.T. Microbiology of the phyllosphere. *Appl. Environ. Microbiol.* **2003**, *69*, 1875–1883. [CrossRef] [PubMed]
33. Bhat, A.; Ryu, C.-M. Plant perceptions of extracellular DNA and RNA. *Mol. Plant* **2016**, *9*, 956–958. [CrossRef] [PubMed]
34. Luziatelli, F.; Ficca, A.G.; Colla, G.; Švecová, E.B.; Ruzzi, M. Foliar application of vegetal-derived bioactive compounds stimulates the growth of beneficial bacteria and enhances microbiome biodiversity in lettuce. *Front. Plant Sci.* **2019**, *10*, 1–16. [CrossRef]
35. Cardinale, M.; Grube, M.; Erlacher, A.; Quehenberger, J.; Berg, G. Bacterial networks and co-occurrence relationships in the lettuce root microbiota. *Environ. Microbiol.* **2015**, *17*, 239–252.
36. Erlacher, A.; Cardinale, M.; Grube, M.; Berg, G. Biotic stress shifted structure and abundance of enterobacteriaceae in the lettuce microbiome. *PLoS ONE* **2015**, *10*, e0118068. [CrossRef]
37. Klerks, M.M.; Franz, E.; Van Gent-Pelzer, M.; Zijlstra, C.; Van Bruggen, A.H.C. Differential interaction of Salmonella enterica serovars with lettuce cultivars and plant-microbe factors influencing the colonization efficiency. *ISME J.* **2007**, *1*, 620–631.
38. Mapelli, F.; Marasco, R.; Rolli, E.; Barbato, M.; Cherif, H.; Guesmi, A.; Ouzari, I.; Daffonchio, D.; Borin, S. Potential for Plant Growth Promotion of Rhizobacteria Associated with Salicornia Growing in Tunisian Hypersaline Soils. *BioMed Res. Int.* **2013**, *2013*, 248078. [CrossRef]
39. Riva, F.; Riva, V.; Eckert, E.M.; Colinas, N.; Di Cesare, A.; Borin, S.; Mapelli, F.; Crotti, E. An environmental Escherichia coli strain is naturally competent to acquire exogenous DNA. *Front. Microbiol.* **2020**, *11*, 1–13. [CrossRef]
40. Li, J.; McLellan, S.; Ogawa, S. Accumulation and fate of green fluorescent labeled Escherichia coli in laboratory-scale drinking water biofilters. *Water Res.* **2006**, *40*, 3023–3028.
41. Zhang, D.; Zhu, L.; Li, F. Influences and mechanisms of surfactants on pyrene biodegradation based on interactions of surfactant with a Klebsiella oxytoca strain. *Bioresour. Technol.* **2013**, *142*, 454–461. [CrossRef] [PubMed]
42. Halder, S.K.; Yadav, K.K.; Sarkar, R.; Mukherjee, S.; Saha, P.; Haldar, S.; Karmakar, S.; Sen, T. Alteration of Zeta potential and membrane permeability in bacteria: A study with cationic agents. *SpringerPlus* **2015**, *4*, 1–14. [CrossRef] [PubMed]

antibiotics

MDPI

Article

Antimicrobial Resistance and β-Lactamase Production in Clinically Significant Gram-Negative Bacteria Isolated from Hospital and Municipal Wastewater

Mohammad Irfan *, Alhomidi Almotiri and Zeyad Abdullah AlZeyadi

Department of Clinical Laboratory Sciences, College of Applied Medical Sciences, Shaqra University, Shaqra 11961, Saudi Arabia; hsalmutiri@su.edu.sa (A.A.); zalzeyadi@su.edu.sa (Z.A.A.)

* Correspondence: mquraish@su.edu.sa

Abstract: Hospital and municipal wastewater contribute to the spread of antibiotic-resistant bacteria and genes in the environment. This study aimed to examine the antibiotic resistance and β-lactamase production in clinically significant Gram-negative bacteria isolated from hospital and municipal wastewater. The susceptibility of bacteria to antibiotics was tested using the disk diffusion method, and the presence of extended-spectrum β-lactamases (ESBL) and carbapenemases was determined using an enzyme inhibitor and standard multiplex PCR. Analysis of antimicrobial resistance of total bacterial strains (n = 23) revealed that most of them were resistant to cefotaxime (69.56%), imipenem (43.47%), meropenem (47.82%) and amoxicillin-clavulanate (43.47%), gentamicin (39.13%), cefepime and ciprofloxacin (34.78%), trimethoprim-sulfamethoxazole (30.43%). A total of 8 of 11 phenotypically confirmed isolates were found to have ESBL genes. The bla_{TEM} gene was present in 2 of the isolates, while the bla_{SHV} gene was found in 2 of the isolates. Furthermore, the $bla_{CTX\text{-}M}$ gene was found in 3 of the isolates. In one isolate, both the bla_{TEM} and bla_{SHV} genes were identified. Furthermore, of the 9 isolates that have been phenotypically confirmed to have carbapenemase, 3 were confirmed by PCR. Specifically, 2 isolates have the $bla_{OXA\text{-}48}$ type gene and 1 have the $bla_{NDM\text{-}1}$ gene. In conclusion, our investigation shows that there is a significant rate of bacteria that produce ESBL and carbapenemase, which can promote the spread of bacterial resistance. Identifying ESBL and carbapenemase production genes in wastewater samples and their resistance patterns can provide valuable data and guide the development of pathogen management strategies that could potentially help reduce the occurrence of multidrug resistance.

Keywords: wastewater; sewage; ESBL; carbapenemase; antibiotic resistance; antibiotic-resistant bacteria

check for updates

Citation: Irfan, M.; Almotiri, A.; AlZeyadi, Z.A. Antimicrobial Resistance and β-Lactamase Production in Clinically Significant Gram-Negative Bacteria Isolated from Hospital and Municipal Wastewater. *Antibiotics* **2023**, *12*, 653. https://doi.org/10.3390/antibiotics12040653

Academic Editor: Akebe Luther King Abia

Received: 28 February 2023
Revised: 19 March 2023
Accepted: 23 March 2023
Published: 26 March 2023

1. Introduction

Hospital wastewater is considered potentially hazardous due to the presence of pharmaceutical residues, radioisotopes, and microbes, which could pose risks to human and environmental health. Antibiotics used in hospitals can end up in wastewater through patient urine and feces, selecting multidrug resistant (MDR) bacteria to thrive. This is because the human body is unable to fully metabolize some of the active ingredients in these drugs [1]. The sewer system in metropolitan areas transports antibiotic residues and resistant bacteria from people and/or animals to discharge sites, such as wastewater treatment facilities [2]. The MDR bacteria that produce hydrolyzing enzymes are found regularly in hospitals but have also been found in environmental sources such as rivers, seawater, and wastewater from both urban and hospital sources [3–6]. Studies have found that municipal wastewater treatment plants can harbor MDR bacteria that can spread to the environment [7,8]. The prevalence of antibiotic-resistant bacteria (ARB) varies over time and between hospitals and wastewater treatment plants (WWTP) in different locations [9]. The spread of extended-spectrum β-lactamases (ESBL) has become an important factor in the emergence of gram-negative MDR bacteria in hospitals, identified in Europe and then worldwide [10]. The β-lactam class of antibiotics is the most commonly prescribed group of antibacterial agents, accounting for approximately 70% of prescriptions, due to their ability to effectively target a wide range of bacteria [11]. These antibiotics are commonly used to treat severe infections, but their effectiveness has been compromised by the emergence of ESBL and carbapenemase, which have a negative impact on their clinical use [12].

The World Health Organization (WHO) has identified carbapenemase-producing *Enterobacteriaceae* (CRE) as a critical threat to human health and has included it in its list of priority diseases for which new treatments are urgently needed. CRE has become a major concern in recent years due to its resistance to antibiotics and the proliferation of antibiotic-resistant pathogens, which poses a significant challenge for Saudi Arabia [13]. The transmission of antibiotic-resistant strains of *Enterobacteriaceae* is a significant concern, and the large volume of human movement (pilgrim, tourism, work) within and outside the Gulf region is a major risk factor for their spread. These strains have been documented in several studies in various regions of Saudi Arabia [14–19]. There is a lack of data on the prevalence and patterns of antimicrobial resistant bacteria in hospital and municipal wastewater in Saudi Arabia. Therefore, we conducted this study to determine the resistance patterns of clinically significant isolates to various antibiotics and to investigate the presence of ESBL and carbapenemase-producing bacteria. The study also aimed to determine the presence of specific ESBL and carbapenemase genes in isolated organisms.

2. Results

2.1. Bacterial Isolation

In this study, 23 bacterial isolates from MacConkey agar containing 2 μg of meropenem were selected (as shown in Table 1). Of these isolates, 7 were obtained from hospital wastewater samples, 14 were obtained from municipal wastewater samples, and 2 were obtained from municipal treated wastewater samples. No isolates were obtained from treated wastewater samples collected from the hospital.

Table 1. List of bacteria isolated.

<table>
<tr><th></th><th colspan="4">Bacteria Isolated/Number of Isolates</th></tr>
<tr><th></th><th>Hospital (Wastewater)</th><th>Hospital (Treated Wastewater)</th><th>Municipal (Wastewater)</th><th>Municipal (Treated Wastewater)</th></tr>
<tr><td rowspan="5">Enterobacteriaceae</td><td>Klebsiella spp. (2)</td><td rowspan="5">No growth</td><td>E. coli (3)</td><td rowspan="5">Enterobacter spp. (1)</td></tr>
<tr><td rowspan="4">Enterobacter spp. (1)</td><td>Klebsiella spp. (2)</td></tr>
<tr><td>Enterobacter spp. (1)</td></tr>
<tr><td>Citrobacter spp. (2)</td></tr>
<tr><td>Proteus spp. (1)</td></tr>
<tr><td rowspan="2">Non-Enterobacteriaceae</td><td>Acinetobacter spp. (3)</td><td rowspan="2">No growth</td><td>Acinetobacter spp. (2)</td><td rowspan="2">Pseudomonas spp. (1)</td></tr>
<tr><td>Pseudomonas spp. (1)</td><td>Pseudomonas spp. (3)</td></tr>
</table>

2.2. Identification of Isolates

Of 23 isolates, 13 were found to belong to the *Enterobacteriaceae* family, including 3 *E. coli*, 4 *Klebsiella* spp., 3 *Enterobacter* spp., 2 *Citrobacter* spp. and 1 *Proteus* spp. The remaining 11 strains were identified as non-*Enterobacteriaceae*, including 5 *Acinetobacter* spp. and 5 *Pseudomonas* spp. Of the total of seven isolates from hospital wastewater, the most predominant taxa were *Acinetobacter* spp. followed by *Klebsiella* spp., *Enterobacter* spp. and *Pseudomonas* spp. In the wastewater and treated wastewater samples collected from the municipality, we identified 16 strains of bacteria. The most common strains were *Pseudomonas* spp. followed by *E. coli*, *Klebsiella* spp., *Acinetobacter* spp., *Enterobacter* spp., *Citrobacter* spp., and *Proteus* spp. (Table S1, supplementary materials).

2.3. Determination of the Antimicrobial Susceptibility Pattern of the Isolates

In our study, the antibiotic susceptibility patterns of the *Enterobacteriaceae* strains were as follows: *Enterobacter* spp. (n = 3) Isolated from the hospital and municipal wastewater and treated wastewater were found resistant to amoxicillin-clavulanate (66.66%), cefotaxime (100%), imipenem (33.33%), meropenem (33.33%), gentamicin (66.66%), ciprofloxacin (33.33%) and trimethoprim-sulfamethoxazole (33.33%). *Klebsiella* spp. (n = 4) isolated from hospital and municipal wastewater showed resistance to amoxicillin-clavulanate (50%), cefotaxime (75%), cefepime (25%), imipenem (75%), meropenem (50%), ciprofloxacin (25%), gentamicin (25%) and trimethoprim-sulfamethoxazole (50%). *E. coli* spp. (n = 3) isolated from municipal wastewater showed resistance to ceftazidime (33.33%), cefotaxime (100%), imipenem (33.33%), meropenem (33.33%), ciprofloxacin (66.66%), gentamicin (33.33%) and trimethoprim-sulfamethoxazole (33.33%). *Citrobacter* spp. (n = 2) isolated from municipal wastewater were found to be resistant to amoxicillin-clavulanate (100%), ceftazidime (50%), cefepime (50%), cefotaxime (50%), imipenem (50%), meropenem (50%), ciprofloxacin (50%) and trimethoprim-sulfamethoxazole (50%). *Proteus* spp. (n = 1) isolated from municipal wastewater were resistant to amoxicillin-clavulanate (100%), ceftazidime (100%), cefotaxime (100%), cefepime (100%), meropenem (100%) and trimethoprim-sulfamethoxazole (100%). Analysis of 13 *Enterobacteriaceae* strains for antimicrobial resistance (AMR) showed that most of them were resistant to cefotaxime (84.61%), followed by amoxicillin-clavulanate (53.84%), imipenem and meropenem (46.15% each), trimethoprim-sulfamethoxazole (38.46%) and ciprofloxacin (30.76%).

The antibiotic susceptibility pattern of strains other than *Enterobacteriaceae* in our study was recorded as *Acinetobacter* spp. (n = 5) isolated from hospital and municipal wastewater were found to be resistant to cefotaxime (80%), cefepime (60%), imipenem (40%), meropenem (40%), ciprofloxacin (20%), gentamicin (20%) and trimethoprim-sulfamethoxazole (40%). *Pseudomonas* spp. (n = 5) isolated from hospital and municipal wastewater and from treated municipal wastewater were resistant to ceftazidime (40%), cefotaxime (20%), cefepime (40%), imipenem (40%), meropenem (60%), ciprofloxacin (60%) and gentamicin (80%). The AMR patterns of 10 strains of *non-Enterobacteriaceae* were also examined, and it was found that most showed resistance to cefotaxime, cefepime, Gentamicin, and Meropenem (50.00%), Imipenem and ciprofloxacin (40%).

An analysis of 23 bacterial strains found that most were resistant to cefotaxime (69.56%), followed by meropenem (47.82%), imipenem and amoxicillin-clavulanate (43.47%), gentamicin (39.13%), cefepime and ciprofloxacin (34.78%), and trimethoprim-sulfamethoxazole (30.43%). No bacteria were found to be resistant to colistin (Table S2, supplementary materials).

2.4. Screening for β-Lactamases

Of the 23 bacterial strains isolated from municipal and hospital wastewater and treated wastewater, 18 were resistant to cefotaxime/ceftazidime or both antibiotics. The 18 potential ESBL strains were further tested for confirmation of ESBL. 11 were confirmed to be producers of ESBL belonging to species *Acinetobacter, Enterobacter, Pseudomonas, E. coli, Citrobacter,* and *Proteus.* 13 isolates were found to be resistant to imipenem and/or meropenem; out of which 9 isolates were positive for Modified Hodge Test (MHT). The isolates were belonging to *Klebsiella, Citrobacter, Enterobacter, Acinetobacter* and *Pseudomonas* species (Figure S1 and S2, supplementary materials).

2.5. Detection of Resistance Genes by PCR

Of the 11 phenotypically confirmed ESBL isolates, 8 carried ESBL genes. The bla_{TEM} gene was identified in a total of 2 strains, mainly harbored in the *Pseudomonas and Enterobacter* species. Furthermore, the bla_{SHV} gene was identified in 2 strains mainly harbored by *Citrobacter and Proteus* species. The $bla_{CTX\text{-}M}$ gene was identified in 3 strains mainly harbored by *Acinetobacter* species. Of the total PCR-positive ESBL isolates, the coexistence of two different genes, that is, bla_{TEM} and bla_{SHV}, in a single isolate was revealed in a *E. coli.* The most common carbapenemase encoding gene found in this study was $bla_{OXA\text{-}48}$ and *bla*$_{\text{NDM-1}}$. It was present in 3 of the 9 phenotypically confirmed carbapenemase producing isolates. 2 of *Klebsiella* species were found to harbor *bla*$_{\text{OXA-48}}$. These isolates came from the hospital and municipal wastewater. The second prevalent carbapenemase encoding gene found was *bla*$_{\text{NDM-1}}$, which was present in 1 of *Acinetobacter* spp. which was isolated from municipal wastewater (Figures S3 and S4 Supplementary Materials).

3. Discussion

The overuse and abuse of antimicrobials in human and veterinary medicine, as well as environmental contamination, have contributed significantly to the emergence of AMR as a major threat to public health. The most common causes of AMR in healthcare facilities are the inappropriate use of antimicrobials and an inadequate infection control program. It has been recognized that aquatic environments can serve as a means of transmission of infection, and this is often related to the discharge of wastewater effluents from medical facilities, animal breeding farms, and sewer systems [20]. Despite this, there is a lack of conclusive information on the conditions or mechanisms that contribute to the development of drug-resistant strains in individuals [21]. Recent research has shown that bacteria and their genetic material can be easily transferred between humans, animals, and the environment [22–24].

In our study, the most predominant species identified in hospital wastewater were *Klebsiella* spp., *Acinetobacter* spp. *Enterobacter* spp. and *Pseudomonas* spp. The strains identified in municipal wastewater and treated wastewater samples were dominated by *Pseudomonas* spp., *E. coli, Enterobacter* spp., *Citrobacter* spp., *Klebsiella* spp., *Acinetobacter* spp. and *Proteus* species at the lowest abundance. Similarly, a study by Khaled et al. characterized bacterial species isolated from domestic wastewater treatment plants in Jazan, KSA, describing several enteric and non-enteric Gram-negative strains [25]. A study by Röderová et al. also found human and environmental bacteria in wastewater from hospitals and urban wastewater treatment plants [26].

We found that isolates from hospital wastewater, as well as municipal wastewater and treated wastewater, showed resistance to various antibiotics. The results of our analysis of the AMR of *Enterobacteriaceae* strains showed that most of them were resistant to cefotaxime (84.61%), amoxicillin-clavulanate (53.84%), imipenem and meropenem (46.15%) and trimethoprim-sulfamethoxazole (38.46%). Ciprofloxacin had a lower resistance level of 30.76%. The results of our study are consistent with previous research on resistance patterns of *Enterobacteriaceae* strains, such as a study conducted in Germany that found a high level of resistance to cefotaxime (89%), ceftazidime (95%) and ciprofloxacin (53%) [27]. The resistance pattern of the *non-Enterobacteriaceae* strains revealed that most of them showed resistance to cefotaxime, cefepime, Gentamicin and Meropenem (50.00%), Imipenem and ciprofloxacin (40%), and many studies have found carbapenem-resistant *Acinetobacter* spp. in hospital wastewater [28–30], but resistance to carbapenems has rarely been studied in isolates obtained from municipal wastewater [31].

A major concern for global public health is the rapid increase in the incidence of *Enterobacteriaceae* producing ESBL and its subsequent spread to the general population. The frequency of ESBL production was highest among *Acinetobacter*, followed by *Enterobacter, Pseudomonas, E. coli, Citrobacter and Proteus.* A study by Bréchet et al. found a high prevalence of *Enterobacteriaceae* producing ESBL in hospital wastewater [32]. Furthermore, global studies have found significant variations in the prevalence and percentage of strains that produce ESBL between different nations [33]. It appears that the production of ESBL by *Enterobacteriaceae* and non-*Enterobacteriaceae* strains may restrict the treatment options for infections caused by this group of bacteria. Therefore, the bacteria that produce ESBL pose a significant problem that requires proactive efforts to prevent their occurrence.

In our study, carbapenemase producers were phenotypically identified among *Klebsiella, Citrobacter, Enterobacter, Acinetobacter, and Pseudomonas species.* Two separate phenotypic studies conducted in Mecca found that 48.4% and 38% of the samples were positive for carbapenemase production in *Klebsiella pneumoniae* [34,35]. Wastewater serves as a reservoir of antibiotic resistant bacteria that reflects the composition of bacterial populations carried out by the general population, and wastewater is a hotspot for the exchange of resistant genes among bacteria [36]. Isolates that were found to produce ESBL or carbapenemase by any phenotypic method were further characterized by molecular analysis. The bla_{TEM}-type gene was detected in 2 strains of *Pseudomonas* spp. and *Enterobacter* spp. isolated from municipal wastewater and treated wastewater, respectively. The bla_{SHV}-type gene was also found in 2 strains, mainly in *Citrobacter* and *Proteus* spp. isolates from municipal wastewater. The $bla_{CTX\text{-}M}$ type gene was identified in 3 strains, mainly in *Acinetobacter* spp. isolates from the hospital and municipal wastewater. The prevalence of the bla_{TEM} gene in this study is similar to the findings of a study conducted in Portugal, where the most commonly identified genes were bla_{TEM} (24.1%) and $bla_{CTX\text{-}M}$ (5.6%) [37]. In a separate study, the bla_{TEM} gene was found to be the most prevalent in wastewater samples collected during biological treatment, including treated wastewater. However, in another study, the bla_{SHV} gene was the least prevalent among the genes tested [38]. A recent study revealed that a small percentage of ESBL genes were found in isolates obtained from wastewater effluent. Among these samples, 9.2% carried the bla_{TEM} gene, 1.4% carried the $bla_{SHV\text{-}12}$ gene, 0.2% carried the $bla_{CTX\text{-}M\text{-}1}$ gene, and 1% carried the $bla_{CTX\text{-}M\text{-}15}$ gene [39]. In WWTP, the genes $bla_{CTX\text{-}M}$, bla_{TEM}, bla_{SHV}, and bla_{OXA} have been identified in multiple species within the *Enterobacteriaceae* species group. Our study identified a combination of bla_{TEM} and bla_{SHV} genes in 1 *E. coli* spp. isolated from municipal wastewater. In other studies, bla_{SHV} and/or bla_{TEM} were also frequently found [40–42]. Furthermore, we found that the genes $bla_{OXA\text{-}48}$ and $bla_{NDM\text{-}1}$ were prevalent among carbapenemase genes. Specifically, the $bla_{OXA\text{-}48}$ gene was the most identified in *Klebsiella* spp. isolated from hospital and municipal wastewater. The presence of $bla_{OXA\text{-}48}$ has also been detected in Saudi Arabian clinical samples from Saudi Arabia [43]. Studies also reported the prevalence of $bla_{OXA\text{-}48}$ in wastewater [44,45]. Meanwhile, the $bla_{NDM\text{-}1}$ gene was detected in *Acinetobacter* spp. recovered from municipal wastewater. Our results are consistent with those of previous studies showing that the $bla_{NDM\text{-}1}$ gene has been found in a wide variety of species and is spreading rapidly in various environments [28,46,47]. In this study, none of the isolates tested positive for carbapenemase encoding genes of type bla_{IMP}, bla_{VIM} or bla_{KPC}.

Our research had some limitations, including the fact that we only tested β lactamase genes in bacteria that were phenotypically confirmed, the list of resistance testing primers did not cover everything, and we did not test the mechanism of resistance to carbapenems other than the production of carbapenemase. Resistance genes could be present in bacteria that do not show resistance phenotypically. The only way to overcome this is to perform whole genome sequencing for all isolates. Furthermore, our sample size was relatively small, so future studies with more samples from various sources will provide a more comprehensive understanding of pathogens and β-lactam genes. Another limitation was that our study only looked at a hospital and a municipal wastewater treatment plant in a specific location, so the results may not apply to other locations.

4. Materials and Methods

4.1. Sample Collection

Six samples, consisting of three wastewater samples and three treated wastewater samples, were collected from a hospital and municipal wastewater treatment plant in the central region of Saudi Arabia between October 2021 and December 2021. The samples were collected between 8 am and 11 am and placed in 1-L plastic containers that had been sterilized with 70% alcohol and rinsed with deionized water. After collection, the samples were transported in an insulated box with ice packs to the laboratory for processing. All samples were stored at a temperature of 4 °C and analyzed within 24 h after collection.

4.2. Bacterial Isolates

10 mL of wastewater and 100 mL of treated wastewater were centrifuged at 5000× *g* for 10 min. The samples were then serially diluted with normal sterile saline (10^{-1}, 10^{-2}, 10^{-3})

and 100 µL of each aliquot was spread on MacConkey agar with 2 µg/mL of meropenem added. The plates were incubated overnight at a temperature of 35 ± 2 °C. To further purify the bacteria, colonies with distinctive color and characteristics were randomly selected and subcultured on MacConkey agar containing 2 µg of meropenem. The isolates were then stored in TSA + 10% glycerol stock at a temperature of −80 °C for further analysis. The identifications of the isolates were confirmed by Gram staining and then further determined by biochemical analysis, as detailed by Mahan et al. [48].

4.3. *Antimicrobial Sensitivity*

The antibiotic sensitivity test (AST) was performed using the disk diffusion method as per the recommendations of the Clinical Laboratory Standard Institute (CLSI) [49]. The disk diffusion test was carried out using the Kirby-Bauer technique with cefotaxime (CTX, 30 µg), cefepime (FEP, 5 µg), imipenem (IMP, 10 µg), meropenem (MEM, 10 µg), ciprofloxacin (CIP, 5 µg), gentamicin (GEN, 10 µg), trimethoprim/sulfamethoxazole (SXT, 23.75 µg + 1.25 µg), ceftazidime (CAZ, 30 µg), amoxicillin-clavulanate (AMC, 30 µg), and colistin (CST) (30 µg). All antibiotics were obtained from Oxide Pvt. Ltd. The quality control process included the use of strains from the American Type Culture Collection (ATCC) *Escherichia coli* (*E. coli*) 25,922 and *P. aeruginosa* 27,953.

4.4. *Phenotypic Detection of β-Lactamases*

A double disc diffusion test [49] was carried out to verify the presence of ESBL, discs containing ceftazidime (30 µg), cefotaxime (30 µg), and a combination of clavulanic acid (30 µg)/10 µg) were used. The disks were placed at the appropriate distance on MHA plates that had been inoculated with a bacterial suspension of 0.5 McFarland turbidity standards. The plates were left to incubate for 18–20 h at 37 °C. The isolates were determined to be producers of ESBL if the difference in the zone of inhibition of the drug and inhibitor was at least 5 mm compared to cephalosporin alone.

Modified Hodge Test [49] was performed to determine carbapenemase production according to CLSI standards. A suspension of *E. coli* ATCC 25,922 was adjusted to the 0.5 McFarland standard and swabbed on MHA plates. After drying, a disc containing 10 µg of meropenem was left in the middle of the plate and then the isolates were spread in a thin line from the edge of the disc that extended to the edge of the plate. The plates were incubated overnight at 37 °C. A distorted inhibitory zone in the shape of a clover leaf on the meropenem disc around the growth of *E. coli* ATCC 25,922 indicated a positive result.

4.5. *Analysis of Gene Molecules of ESBL and Carbapenemase*

4.5.1. DNA Extraction

Fresh colonies of all phenotypically verified ESBL and carbapenemase isolates were processed for DNA extraction using the boiling method [50]. Briefly, a suspension was made by suspending 2–4 fresh colonies of each isolate in 500 µL of nuclease-free distilled water. The suspension was heated to 95 °C for 10 min, followed by cooling and then centrifugation at 10,000 rpm for 10 min. Finally, 150 µL of the supernatant was stored at −20 °C and used as a template for subsequent amplification.

4.5.2. Detection of Genes Encoding ESBL and Carbapenemase

The multiplex polymerase chain reaction (PCR) was performed in two separate reactions using the BIO-RAD T100 thermal cycler (Applied Biosystems, Waltham, MA, USA). In the first reaction, the genes $bla_{CTX\text{-}M}$, bla_{TEM}, and bla_{SHV} were multiplexed in a single tube to detect ESBL. In the second reaction, the genes bla_{IMP}, bla_{VIM}, bla_{KPC}, bla_{NDM}, and $bla_{OXA\text{-}48}$ were multiplexed to detect carbapenemase. The PCR procedures were performed in a total volume of 20 µL, including 4 µL of 5× FIREPol® Master Mix (Solis Biodyne, Tartu, Estonia), 0.2 µL of each primer, 1 µL of DNA template and 14.6 µL of nuclease-free water. The amplification cycle consisted of initial denaturation at 95 °C for 3 min, followed by 30 cycles of denaturation at 95 °C for 15 s, annealing at the temperature specified in Table 2 for 30 s, extension at 72 °C for 1 min, and final extension at 72 °C for 5 min. The PCR results were analyzed by gel electrophoresis on 1.5% agarose gel. The size of the amplicon was calculated compared to the 100 bp ladder marker (Solis Biodyne, Tartu, Estonia).

Table 2. List of primers used.

Targeted Genes	Nucleotide Sequence (5′to 3′)	Amplicon Size (bp)	Annealing Temp	References
bla$_{\text{CTX-M}}$	Forward—GTGATACCACTTCACCTC Reverse-AGTAAGTGACCAGAATCAG	255	56	[51]
bla$_{\text{SHV}}$	Forward—ACTATCGCCAGCAGGATC Reverse—ATCGTCCACCATCCACTG	356	53	[51]
bla$_{\text{TEM}}$	Forward—GATCTCAACAGCGGTAAG Reverse—CAGTGAGGCACCTATCTC	786	58	[51]
bla$_{\text{KPC}}$	Forward—CATTCAAGGGCTTTCTTGCTGC Reverse—ACGACGGCATAGTCATTTGC	538	55	[52]
bla$_{\text{IMP}}$	Forward—TTGACACTCCATTTACDG Reverse—GATYGAGAATTAAGCCACYCT	139	55	[52]
bla$_{\text{VIM}}$	Forward—GATGGTGTTTGGTCGCATA Reverse—CGAATGCGCAGCACCAG	390	55	[52]
bla$_{\text{OXA-48}}$	Forward—GCTTGATCGCCCTCGATT Reverse—GATTTGCTCCGTGGCCGAAA	281	57	[52]
bla$_{\text{NDM-1}}$	Forward—GGTTTGGCGATCTGGTTTTC Reverse—CGGAATGGCTCATCACGATC	621	52	[53]

5. Conclusions and Future Perspectives

Our data indicate that that hospital and municipal wastewater contained a range of resistant bacteria dominated by *Klebsiella, Acinetobacter, Enterobacter, and Pseudomonas* species. These isolates showed resistance to various antibiotics, particularly cefotaxime, amoxicillin-clavulanate, imipenem, meropenem, and trimethoprim-sulfamethoxazole. Furthermore, Enterobacteriaceae and non-Enterobacteriaceae strains producing ESBL and carbapenemase were also identified. To address this issue, it is important to identify the genes responsible for producing ESBL and carbapenemase in nonclinical samples, such as wastewater. So, we can gain valuable information to help develop effective strategies for managing pathogens, which can help reduce the occurrence of multidrug resistance. Additionally, there is a practice of reusing wastewater for agricultural purposes, and the potential use of wastewater sludge for other applications. Given the high levels of resistant bacteria found in wastewater, we must take additional measures to remove these bacteria before releasing the water back into the environment or reusing it for other purposes. Therefore, it is essential to regularly evaluate wastewater systems in hospitals and municipalities. Furthermore, more research is needed to understand the risks associated with wastewater disposal and recycling. We must assess the extent of ecosystem pollution that occurs because of these practices. By doing so, we can develop more effective methods to manage wastewater and ensure that it does not contribute to the spread of antibiotic resistance in the environment.

Supplementary Materials: The following supporting information can be downloaded at: https://www.mdpi.com/article/10.3390/antibiotics12040653/s1, Table S1. Biochemical analyses of isolates; Table S2. Antibiotic resistance profile; Figure S1. Double disc diffusion test for ESBLs; Figure S2. Modified Hodge test; Figure S3. Detection of ESBL genes (multiplex PCR); Figure S4. Detection of Carbapenemase genes (multiplex PCR).

Author Contributions: Conceptualization, M.I.; methodology, M.I, A.A. and Z.A.A.; analysis, M.I, A.A. and Z.A.A.; writing and editing all authors. All authors have read and agreed to the published version of the manuscript.

Funding: This research was funded by the "Deputyship for Research and Innovation, Ministry of Education in Saudi Arabia" (project IFP2021-085).

Institutional Review Board Statement: The research plan was examined and authorized by the Ethical Research Committee of Shaqra University, and its approval number is ERC_SU 20210031.

Informed Consent Statement: Not applicable.

Data Availability Statement: The data are contained within the article.

Acknowledgments: The authors extend their appreciation to the "Deputyship for Research and Innovation, Ministry of Education in Saudi Arabia" for funding this research work through the project number IFP2021-085. In addition, the authors extend their appreciation to Deanship of scientific research at Shaqra University for supporting this work.

Conflicts of Interest: The authors declare no conflict of interest. The funders had no role in the design of the study; in the collection, analyses, or interpretation of the data; in the writing of the manuscript; or in the decision to publish the results.

References

1. Jelic, A.; Rodriguez-Mozaz, S.; Barceló, D.; Gutierrez, O. Impact of In-Sewer Transformation on 43 Pharmaceuticals in a Pressurized Sewer under Anaerobic Conditions. *Water Res.* **2015**, *68*, 98–108. [CrossRef]
2. Karkman, A.; Pärnänen, K.; Larsson, D.G.J. Fecal Pollution Can Explain Antibiotic Resistance Gene Abundances in Anthropogenically Impacted Environments. *Nat. Commun.* **2019**, *10*, 80. [CrossRef]
3. Aldrazi, F.A.; Rabaan, A.A.; Alsuliman, S.A.; Aldrazi, H.A.; Alabdalslam, M.J.; Alsadiq, S.A.; Alhani, H.M.; Bueid, A.S. ESBL Expression and Antibiotic Resistance Patterns in a Hospital in Saudi Arabia: Do Healthcare Staff Have the Whole Picture? *J. Infect. Public Health* **2020**, *13*, 759–766. [CrossRef]
4. Liu, H.; Zhou, H.; Li, Q.; Peng, Q.; Zhao, Q.; Wang, J.; Liu, X. Molecular Characteristics of Extended-Spectrum β-Lactamase-Producing Escherichia Coli Isolated from the Rivers and Lakes in Northwest China. *BMC Microbiol.* **2018**, *18*, 125. [CrossRef]
5. Čornejová, T.; Venglovsky, J.; Gregova, G.; Kmetova, M.; Kmet, V. Extended Spectrum Beta-Lactamases in *Escherichia Coli* from Municipal Wastewater. *Ann. Agric. Environ. Med.* **2015**, *22*, 447–450. [CrossRef]
6. Lépesová, K.; Olejníková, P.; Mackuľak, T.; Cverenkárová, K.; Krahulcová, M.; Bírošová, L. Hospital Wastewater—Important Source of Multidrug Resistant Coliform Bacteria with ESBL-Production. *Int. J. Environ. Res. Public Health* **2020**, *17*, 7827. [CrossRef]
7. Mustafa, S.S.; Batool, R.; Kamran, M.; Javed, H.; Jamil, N. Evaluating the Role of Wastewaters as Reservoirs of Antibiotic-Resistant ESKAPEE Bacteria Using Phenotypic and Molecular Methods. *Infect. Drug Resist.* **2022**, *15*, 5715–5728. [CrossRef]
8. Rizzo, L.; Manaia, C.; Merlin, C.; Schwartz, T.; Dagot, C.; Ploy, M.C.; Michael, I.; Fatta-Kassinos, D. Urban Wastewater Treatment Plants as Hotspots for Antibiotic Resistant Bacteria and Genes Spread into the Environment: A Review. *Sci. Total Envron.* **2013**, *447*, 345–360. [CrossRef]
9. Chau, K.K.; Barker, L.; Budgell, E.P.; Vihta, K.D.; Sims, N.; Kasprzyk-Hordern, B.; Harriss, E.; Crook, D.W.; Read, D.S.; Walker, A.S.; et al. Systematic Review of Wastewater Surveillance of Antimicrobial Resistance in Human Populations. *Environ. Int.* **2022**, *162*, 107171. [CrossRef]
10. Sirot, D. Extended-Spectrum Plasmid-Mediated Beta-Lactamases. *J. Antimicrob. Chemother.* **1995**, *36* (Suppl. SA), 19–34. [CrossRef]

11. Bush, K.; Bradford, P.A. β-Lactams and β-Lactamase Inhibitors: An Overview. *Cold Spring Harb. Perspect. Med.* **2016**, *6*, a025247. [CrossRef]
12. Bush, K. The ABCD's of β-Lactamase Nomenclature. *J. Infect. Chemother.* **2013**, *19*, 549–559. [CrossRef]
13. Hussein, K.; Raz-Pasteur, A.; Finkelstein, R.; Neuberger, A.; Shachor-Meyouhas, Y.; Oren, I.; Kassis, I. Impact of Carbapenem Resistance on the Outcome of Patients' Hospital-Acquired Bacteraemia Caused by Klebsiella Pneumoniae. *J. Hosp. Infect.* **2013**, *83*, 307–313. [CrossRef]
14. Alhumaidy, A.; Alahmadi, R.; Eisa, S.; Alotaibi, M.; Filfilan, S.; Alzayer, M.; Okdah, L.; Doumith, M.; Taha, O.; Albishri, B.; et al. Molecular Characterization of Carbapenemase Producing *Acinetobacter Baumannii* and *Pseudomonas Aeruginosa* from Tertiary Care Hospitals in Mecca—Saudi Arabia. *J. Infect. Public Health* **2020**, *13*, 335. [CrossRef]
15. Alahmadi, R.; Alhumaidy, A.; Eisa, S.; Alotaibi, M.; Filfilan, S.; Taha, O.; Albishri, B.; Mulana, A.; Alshelgani, A.; Alzeyadi, Z. Molecular Detection of Common Carbapenemase Resistance Genes in Nosocomial Pathogens Isolated from Neonatal ICU at a Major Tertiary Care Hospital in Mecca. *J. Infect. Public Health* **2020**, *13*, 332. [CrossRef]
16. Yezli, S.; Shibl, A.M.; Memish, Z.A. The Molecular Basis of β-Lactamase Production in Gram-Negative Bacteria from Saudi Arabia. *J Med Microbiol* **2015**, *64*, 127–136. [CrossRef]
17. Al-Agamy, M.H.; Shibl, A.M.; Elkhizzi, N.A.; Meunier, D.; Turton, J.F.; Livermore, D.M. Persistence of *Klebsiella Pnemoniae* Clones with OXA-48 or NDM Carbapenemases Causing Bacteraemias in a Riyadh Hospital. *Diagn Microbiol. Infect Dis.* **2013**, *76*, 214–216. [CrossRef]
18. Garbati, M.A.; Sakkijha, H.; Abushaheen, A. Infections Due to Carbapenem Resistant Enterobacteriaceae among Saudi Arbian Hospitalized Patients: A Matched Case-Control Study. *BioMed. Res. Int.* **2016**, *2016*, e3961684. [CrossRef]
19. Al-Zahrani, I.A.; Alasiri, B.A. The Emergence of Carbapenem-Resistant Klebsiella Pneumoniae Isolates Producing OXA-48 and NDM in the Southern (Asir) Province, Saudi Arabia. *Saudi Med. J.* **2018**, *39*, 23–30. [CrossRef]
20. Irfan, M.; Almotiri, A.; AlZeyadi, Z.A. Antimicrobial Resistance and Its Drivers—A Review. *Antibiotics* **2022**, *11*, 1362. [CrossRef]
21. Galler, H.; Feierl, G.; Petternel, C.; Reinthaler, F.F.; Haas, D.; Habib, J.; Kittinger, C.; Luxner, J.; Zarfel, G. Multiresistant Bact ria Isolated from Activated Sludge in Austria. *Int. J. Environ. Res. Public Health* **2018**, *15*, 479. [CrossRef]
22. Manaia, C.M. Assessing the Risk of Antibiotic Resistance Transmission from the Environment to Humans: Non-Direct Proportionality between Abundance and Risk. *Trends Microbiol.* **2017**, *25*, 173–181. [CrossRef]
23. Oliveira, P.H.; Touchon, M.; Cury, J.; Rocha, E.P.C. The Chromosomal Organization of Horizontal Gene Transfer in Bacteria. *Nat. Commun.* **2017**, *8*, 841. [CrossRef]
24. Martínez, J.L. Ecology and Evolution of Chromosomal Gene Transfer between Environmental Microorganisms and Pathogens. *Microbiol. Spectr.* **2018**, *6*, 6.1.06. [CrossRef]
25. Elgayar, K.E.; Essa, A.M. Characterization of Bacteria Isolated from Domestic Wastewater In Jazan, Saudi Arabia. *Egypt. J. Exp. Biol.* **2018**, *14*, 331. [CrossRef]
26. Röderová, M.; Sedláková, M.H.; Pudová, V.; Hricová, K.; Silová, R.; Imwensi, P.E.O.; Bardoň, J.; Kolář, M. Occurrence of Bacteria Producing Broad-Spectrum Beta-Lactamases and Qnr Genes in Hospital and Urban Wastewater Samples. *New Microbiol.* **2016**, *39*, 124–133.
27. Homeier-Bachmann, T.; Heiden, S.E.; Lübcke, P.K.; Bachmann, L.; Bohnert, J.A.; Zimmermann, D.; Schaufler, K. Antibiotic-Resistant Enterobacteriaceae in Wastewater of Abattoirs. *Antibiotics* **2021**, *10*, 568. [CrossRef]
28. Marathe, N.P.; Berglund, F.; Razavi, M.; Pal, C.; Dröge, J.; Samant, S.; Kristiansson, E.; Larsson, D.G.J. Sewage Effluent from an Indian Hospital Harbors Novel Carbapenemases and Integron-Borne Antibiotic Resistance Genes. *Microbiome* **2019**, *7*, 97. [CrossRef]
29. Qin, J.; Maixnerová, M.; Nemec, M.; Feng, Y.; Zhang, X.; Nemec, A.; Zong, Z. Acinetobacter Cumulans Sp. Nov., Isolated from Hospital Sewage and Capable of Acquisition of Multiple Antibiotic Resistance Genes. *Syst. Appl. Microbiol.* **2019**, *42*, 319–325. [CrossRef]
30. Wang, Q.; Wang, P.; Yang, Q. Occurrence and Diversity of Antibiotic Resistance in Untreated Hospital Wastewater. *Sci. Total Environ.* **2018**, *621*, 990–999. [CrossRef]
31. Higgins, P.G.; Hrenovic, J.; Seifert, H.; Dekic, S. Characterization of *Acinetobacter Baumannii* from Water and Sludge Line of Secondary Wastewater Treatment Plant. *Water Res.* **2018**, *140*, 261–267. [CrossRef]
32. Bréchet, C.; Plantin, J.; Sauget, M.; Thouverez, M.; Talon, D.; Cholley, P.; Guyeux, C.; Hocquet, D.; Bertrand, X. Wastewater Treatment Plants Release Large Amounts of Extended-Spectrum β-Lactamase–Producing *Escherichia Coli* Into the Environment. *Clin. Infect. Dis.* **2014**, *58*, 1658–1665. [CrossRef]
33. Pfaller, M.A.; Jones, R.N.; Doern, G.V. Multicenter Evaluation of the Antimicrobial Activity for Six Broad-Spectrum Beta-Lactams in Venezuela: Comparison of Data from 1997 and 1998 Using the Etest Method. Venezuelan Antimicrobial Resistance Study Group. *Diagn Microbiol. Infect Dis.* **1999**, *35*, 153–158. [CrossRef]
34. Faidah, H.S.; Momenah, A.M.; El-Said, H.M.; Barhameen, A.A.A.; Ashgar, S.S.; Johargy, A.; Elsawy, A.; Almalki, W.; Qurashi, S.A. Trends in the Annual Incidence of Carbapenem Resistant among Gram Negative Bacilli in a Large Teaching Hospital in Makah City, Saudi Arabia. *J. Tuberc. Res.* **2017**, *5*, 229–236. [CrossRef]
35. Khan, M.; Faiz, A. Frequency of Carbapenemase Producing Klebsiella Pneumoniae in Makkah, Saudi Arabia. *J. Microbiol. Infect. Dis.* **2016**, *6*, 121–127. [CrossRef]

36. Korzeniewska, E.; Harnisz, M. Beta-Lactamase-Producing Enterobacteriaceae in Hospital Effluents. *J. Env. Manag.* **2013**, *123*, 1–7. [CrossRef]
37. Amador, P.P.; Fernandes, R.M.; Prudêncio, M.C.; Barreto, M.P.; Duarte, I.M. Antibiotic Resistance in Wastewater: Occurrence and Fate of Enterobacteriaceae Producers of Class A and Class C β-Lactamases. *J. Env. Sci. Health A Tox Hazard Subst Env. Eng.* **2015**, *50*, 26–39. [CrossRef]
38. Zieliński, W.; Buta, M.; Hubeny, J.; Korzeniewska, E.; Harnisz, M.; Nowrotek, M.; Płaza, G. Prevalence of Beta Lactamases Genes in Sewage and Sludge Treated in Mechanical-Biological Wastewater Treatment Plants. *J. Ecol. Eng.* **2019**, *20*, 80–86. [CrossRef]
39. Smyth, C.; O'Flaherty, A.; Walsh, F.; Do, T.T. Antibiotic Resistant and Extended-Spectrum β-Lactamase Producing Faecal Coliforms in Wastewater Treatment Plant Effluent. *Env. Pollut* **2020**, *262*, 114244. [CrossRef]
40. Zieliński, W.; Korzeniewska, E.; Harnisz, M.; Drzymała, J.; Felis, E.; Bajkacz, S. Wastewater Treatment Plants as a Reservoir of Integrase and Antibiotic Resistance Genes—An Epidemiological Threat to Workers and Environment. *Env. Int.* **2021**, *156*, 106641. [CrossRef]
41. Osińska, A.; Korzeniewska, E.; Harnisz, M.; Felis, E.; Bajkacz, S.; Jachimowicz, P.; Niestępski, S.; Konopka, I. Small-Scale Wastewater Treatment Plants as a Source of the Dissemination of Antibiotic Resistance Genes in the Aquatic Environment. *J. Hazard. Mater.* **2020**, *381*, 121221. [CrossRef]
42. Surleac, M.; Czobor Barbu, I.; Paraschiv, S.; Popa, L.I.; Gheorghe, I.; Marutescu, L.; Popa, M.; Sarbu, I.; Talapan, D.; Nita, M.; et al. Whole Genome Sequencing Snapshot of Multi-Drug Resistant *Klebsiella Pneumoniae* Strains from Hospitals and Receiving Wastewater Treatment Plants in Southern Romania. *PLoS ONE* **2020**, *15*, e0228079. [CrossRef]
43. Khan, M.A.; Mohamed, A.M.; Faiz, A.; Ahmad, J. Enterobacterial Infection in Saudi Arabia: First Record of Klebsiella Pneumoniae with Triple Carbapenemase Genes Resistance. *J. Infect Dev. Ctries.* **2019**, *13*, 334–341. [CrossRef] [PubMed]
44. Teban-Man, A.; Farkas, A.; Baricz, A.; Hegedus, A.; Szekeres, E.; Pârvu, M.; Coman, C. Wastewaters, with or without Hospital Contribution, Harbour MDR, Carbapenemase-Producing, but Not Hypervirulent *Klebsiella pneumoniae. Antibiotics* **2021**, *10*, 361. [CrossRef]
45. Gibbon, M.J.; Couto, N.; David, S.; Barden, R.; Standerwick, R.; Jagadeesan, K.; Birkwood, H.; Dulyayangkul, P.; Avison, M.B.; Kannan, A.; et al. A High Prevalence of BlaOXA-48 in *Klebsiella* (Raoultella) Ornithinolytica and Related Species in Hospital Wastewater in South West England. *Microb. Genom.* **2021**, *7*, mgen000509. [CrossRef] [PubMed]
46. Parvez, S.; Khan, A.U. Hospital Sewage Water: A Reservoir for Variants of New Delhi Metallo-β-Lactamase (NDM)- and Extended-Spectrum β-Lactamase (ESBL)-Producing Enterobacteriaceae. *Int. J. Antimicrob. Agents* **2018**, *51*, 82–88. [CrossRef] [PubMed]
47. Haller, L.; Chen, H.; Ng, C.; Le, T.H.; Koh, T.H.; Barkham, T.; Sobsey, M.; Gin, K.Y.-H. Occurrence and Characteristics of Extended-Spectrum β-Lactamase- and Carbapenemase- Producing Bacteria from Hospital Effluents in Singapore. *Sci. Total Env.* **2018**, *615*, 1119–1125. [CrossRef]
48. Mahon, C.; Lehman, D. *Textbook of Diagnostic Microbiology—7th Edition*, 7th ed; Elsevier: Amsterdam, The Netherlands, 2022; ISBN 978-0-323-82997-7.
49. *M100Ed30*; Performance Standards for Antimicrobial Susceptibility Testing, 30rd Edition. Clinical and Laboratory Standards Institute: Wayne, PA, USA, 2020; ISBN 978-1-68440-067-6.
50. Mashwal, F.A.; Safi, S.H.E.; George, S.K.; Adam, A.A.; Jebakumar, A.Z. Incidence and Molecular Characterization of the Extended Spectrum Beta Lactamase-Producing *Escherichia Coli* Isolated from Urinary Tract Infections in Eastern Saudi Arabia. *Saudi Med. J.* **2017**, *38*, 811–815. [CrossRef]
51. Gharrah, M.M.; Mostafa El-Mahdy, A.; Barwa, R.F. Association between Virulence Factors and Extended Spectrum Beta-Lactamase Producing *Klebsiella Pneumoniae* Compared to Nonproducing Isolates. *Interdiscip Perspect Infect Dis.* **2017**, *2017*, 7279830. [CrossRef]
52. Dallenne, C.; Da Costa, A.; Decré, D.; Favier, C.; Arlet, G. Development of a Set of Multiplex PCR Assays for the Detection of Genes Encoding Important β-Lactamases in Enterobacteriaceae. *J. Antimicrob. Chemother.* **2010**, *65*, 490–495. [CrossRef]
53. Nordmann, P.; Poirel, L.; Carrër, A.; Toleman, M.A.; Walsh, T.R. How To Detect NDM-1 Producers. *J. Clin. Microbiol.* **2011**, *49*, 718–721. [CrossRef] [PubMed]

antibiotics MDPI

Article

Comparative Genomics Revealed a Potential Threat of *Aeromonas rivipollensis* G87 Strain and Its Antibiotic Resistance

Esther Ubani K. Fono-Tamo [1], Ilunga Kamika [2], John Barr Dewar [1] and Kgaugelo Edward Lekota [3,*]

1 Department of Life and Consumer Sciences, College of Agriculture and Environmental Sciences, University of South Africa, Florida Campus, Johannesburg 1709, South Africa
2 Institute for Nanotechnology and Water Sustainability (iNanoWS), School of Science, College of Science, Engineering and Technology (CSET), University of South Africa, Florida Campus, Johannesburg 1709, South Africa
3 Unit for Environmental Sciences and Management: Microbiology, North-West University, Potchefstroom Campus, Private Bag X6001, Potchefstroom 2520, South Africa
* Correspondence: 37747959@nwu.ac.za; Tel.: +27-18-299-2381

Abstract: *Aeromonas rivipollensis* is an emerging pathogen linked to a broad range of infections in humans. Due to the inability to accurately differentiate *Aeromonas* species using conventional techniques, in-depth comparative genomics analysis is imperative to identify them. This study characterized 4 *A. rivipollensis* strains that were isolated from river water in Johannesburg, South Africa, by whole-genome sequencing (WGS). WGS was carried out, and taxonomic classification was employed to profile virulence and antibiotic resistance (AR). The AR profiles of the *A. rivipollensis* genomes consisted of betalactams and cephalosporin-resistance genes, while the tetracycline-resistance gene (*tetE*) was only determined to be in the G87 strain. A mobile genetic element (MGE), transposons *TnC*, was determined to be in this strain that mediates tetracycline resistance MFS efflux *tetE*. A pangenomic investigation revealed the G87 strain's unique characteristic, which included immunoglobulin A-binding proteins, extracellular polysialic acid, and exogenous sialic acid as virulence factors. The identified polysialic acid and sialic acid genes can be associated with antiphagocytic and antibactericidal properties, respectively. MGEs such as transposases introduce virulence and AR genes in the *A. rivipollensis* G87 genome. This study showed that *A. rivipollensis* is generally resistant to a class of beta-lactams and cephalosporins. MGEs pose a challenge in some of the *Aeromonas* species strains and are subjected to antibiotics resistance and the acquisition of virulence genes in the ecosystem.

Keywords: *Aeromonas rivipollensis*; whole-genome sequencing; pangenomics; antibiotic resistance; mobile genetic elements

check for updates

Citation: Fono-Tamo, E.U.K.; Kamika, I.; Dewar, J.B.; Lekota, K.E. Comparative Genomics Revealed a Potential Threat of *Aeromonas rivipollensis* G87 Strain and Its Antibiotic Resistance. *Antibiotics* **2023**, *12*, 131. https://doi.org/10.3390/antibiotics12010131

Academic Editor: Norbert Solymosi

Received: 26 November 2022
Revised: 5 January 2023
Accepted: 6 January 2023
Published: 9 January 2023

1. Introduction

Aeromonas species are considered autochthonous to aquatic environments and cause a range of opportunistic infections in humans [1]. They are emerging, opportunistic pathogens that frequently transmit from the environment to humans, causing a wide spectrum of infections [2]. They are characterized as ubiquitous Gram-negative bacilli that consist of a genetic population structure with several characteristics that favor an evolutionary mode of species complexes that are heterogeneous [3]. This group comprises closely related species of distinct strains that are influenced by horizontal gene transfer (HGT) [4].

In previous studies, *Aeromonas* species have been detected in marine, estuarine, and freshwater systems [1,5]. They have also been identified as etiological agents of infections in aquatic animals and humans [6] and are often associated with gastroenteritis and wound infections in humans [7,8]. Several reports linked *Aeromonas* spp. to fish and cold-blooded aquatic animal infections, such as septicaemia, keratitis, open wounds, and ulcers [2,9]. However, in recent times, new potentially pathogenic species such as *A. rivipollensis* have been detected [10]. Marti and Balcázar [11] described *A. rivipollensis* for the first time and classified it as closely related to *A. media* based on the multilocus sequence typing of five housekeeping genes (*gyrA*, *gyrB*, *recA*, *dnaJ*, and *rpoD*). However, it is closely related to both *A. media* and *A. hydrophila* when 16S rRNA phylogenetic analysis is employed. Nevertheless, its genotypic characterization is still incomplete and not fully exploited. A complete genome of *A. rivipollensis* is well described and suggests a zoonotic potential like that of other aeromonads [10].

In most bacterial species, insertion sequences (IS) and transposons (Tn) are examples of mobile genomic elements (MGEs) that promote the spread of antibiotic and virulence genes [12]. The mediation of MGEs often leads to bacterial evolution and also alters phenotypes [13]. This poses a threat, as *Aeromonas* species show a complex heterogeneous strains because they show various metabolic capabilities to adapt to their environmental change, which results in the acquisition of numerous virulence factors [4,14,15]. The *Aeromonas* species comprises a wide range of virulence factors that are involved in biofilm formation, invasion, cell adherence, and cytotoxicity in polar and lateral flagella [16,17], lipopolysaccharides [18], adhesins [19] iron-binding systems [20], and other extracellular toxins and enzymes [21,22].

Although *A. rivipollensis* is considered an emerging species, it is possible that the inability of current conventional identification methods to efficiently differentiate *Aeromonas* species might have masked the reported prevalence as well as the characterization of this organism [5]. The use of mass spectrometry–time of flight (MALDI–TOF MS) and 16S rRNA gene sequencing has proven to be inadequate in differentiating some of the *Aeromonas* species [23]. The reliability of using whole-genome sequencing fully examines the antibiotic resistance and virulence genes, especially in this heterologous species of *Aeromonas* spp. The evolution of this genus also shows limited information about the phylogenomic structure in *A. rivipollensis*, as few genomes are available. The genetic structure of *A. rivipollensis* is unknown, and this species appears to be a heterogeneous phylogenetic cluster that could pose a threat to humans. Thus, studying its genomic features is imperative to understanding its antibiotic resistance and virulence genes. This study sequenced four *A. rivipollensis* genomes to determine the virulence and antibiotic-resistance genes, as well as to define its genetic population structure.

2. Results

2.1. Genome Features of *Aeromonas rivipollensis*

Prior to genomic assessment, isolated strains were identified as *Aeromonas* spp. based on their morphological characteristics on the selective *Aeromonas* isolation agar. The MALDI–TOF method was used to further identify the isolates designated as G36, G42, G78, and G87 strains, which were then determined to be closely related to *A. media*. However, when whole-genome sequencing was employed, the isolates were identified as *A. rivipollensis*. The assembled genomes' quality assessment revealed these isolates had an estimated completeness of more than 99%. The genome sizes (Mb) of the G36, G42, and G78 strains were approximately 4.53, 4.58, and 4.53 Mb, respectively (Table 1). The genome size of the *A. rivipollensis* G87 strain is 4.66 Mb, which is slightly higher than the compared genomes in this study. The protein coding sequences (CDS) of the G36, G42, G78, and G87 genomes consist of 4,239, 4,273, 4,205, and 4,319, respectively. The G + C content of the sequenced *A. rivipollensis* genomes is 61%, identical to *A. rivipollensis* KN-Mc-11N1. The high number of CDSs in *A. rivipollensis* G87 included transposon *Tn7* transposition proteins (*TnsA*, *TnsB*, and *TnsC*), ribosomal protein S12 methylthiotransferase (*RimO*), galactokinase (*GalK*), plastocyanin (*PetE*), copper-resistance protein *CopA*, and cobalt–zinc–cadmium resistance protein *CzcA*. The high number of tRNAs ($n = 98$) was also observed in the *A. rivipollensis* G87 genome.

Table 1. Genome features of the sequenced *A. rivipollensis* strains used in this study compared to KN-Mc-11N1 as a reference strain.

Feature	G36	G42	G78	G87	KN-Mc-11N1 *
Genome size (bp)	4,530,639	4,584,495	4,531,506	4,663,030	4,508,901
CDSs (protein coding sequences)	4,239	4,273	4,205	4,319	4,025
Number of tRNAs	115	109	101	108	124
Number of total rRNAs	5	3	7	4	31
GC%	61,48	61,3	61,48	61,08	61,9
Number of contigs	93	55	57	71	1
N50	94,736	184,598	194,165	160,487	-
Sequence reads archive (SRA) or GenBank	SRR13249124	SRR13249123	SRR13249122	SRR13249121	CP027856.1

* Complete genome of *A. rivipollensis*—Not applicable.

2.2. Taxonomic Classification Using gyrB and Whole-Genome-Based Species Tree

The *gyrB* marker was used to identify the *Aeromonas* spp. isolates investigated in this study (Figure S1). The isolates were identified as *A. rivipollensis* (Figure S1) and grouped with *A. rivipollensis* strain KN-Mc-11N1. The 94-bootstrap value of *A. rivipollensis* distinguishes it from the other *Aeromonas* species. The use of 16S rRNA gene sequencing did not significantly classify the *A. rivipollensis* strains. This species is heterologous since the genus *Aeromonas* contains many phylogroups. Using the whole-genome species tree (Figure 1), it was shown that *Aeromonas* spp. clustered apart from the Enterobactericeae family, which includes *E. coli*, *Salmonella* serovars, and other species. The isolates grouped with previously sequenced genome *A. rivipollensis* KN-Mc-11N1. This demonstrates that the genomes of *A. rivipollensis*, *A. eucroniphilla* strain CECT 4224, *A. salmonicida* subsp. *salmonicida* strain A449, and *A. mulluscorum* strain 848 share some of the core genes.

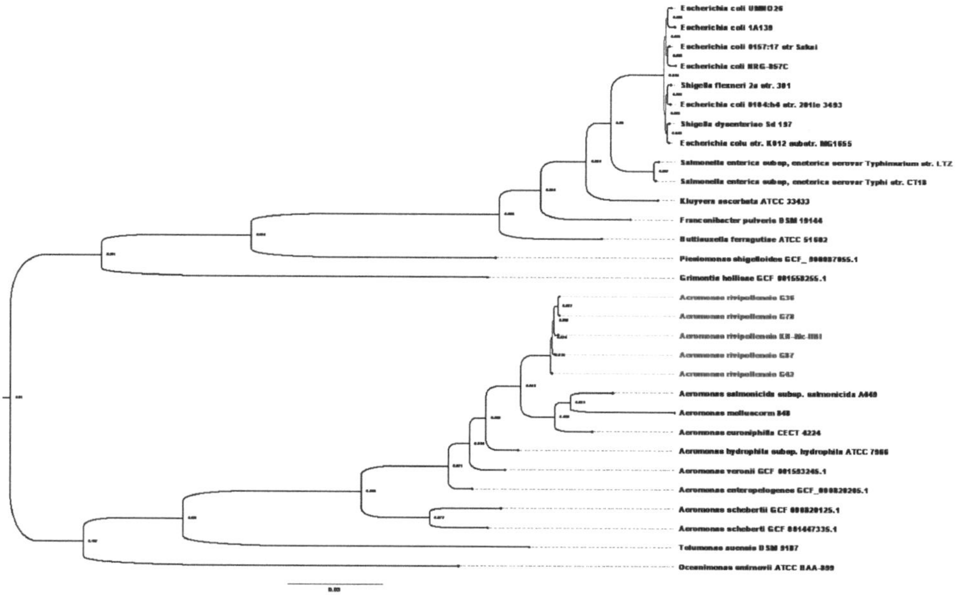

Figure 1. Whole-genome-based species tree showing the clustering of the sequenced *Aeromonas rivipollensis* genomes and KN-Mc-11N1 strain (green annotation) with the closely related genome species of *A. salmonicida* subsp. *salmonicida* A449, *A. molluscorum* 949, and *A. euroniphilla* CECT 4224.

2.3. Pangenome Analysis of the Aeromonas Species

A total of 23,119 genes were examined and defined by the pangenome analysis of the 15 *Aeromonas* spp., with 375 core genes (found in >99% of genomes) shared by the *Aeromonas* species of *rivipollensis, salmonicida, molluscorum,* and *euroniphilla* (Figure 2A). Most genes were identified as accessories and consisted of 8899 and 13,845 shell and cloud genes, respectively. This indicates that *Aeromonas* is a heterogeneous species that consists of many cloud genes (Figure S2). *A. rivipollensis* strains clustered significantly in their own sub-clade (Figure 2 and Figure S2). The different strains of *A. rivipollensis* are shown by their distinctive average nucleotide identity (ANI) profiles identified using accessory genes (Figure 2B). This observation is also an augment as determined by whole-genome species tree. *Aeromonas* species genomes contained core metabolic enzymes, such as amidophosphoribosyltransferase (*purF*), ATP-dependent 6-phosphofructokinase isozyme 1 (*pfka*), nitrogen regulatory protein (*ptsN*), glutamate-pyruvate aminotransferase (*alaA*), UDP-3-O-acyl-N-acetylglucosamine deacetylase (*ipxC*), peptidyl-prolyl cis-trans isomerase B (*ppiB*), maltose transport system permease (*malG*), cysteine desulfurase (*iscS*), dihydrolipoyl dehydrogenase (*ipdA*), UDP-N-acetylglucosamine 1-carboxyvinyltransferase (*murA*), and oligopeptide transport system permease (*oppC*). The accessory binary genes (Figure 2B) found in *A. rivipollensis* strain G87 were biosynthetic genes for polysialic acid, which is responsible for capsulation and is also found in the KN-Mc-11N1 strain.

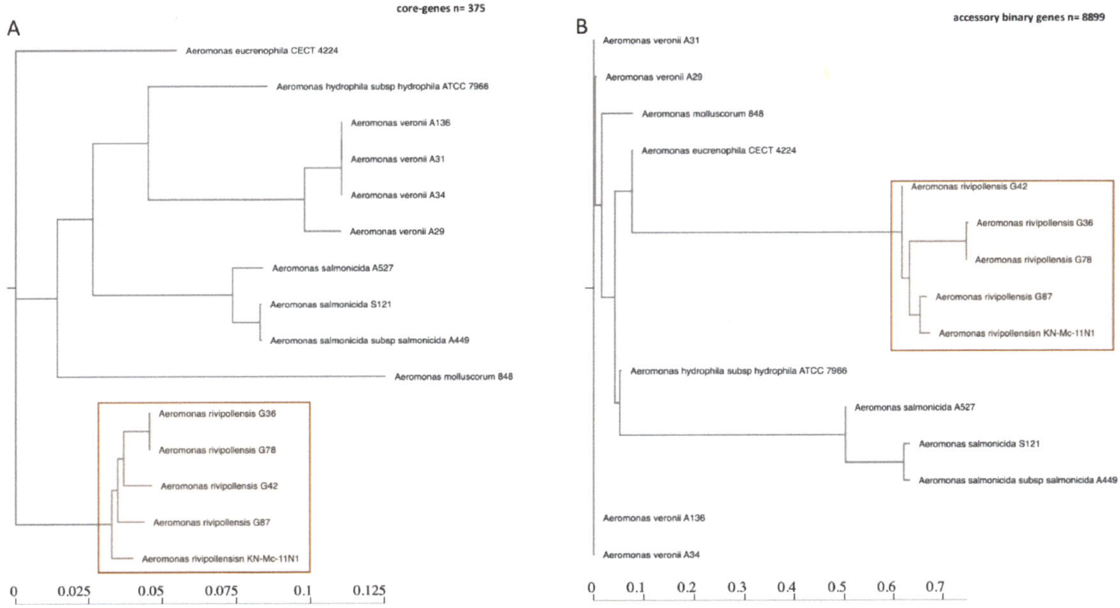

Figure 2. Phylogeny of the compared *Aeromonas* species using 375 core genes (**A**) and 8899 accessory binary genes (**B**). The tree shows phylogenetic tree of the 4 *Aeromonas* species as highlighted with orange color. About 375 core-genes (**A**) and 8899 accessory binary genes (**B**) were used to construct the phylogenetic tree.

The accessory metabolic genes on *A. rivipollensis* strain G87 included genes such as taurine import ATP-binding protein (*tauB*) and taurine-binding periplasmic proteins, cellulose synthase operon protein C (*bcsC*), beta-xylosidase (*xynB*), glucose-6-phosphate isomerase (*pgiA*), unsaturated chondroitin disaccharide hydrolase (*ugi*), p-aminobenzoyl-glutamate transport protein (*abgT*), morphine 6-dehydrogenase (*morA*), beta-glucoside kinase (*bglK*), and aryl-phospho-beta-D-glucosidase (*bglC1* and *bglC2*).

2.4. Polysialic Acid and Sialic Acid Biosynthesis Genes

In the *A. rivipollensis* G87 and KN-Mc11N1 phylogroup, we have identified a polysialic acid operon that consists of kpsM, kpsT, kpsE, kpsD, and KpsFS (Table 2). These are capsular polysaccharide genes that are associated with polysialic acid in the outer membrane. The gene cluster organisation (Figure 3) is also outlined, which shows different kps genes and precursor components (neuABC) for the biosynthesis of extracellular polysialic acid. The kps cluster comprises two different regions, namely: region 1 (kpsDMTE) and region 3 (neuC and kpsFS) (Figure 3). The extracellular kpsDMTE genes and kpsFS are required for the polysaccharide capsule formation in the bacteria (blue and red). The kpsFS genes participate in the translocation of the polysaccharide capsule. Pangenome analysis showed that these genes are absent in the other sequenced *A. rivipollensis* in this study. Genome strain G87 can be separated from the KN-Mc-11N1 strain based on genes responsible for exogenous sialic acid production.

Table 2. Gene annotation of the polysaccharide (polysialic acid) capsular and sialic acid genes involved in biosynthesis present in the genome of *A. rivipollensis* strain G87.

Gene Annotation	Abbreviation	Subsystem Assigned
Capsular polysaccharide export system periplasmic protein	*kpsD*	Capsular polysaccharide (CPS) of *Campylobacter* CPS biosynthesis and assembly
Capsular polysaccharide ABC transporter, permease protein	*kpsM*	Rhamnose containing glycans, CPS of Campylobacter, CPS biosynthesis and assembly
Capsular polysaccharide ABC transporter, ATP-binding protein	*kpsT*	CPS biosynthesis and assembly
Capsular polysaccharide export system inner membrane protein	*kpsE*	CPS of *Campylobacter;* CPS biosynthesis and assembly
COG3563: Capsule polysaccharide export protein	*KpsF*	CPS biosynthesis and assembly
Capsular polysaccharide export system protein	*kpsS*	CPS biosynthesis and assembly
N-Acetylneuraminate cytidylyltransferase (EC 2.7.7.43)	*neuA*	CMP-N-acetylneuraminate_biosynthesis; Sialic acid metabolism
N-acetylneuraminate synthase (EC 2.5.1.56)	*neuB*	CMP-N-acetylneuraminate biosynthesis; Sialic acid metabolism
dTDP-4-dehydrorhamnose 3,5-epimerase (EC 5.1.3.13)	*neuC*	dTDP-rhamnose_synthesis; Rhamnose containing glycans; Capsular_heptose_biosynthesis
Transcriptional regulator NanR	*nanR*	Sialic acid metabolism
N-acetylneuraminate lyase (EC 4.1.3.3)	*nanA2*	Sialic acid metabolism
TRAP-type C4-dicarboxylate transport system, periplasmic component	*nanTp* or *siaM*	TRAP Transporter collection
TRAP-type C4-dicarboxylate transport system, large permease component	*nanTI*	TRAP Transporter collection
Sialidase (EC 3.2.1.18)	*nanH*	Galactosylceramide and sulfatide metabolism; Sialic acid metabolism
N-acetylneuraminate lyase (EC 4.1.3.3)	*nanA1*	Sialic acid metabolism
Sialic acid utilization regulator, RpiRfamily	*nanX*	Sialic acid metabolism
N-acetylmannosamine-6-phosphate 2-epimerase (EC 5.1.3.9)	*nanE*	Sialic acid metabolism
N-acetylmannosamine kinase (EC 2.7.1.60)	*nanK*	Sialic acid metabolism
Predicted sialic acid transporter	*nanP*	Sialic acid metabolism
Putative sugar isomerase involved in processing of exogenous sialic acid	*yhcH*	Sialic acid metabolism

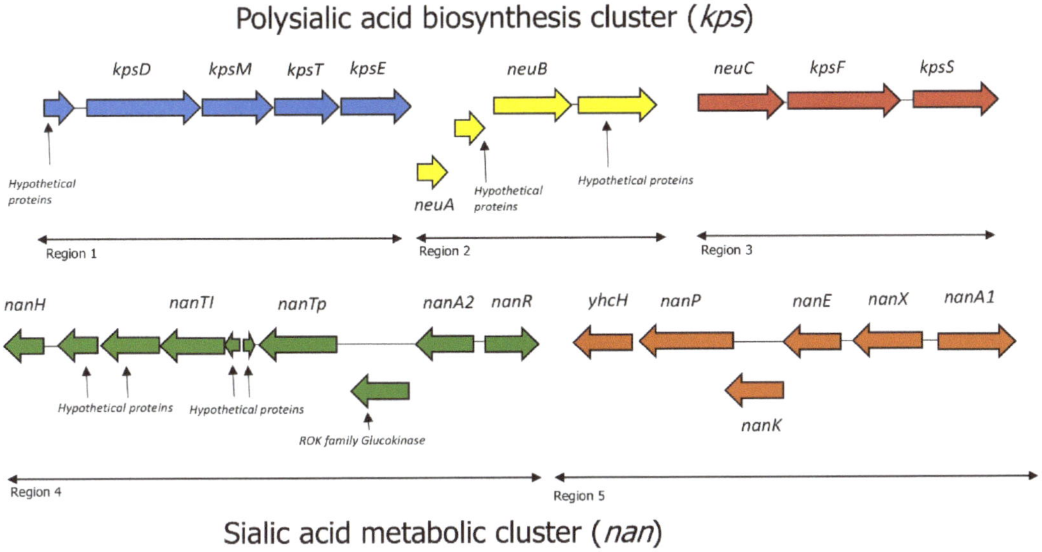

Figure 3. *Aeromonas rivipollensis* strain G87 organization gene clusters for capsular polysialic acids and an exogeneous sialic acid metabolic cluster. The *kpsDMTE* and *kpsFS* genes are required for capsulation (region 1, blue, and region 3, red). The *kpsFS* genes participate in the translocation of the polysaccharide. The precursors of polysialic acid biosynthesis are *neuABC* (region 2, yellow, and region 3, red). The *nanARH* with TRAP transporters in region 4, and *nanTp-TI* genes (green) are responsible for exogenous sialic acid, while the *nanAXEKP* and *yhcH* genes (orange) are responsible for the degradation or catabolism of salic acid.

A. rivipollensis strain G87 was the only genome with an exogenous sialic acid metabolism. This was further confirmed by the RAST annotation server, which assigned the subsystem a score of 2.0. The metabolic cluster for sialic acid is composed of different nan-genes (Figure 3). The annotation names for the polysialic acid biosynthesis cluster (kps) and sialic acid metabolic cluster were assigned to the *A. rivipollensis* strain G87 (Table 2). The nanARH and TRAP transporters (nanTp-TI) (green) are responsible for exogenous sialic acid, while the nanAXEKP and yhcH genes (orange) are responsible for the degradation or catabolism of salic acid.

2.5. Antibiotics and Virulence Genes of Aeromonas rivipollensis Genomes

In this study, several core-virulence genes ($n = 7$) from the sequenced *Aeromonas rivipollensis* were identified (Figure 4). The chemoreceptor tsr gene, flagellar biosynthesis proteins *fliACN*, and twitching motility proteins *pilBJT* were among them. The antibiotic resistance genes shared by the *A. rivipollensis* genomes included cephalosporins (*ampH*) and beta-lactams (*blaCMY*) genes. Tetracycline resistance (*tetE*) gene was the unique antibiotic-resistance gene present in the *A. rivipollensis* G87 genome.

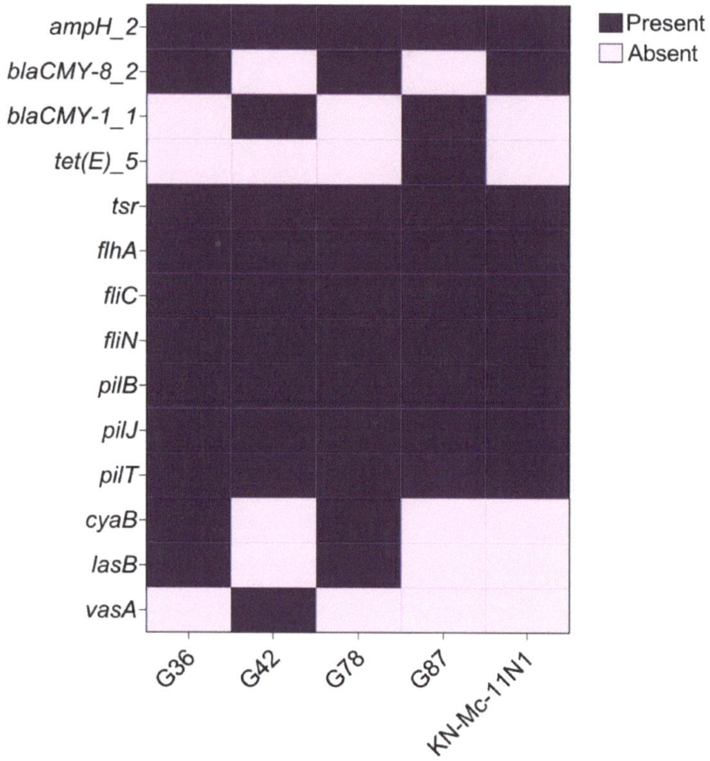

Figure 4. Heat map showing the antibiotic resistance and virulence genes detected among the 4 sequenced and the compared *A. rivipollensis* strain KN-Mc-11N1.

2.6. Mobile Genetic Elements

In this G87 strain containing the transposition protein TnsC, a tetracycline-resistance MFS efflux pump known as tetE and a tetracycline-resistance regulatory protein tetR were discovered (Figure S3). The transposition protein TnsC had a BLAST nucleotide homology of 98.70% with *A. veronii* strain wp8-s18-ESNL-11. The hypothetical proteins identified in this gene cluster also had a 100% nucleotide identity with *A. veronii* strain wp8-s18-ESNL-11. In the upstream region in this operon, a Type I restriction–modification system specific subunit S and DNA–methyltransferase subunit-M were determined to influence genomic evolution by horizontal gene transfer. A transposase, InsH for insertion sequence element IS5, was also determined to be in *A. rivipollensis* strain G87. In the downstream part of the gene arrangement cluster, this InsH transposase also features a secretory immunoglobulin A-binding protein (esiB1) of 726 bp (242 aa). The second esiB2 gene of about 1656 bp (522 aa) was also found lying downstream with other mobile genetic elements. The IS3 family transposase ISAs7 (618 bp) was also found that had a BLASTn of 98.54% and 98.22% with A. media strain T0.1-19 and *A. rivipollensis* strain KN-Mc-11N1, respectively. Other MGEs identified were two transposon Tn3 resolvase proteins (tnpR1 and tnpR2) and Tn7 found in the G87 strain.

3. Materials and Methods

3.1. Sample Isolation and Classical Microbiological Tests

We collected water samples from the Jukskei River continuum in Johannesburg (25.948156 S, 27.957528 E) in 2018. Water samples were aseptically collected in duplicates of approximately 1 L in a sterile container. Water samples were immediately placed in a cooler box at 4 °C and transported to the laboratory for further analysis. For bacterial isolation, 100 mL of the sample was filtered through a nitrocellulose filter membrane (0.22 µm), and the filters were then placed on *Aeromonas* isolation agar (Merck, Millipore) and incubated at 37 °C for 24 h. Four distinct isolates were coded as G36, G42, G78, and G87 and were presumptive *Aeromonas* species. The presumptive isolates were further identified using matrix-assisted laser desorption ionization–time-of-flight mass spectrometry (MALDI–TOF) (Bruker, Bremen, Germany). Briefly, a single colony was transferred into an Eppendorf tube containing 300 µL of sterile distilled water and 900 µL of absolute ethanol, mixed thoroughly, and later centrifuged for 2 min at 13,000 rpm. The supernatant was discarded, and the Eppendorf tube was later filled with 5 µL of 70% formic acid and thoroughly mixed.

3.2. DNA Extractions

The genomic DNA of the *Aeromonas* species strains was extracted using the High Pure PC Template preparation kit (Roche, Germany). The DNA was quantified on qubit fluorometric quantization using the Broad Range assay kit (Invitrogen™). The quality of the DNA was analyzed by electrophoresis on a 0.8% agarose gel using ethidium bromide and visualized under UV-light.

3.3. Whole-Genome Sequencing, Quality Control and Assembly

The sequencing libraries of the *Aeromonas* isolates ($n = 4$) were generated using the NEBNext® Ultra™ II FS DNA library prep kit (New England Biolabs). The 150 bp paired-end sequence reads were generated with the Illumina MiSeq sequencer (Illumina, USA). FastQC v. 0.11.52 (http://www.bioinformatics.babraham.ac.uk/projects/fastqc (accessed on 6 February 2022)) was used to assess the quality of the paired-end reads associated with each isolate. Sequence coverage of the genomes of *Aeromonas* isolates G36, G42, G78, and G87 was 39X, 144X, 54, and 294X, respectively. Trimmomatic v. 0.33 [24] was used to remove the sequenced adapters and the leading and trailing ambiguous bases. The trimming parameters included LEADING:3 and TRAILING:3; reads with average per-base quality scores of <15 within a 4 bp sliding window. The SLIDINGWINDOW:4:15; reads with length < 36 bp were removed. Trimmed reads were de novo assembled using the CLC Genomics Workbench v. 11.01 (Qiagen). QUAST v. 4.5 [25] was used to assess the quality of the associated assembled genome using default parameters. CheckM [26] was additionally used to assess the potential contaminants in each assembled genome of *Aeromonas* isolates using default parameters. BLASTn [27] was used to align the assembled contigs using *A. rivipollensis* KN-Mc-11N1 [10] as a reference. For consistency and the removal of contaminants, multiple genome alignments were constructed using the progressive MAUVE tool [28]. The feature prediction and annotation of the sequenced genomes were performed using the NCBI prokaryotic Genome Annotation pipeline (PGAP) [29] and rapid annotation RAST [30].

3.4. Phylogenetic Analysis Using gyraseB and Whole-Genome Species Tree

The gyraseB (*gryB*) gene sequences were extracted from the assembled genomes of the *A. rivipollensis* strains. The nucleotide sequence queries of the *Aeromonas* isolates were BLAST-searched and compared with the available sequences of *Aeromonas* species in NCBI (http://www.ncbi.nlm.nih.gov (accessed on 25 April 2022)). This enabled the evaluation of homologous hits to the NCBI's available sequences. Multiple sequence alignments of the extracted gene sequence and mined NCBI sequences were performed using MAFFT [31]. Maximum likelihood phylogenetic analysis of *A. rivipollensis* was performed using 1000 bootstrap iterations in MEGA 11.0 [32]. Utilizing K-base's species tree (https://www.kbase.us/ (accessed on 12 March 2022)), the in silico taxonomic classification of all four sequenced genomes was performed. The assembled genomes were compared to other genomes that were accessible in the NCBI database. The whole-genome phylogenetic tree was visualized using Figtree v1.16.6 (http://tree.bio.ed.ac.uk/software/figtree/ (accessed on 25 March 2022)).

3.5. Pangenomics Analysis

The inclusion of the *Aeromonas* spp. genomes (n = 11) was based on the species tree generated from whole-genome-based taxonomic classification. This study included the *A. veronii* and *A. hydrophilla* genomes based on their completeness status. *A. veronni* genomes included the South African strains isolated from human cases, and none were found from the environment. In total, about 15 *Aeromonas* spp. genomes were used for comparative genomic analysis that includes the 4 sequenced *A. rivipollensis*. Prokka v.1.14.0 [33] was used to annotate the genomes of *Aeromonas* species using the default parameters. The pan-genome composition was extracted using Roary [34]. Pan-genome clusters were defined as follows: Core-genes were present in all isolates; soft core-genes present in at least 95% of isolates; shell-genes were present between 15% and 95% of isolates; cloud-genes were present in less than 15% of isolates. IQ-TREE v.2 [35] was used to construct the phylogenetic tree of the aligned core-genes using default parameters. The core genome phylogenetic tree was visualized using the Newick tree display [36]. Additionally, phandango v1.3.0 (https://jameshadfield.github.io/phandango/#/ (accessed on 25 April 2022)) was used for the interactive visualization of the genome phylogeny.

3.6. Antibiotics Resistance, Plasmid Replicon, Mobile Genetic Elements, and Virulence Factor Determinants

Antibiotic-resistance genes were identified in four sequenced *Aeromonas* genome sequences and the reference strain. In the ABRicate pipeline, AMR determinants were identified in each assembled genome using the ResFinder database (–db ResFinder; accessed 23 April 2022) [37], which has minimum identity and coverage thresholds of 75 (–minid 75) and 50% (–mincov 50), respectively. Plasmid replicons were identified on the sequenced genomes using the PlasmidFinder database [38]. Resistance genes were determined using the Virulence Factor Database (VFDB; –db vfdb, accessed 19 April 2022) [39], using minimum identity and coverage thresholds of 70 (–minid 70) and 50% (–mincov 50), respectively. OriTfinder v1.1 [40] was also used to predict the virulence factors and acquired antibiotic resistance genes. Mobile genetic elements (MGEs) were investigated on the sequenced genomes of *Aeromonas* spp. using this tool as well as default parameters. The heatmap of the antibiotics resistance and virulence genes was generated using GraphPad Prism9.

4. Discussion

The identification of *Aeromonas* spp. isolates to the species level remains a challenge using classic microbiological tests. Without a suitably comprehensive database, methods that are most frequently used, like MALDI–TOF, may misidentify samples [23]. However, this study used a high-resolution whole-genome and pangenomics analysis to confirm and identify *A. rivipollensis* genomes. This study showed that *A. rivipollensis* seems to be an emerging pathogen that has not yet been thoroughly characterized. The observation of accessory genes that included polysialic acid and sialic acid, mobile genetic elements, and an antibiotic-resistance profile, especially in the genome of G87, elucidate a unique genetic cluster of *A. rivipollensis*.

The use of *gyrB* was used in this study to fairly classify and identify *A. rivipollensis*. The sequenced *Aeromonas* species could only be correctly identified as *A. rivipollensis* using the high-resolution method of WGS and whole-genome species tree. These isolates were identified as *A. media* using MALDI-TOF. They were grouped with *A. rivipollensis* KN-Mc-11N1 using the WGS species tree (Figure 1), and pangenome analysis. Their genomes are quite closely related to those of *A. eucroniphilla* strain CECT 4224, *A. salmonicida* subsp. *salmonicida* strain A449, and *A. mulluscorum* strain 848. The pangenomic examination of this study's species revealed that the genus *Aeromonas* is diverse when compared to other species, since only a small number (n = 375) of core genes could be identified. Distinct clusters are also observed among *A. rivopollensis* genomes. The genomes of KN-Mc-11N1 and G87, which share several core genes, make up one of the clusters. This cluster contained the polysialic acid (PGA) (*kpsDMTE*) genes responsible for exogenous capsulation, whereas sialic acid was only found in G87, which is associated with virulence and adaptation in the environment [41].

The primary strains for polysialic acid (PSA) biosynthesis and metabolism were A. rivipollensis G87 and KN-Mc-11N1. Many other bacteria, such as *Mannheimia hemolytica* (previously *Pasteurella haemolytica*) [42] and *E. coli* [43,44], have been associated with the production of PSA as their extracellular capsules. In bacteria, the PSA acts as a virulence factor that mimics the mammalian PSA's structure and as an antiphagocytic [45]. The *kps* gene cluster that is involved in the PSA biosynthesis, modification, and transport of the bacteria's PSA chains is outlined in this study for *A. rivipollensis* (Figure 3). The *kps* cluster comprises of two different regions, namely; region 1 (*kpsDMTE*) and region 3 (*neuC* and *kpsFS*), which participate in the translocation of the polysaccharide across the periplasmic space and onto the cell surface [44,46]. PSA metabolism is regulated at a transcriptional level by the transcriptional activator *rfaH* [47]. In *E. coli* K92, *rfaH* enhanced *kps* expression for the synthesis of the polysialic acid capsule [43]. This gene was also present in the genome of *A. rivipollensis* G87 at the downstream end of the operon. The polysialic acid capsule is transported across the outer membrane to the cell surface by the KpsD protein. It functions as the periplasmic binding element of the PSA transport system, in which it transiently interacts with the membrane component of the transporter, binds polysaccharide, and transports the polymer to a component in the outer membrane. This is also observed in bacteria containing poly-gamma-glutamate transpeptidase, responsible for capsulation [48]. Other components reported included the *kpsT* and *kpsM* genes, which are ABC transporters that export PSA from the cytoplasm. These transporters also require *kpsE*, a polysaccharide export system located in the inner membrane protein [46]. However, the mechanism of expressing the polysialic is not well understood and characterized in *A. rivipollensis*, as this is the first report in this phylogroup of G87 and KN-Mc-11N1 genomes that needs further investigation.

A complete nan system was outlined as including at least one ortholog of each of the genes encoding *nanA*, *nanE*, and *nanK*, more especially in the *E. coli* model [49]. These genes were absent from the other sequenced and compared genomes in this study but were present in the *A. rivipollensis* strain G87 genome. This was discovered in the annotation subsystem and was confirmed as an exogenous sialic acid based on the genetic variant code 2.0 assigned to it. Sialic acid is biosynthesized, activated, and polymerized by proteins NeuABCD [50], which are present in the G87 genome with the exception of the *neuD* gene. The *neuD* is a gene found in organisms that can synthesize sialic acid [51].

It is well recognized that the precursor to PSA is the gene for N-acetylneuraminate (Neu5Ac aldolase or *neuC* gene). By mimicking sialic acid, some pathogenic bacteria can circumvent host defenses. The *neuC* is located upstream with other *kpsFS* genes, which is involved in the production of capsular heptose. Exogenous sialic acid nan operon *nanRAHTpTI* (region 4) and degradation nan operon *nanAXEKP-YhcH* (region 5) were assigned in Figure 3. De novo synthetic genes of the sialic acid *neuABC* (region 2/3) were identified in this operon. However, according to the annotation genetic variation code, the G87 strain displayed a non-synthetic sialic acid. Therefore, organisms that can catabolize but not synthesize salic acids are classified as exogenous sialic acids. The sialic acid operon contained the two tripartite ATP-independent periplasmic (TRAP) transporters, *nanTp and nanTI*, respectively. The *nanTp* is a major permease component of the TRAP-type C4-dicarboxylate transport system (Figure 3). The TRAPs are well studied as the key transporters involved in the uptake of sialic acid and are associated with roles in pathogenicity [52,53]. A second N-acetylneuraminate lyase (*nanA2*) was identified in the upstream with transcriptional regulator *nanR*, which controls the expression of proteins involved in sialic acid absorption and metabolism [54,55]. Other salic acid genes that were not well characterized in this study might also be suggested by the region 2 putative proteins. It has now been established beyond doubt that microbial sialic acid metabolism contributes to the pathogenicity of a variety of infectious illnesses. Many vertebrate cells' surfaces include glycan molecules with sialic acid occupying the terminal position. Sialic acid engages in a number of biological processes, such as cell signaling and intercellular adhesion [56]. Pathogenic bacteria that coat themselves with sialic acid, such as Group B *Streptococcus*, offer resistance to components of the host's innate immune response. These bacteria have evolved to utilize this substance to their advantage [41,57]. Two secretory immunoglobulin A-binding proteins EsiB (esiB1) and EsiB2 found in the G87 genome were among the other virulence factors discovered in this study. They have different sequence lengths, with *esiB1* being 726 bp (242 aa) and *esiB2* being 1656 bp (522 aa), respectively. Pathogenic strains are primarily composed of the *esiB* genes, which are known to impair neutrophil activation [58].

Aeromonas species are generally resistant to betalactams (*blaCMY*), and this was also observed in this study. The presence of *blaCMY* and *ampH* genes in all isolated *A. rivipollensis* was not a surprise, as they have been recorded in several bacteria isolates including *Aeromonas* species [59,60]. In addition, the genome of isolate G87 was only one of the sequenced *A. rivipollensis* in this study that showed a multidrug tetracycline-resistance gene. This AR gene was found in this genome because it was linked to a mobile genetic element, *TnC*, with a nucleotide percentage identity similar to that of *A. veronii*. However, tetracycline resistance has previously been reported in *A. veronii* strain MS-17-88 recovered from channel catfish [12,61]. It has also been reported from *Aeromonas* species isolated from South African aquatic environments [62].

Flagellar biosynthesis proteins FliACN and twitching motility proteins PilBJT (Type IV pilus) were found in all *A. rivipollensis* strains sequenced in our study. These genes are commonly found in *Aeromonas* species that are associated with pathogenicity for colonization [63]. The chemoreceptor *tsr* gene was also present in the sequenced *A. rivipollensis* strains. In the study, Oh et al. [64] also detected this gene in *E. coli*. This has also been confirmed in other studies, indicating that *E. coli* and *S. enterica* serovar *Typhimurium* genomes possess many chemoreceptor genes, *tsr* [65]. Many chemoreceptor genes have also been reported in many other microorganisms [65,66]. However, no study has reported the presence of the *tsr* gene in *A. rivipollensis*.

5. Conclusions

Using WGS analysis, we were able to determine the resistome of *Aeromonas rivipollensis*. All *A. rivipollensis* strains show potential resistance to various antibiotic lactamase classes, indicating that these aeromonads are potentially virulent emerging pathogens that can be transmitted by river water. The determined polysialic acid and sialic acid genes in the G87 genome can be associated with antiphagocytic and anti-bactericidal properties, respectively. Mobile genetic elements, such as transposases, introduce virulence and resistance genes, such as secretory immunoglobulin A-binding proteins and multidrug tetracycline genes in the *A. rivipollensis* G87 genome. These genomes will be used as a resource for additional research that may reveal new information on the genes responsible for accurate identification, pathogenic potential, and the relative health risks posed by environmental strains of *A. rivipollensis*.

Supplementary Materials: The following supporting information can be downloaded at: https://www.mdpi.com/article/10.3390/antibiotics12010131/s1, Figure S1: Phylogenetic analysis of the *Aeromonas* species isolates using the *gyrB*. The 4 sequenced *A. rivipollensis* are highlighted in blue as well as the reference strain KN-Mc-11-N1. Bootstrap value of 1000 was used to construct the tree. Figure S2: Pangenome genome of the 15 *Aeromonas* spp. isolates showing the core, shell and cloud genes. A total of 23,119 CDS genes was used to construct the pangenome phylogenetic tree generated using Phandango. The colour coded blue represents compared coding genes amongst the genomes. Figure S3: Gene organization of tetracycline resistance genes (yellow) with transposase *ISAs31* and transposition protein *TnsC* (brown) as well as Type 1 restriction recognition sites subunits (orange) that drives horizontal gene transfer determined in *A. rivipollensis* G87 genome. The CDS were annotated using prokka and visualized on Geneious version 9.0.5.

Author Contributions: Conceptualization, I.K., K.E.L. and J.B.D.; data curation, E.U.K.F.-T. and K.E.L.; formal analysis, K.E.L.; funding acquisition, K.E.L. and J.B.D.; investigation, E.U.K.F.-T., I.K. and K.E.L.; methodology, E.U.K.F.-T.; project administration, J.B.D.; resources, K.E.L. and J.B.D.; bioinformatics analysis, K.E.L.; supervision, I.K. and J.B.D.; validation, I.K. and K.E.L.; visualization, K.E.L.; writing—original draft, E.U.K.F.-T.; writing—review and editing, I.K., K.E.L. and J.B.D. All authors have read and agreed to the published version of the manuscript.

Funding: This research was funded by National Research Foundation (NRF) grant number "TTK200306508304" made available to KEL and supported by University of South Africa (UNISA).

Institutional Review Board Statement: The study was conducted according to the guidelines of the Declaration of Helsinki and approved by the Ethics Committee of the University of South Africa (Ref. no. 2018/CAES/048).

Informed Consent Statement: Not applicable.

Data Availability Statement: *A. rivipollensis* G36, G42, G78, and G87 genome sequences were deposited in NCBI GenBank under the accession numbers JAAILC0000000001, GCA_010974915.1, GCA_010974825.1, and JAAIKZ000000000, respectively. The sequence read achieve (SRA) accession numbers are assigned as G87 (SRR13249121), G78 (SRR13249122), G42 (SRR13249123), or (G36 (SRR13249124).

Conflicts of Interest: The authors declare no conflict of interest.

References

1. Khor, W.C.; Puah, S.M.; Tan, J.A.; Puthucheary, S.D.; Chua, K.H. Phenotypic and Genetic Diversity of Aeromonas Species Isolated from Fresh Water Lakes in Malaysia. *PLoS ONE* **2015**, *10*, e0145933. [CrossRef] [PubMed]
2. Li, T.; Raza, S.H.A.; Yang, B.; Sun, Y.; Wang, G.; Sun, W.; Qian, A.; Wang, C.; Kang, Y.; Shan, X. Aeromonas veronii Infection in Commercial Freshwater Fish: A Potential Threat to Public Health. *Animals* **2020**, *10*, 608. [CrossRef] [PubMed]
3. Vasquez, I.; Hossain, A.; Gnanagobal, H.; Valderrama, K.; Campbell, B.; Ness, M.; Charette, S.J.; Gamperl, A.K.; Cipriano, R.; Segovia, C.; et al. Comparative Genomics of Typical and Atypical Aeromonas salmonicida Complete Genomes Revealed New Insights into Pathogenesis Evolution. *Microorganisms* **2022**, *10*, 189. [CrossRef] [PubMed]
4. Talagrand-Reboul, E.; Colston, S.M.; Graf, J.; Lamy, B.; Jumas-Bilak, E. Comparative and Evolutionary Genomics of Isolates Provide Insight into the Pathoadaptation of *Aeromonas*. *Genome Biol. Evol.* **2020**, *12*, 535–552. [CrossRef] [PubMed]
5. Chaix, G.; Roger, F.; Berthe, T.; Lamy, B.; Jumas-Bilak, E.; Lafite, R.; Forget-Leray, J.; Petit, F. Distinct *Aeromonas* Populations in Water Column and Associated with Copepods from Estuarine Environment (Seine, France). *Front. Microbiol.* **2017**, *8*, 1259. [CrossRef] [PubMed]
6. Puthucheary, S.D.; Puah, S.M.; Chua, K.H. Molecular characterization of clinical isolates of *Aeromonas* species from Malaysia. *PLoS ONE* **2012**, *7*, e30205. [CrossRef]
7. Villari, P.; Crispino, M.; Montuori, P.; Boccia, S. Molecular typing of *Aeromonas* isolates in natural mineral waters. *Appl. Environ. Microbiol.* **2003**, *69*, 697–701. [CrossRef]
8. Rutteman, B.; Borremans, K.; Beckers, J.; Devleeschouwer, E.; Lampmann, S.; Corthouts, I.; Verlinde, P. *Aeromonas* wound infection in a healthy boy, and wound healing with polarized light. *JMM Case Rep.* **2017**, *4*, e005118. [CrossRef]
9. Yang, W.; Li, N.; Li, M.; Zhang, D.; An, G. Complete Genome Sequence of Fish Pathogen *Aeromonas hydrophila* JBN2301. *Genome Announc.* **2016**, *4*, e01615-15. [CrossRef]
10. Park, S.Y.; Lim, S.R.; Son, J.S.; Kim, H.K.; Yoon, S.W.; Jeong, D.G.; Lee, M.S.; Lee, J.R.; Lee, D.H.; Kim, J.H. Complete Genome Sequence of Aeromonas rivipollensis KN-Mc-11N1, Isolated from a Wild Nutria (*Myocastor coypus*) in South Korea. *Microbiol. Resour. Announc.* **2018**, *7*, e00907-18. [CrossRef]
11. Marti, E.; Balcazar, J.L. Aeromonas rivipollensis sp. nov., a novel species isolated from aquatic samples. *J. Basic Microbiol.* **2015**, *55*, 1435–1439. [CrossRef] [PubMed]
12. Tekedar, H.C.; Kumru, S.; Blom, J.; Perkins, A.D.; Griffin, M.J.; Abdelhamed, H.; Karsi, A.; Lawrence, M.L. Comparative genomics of Aeromonas veronii: Identification of a pathotype impacting aquaculture globally. *PLoS ONE* **2019**, *14*, e0221018. [CrossRef] [PubMed]
13. Carr, V.R.; Witherden, E.A.; Lee, S.; Shoaie, S.; Mullany, P.; Proctor, G.B.; Gomez-Cabrero, D.; Moyes, D.L. Abundance and diversity of resistomes differ between healthy human oral cavities and gut. *Nat. Commun.* **2020**, *11*, 693. [CrossRef]
14. Seshadri, R.; Joseph, S.W.; Chopra, A.K.; Sha, J.; Shaw, J.; Graf, J.; Haft, D.; Wu, M.; Ren, Q.; Rosovitz, M.J.; et al. Genome sequence of *Aeromonas hydrophila* ATCC 7966T: Jack of all trades. *J. Bacteriol.* **2006**, *188*, 8272–8282. [CrossRef]
15. Talagrand-Reboul, E.; Jumas-Bilak, E.; Lamy, B. The Social Life of *Aeromonas* through Biofilm and Quorum Sensing Systems. *Front. Microbiol.* **2017**, *8*, 37. [CrossRef] [PubMed]

16. Rabaan, A.A.; Gryllos, I.; Tomas, J.M.; Shaw, J.G. Motility and the polar flagellum are required for *Aeromonas caviae* adherence to HEp-2 cells. *Infect. Immun.* **2001**, *69*, 4257–4267. [CrossRef]
17. Gavin, R.; Merino, S.; Altarriba, M.; Canals, R.; Shaw, J.G.; Tomas, J.M. Lateral flagella are required for increased cell adherence, invasion and biofilm formation by *Aeromonas* spp. *FEMS Microbiol. Lett.* **2003**, *224*, 77–83. [CrossRef]
18. Canals, R.; Jimenez, N.; Vilches, S.; Regue, M.; Merino, S.; Tomas, J.M. Role of Gne and GalE in the virulence of *Aeromonas hydrophila* serotype O34. *J. Bacteriol.* **2007**, *189*, 540–550. [CrossRef]
19. Kirov, S.M.; O'Donovan, L.A.; Sanderson, K. Functional characterization of type IV pili expressed on diarrhea-associated isolates of *Aeromonas* species. *Infect. Immun.* **1999**, *67*, 5447–5454. [CrossRef]
20. Massad, G.; Arceneaux, J.E.; Byers, B.R. Acquisition of iron from host sources by mesophilic *Aeromonas* species. *J. Gen. Microbiol.* **1991**, *137*, 237–241. [CrossRef]
21. Burr, S.E.; Stuber, K.; Wahli, T.; Frey, J. Evidence for a type III secretion system in *Aeromonas salmonicida* subsp. salmonicida. *J. Bacteriol.* **2002**, *184*, 5966–5970. [CrossRef] [PubMed]
22. Sha, J.; Pillai, L.; Fadl, A.A.; Galindo, C.L.; Erova, T.E.; Chopra, A.K. The type III secretion system and cytotoxic enterotoxin alter the virulence of *Aeromonas hydrophila*. *Infect. Immun.* **2005**, *73*, 6446–6457. [CrossRef] [PubMed]
23. Shin, H.B.; Yoon, J.; Lee, Y.; Kim, M.S.; Lee, K. Comparison of MALDI-TOF MS, housekeeping gene sequencing, and 16S rRNA gene sequencing for identification of *Aeromonas* clinical isolates. *Yonsei. Med. J.* **2015**, *56*, 550–555. [CrossRef] [PubMed]
24. Bolger, A.M.; Lohse, M.; Usadel, B. Trimmomatic: A flexible trimmer for Illumina sequence data. *Bioinformatics* **2014**, *30*, 2114–2120. [CrossRef]
25. Gurevich, A.; Saveliev, V.; Vyahhi, N.; Tesler, G. QUAST: Quality assessment tool for genome assemblies. *Bioinformatics* **2013**, *29*, 1072–1075. [CrossRef]
26. Parks, D.H.; Imelfort, M.; Skennerton, C.T.; Hugenholtz, P.; Tyson, G.W. CheckM: Assessing the quality of microbial genomes recovered from isolates, single cells, and metagenomes. *Gen. Res.* **2015**, *25*, 1043–1055. [CrossRef]
27. Altschul, S. Hot papers-Bioinformatics-Gapped BLAST and PSI-BLAST: A new generation of protein database search programs by S.F. Altschul, T.L. Madden, A.A. Schaffer, J.H. Zhang, Z. Zhang, W. Miller, D.J. Lipman-Comments. *Scientist* **1999**, *13*, 15.
28. Darling, A.C.E.; Mau, B.; Blattner, F.R.; Perna, N.T. Mauve: Multiple alignment of conserved genomic sequence with rearrangements. *Gen. Res.* **2004**, *14*, 1394–1403. [CrossRef]
29. Haft, D.H.; DiCuccio, M.; Badretdin, A.; Brover, V.; Chetvernin, V.; O'Neill, K.; Li, W.; Chitsaz, F.; Derbyshire, M.K.; Gonzales, N.R.; et al. RefSeq: An update on prokaryotic genome annotation and curation. *Nucleic Acids Res* **2018**, *46*, D851–D860. [CrossRef]
30. Aziz, R.K.; Bartels, D.; Best, A.A.; DeJongh, M.; Disz, T.; Edwards, R.A.; Formsma, K.; Gerdes, S.; Glass, E.M.; Kubal, M.; et al. The RAST server: Rapid annotations using subsystems technology. *BMC Gen.* **2008**, *9*, 75. [CrossRef]
31. Katoh, K.; Rozewicki, J.; Yamada, K.D. MAFFT online service: Multiple sequence alignment, interactive sequence choice and visualization. *Brief. Bioinform.* **2019**, *20*, 1160–1166. [CrossRef]
32. Tamura, K.; Stecher, G.; Kumar, S. MEGA11 Molecular Evolutionary Genetics Analysis Version 11. *Mol. Biol. Evol.* **2021**, *38*, 3022–3027. [CrossRef]
33. Seemann, M. *Das neue Spiel: Strategien fur die Welt nach dem digitalen Kontrollverlust;* Orange-Press: Freiburg, Germany, 2014; p. 255.
34. Page, A.J.; Cummins, C.A.; Hunt, M.; Wong, V.K.; Reuter, S.; Holden, M.T.G.; Fookes, M.; Falush, D.; Keane, J.A.; Parkhill, J. Roary: Rapid large-scale prokaryote pan genome analysis. *Bioinformatics* **2015**, *31*, 3691–3693. [CrossRef]
35. Minh, B.Q.; Schmidt, H.A.; Chernomor, O.; Schrempf, D.; Woodhams, M.D.; von Haeseler, A.; Lanfear, R. IQ-TREE 2: New Models and Efficient Methods for Phylogenetic Inference in the Genomic Era. *Mol. Biol. Evol.* **2020**, *37*, 2461. [CrossRef]
36. Junier, T.; Zdobnov, E.M. The Newick utilities: High-throughput phylogenetic tree processing in the UNIX shell. *Bioinformatics* **2010**, *26*, 1669–1670. [CrossRef]
37. Feldgarden, M.; Brover, V.; Haft, D.H.; Prasad, A.B.; Slotta, D.J.; Tolstoy, I.; Tyson, G.H.; Zhao, S.; Hsu, C.H.; McDermott, P.F.; et al. Validating the AMRFinder Tool and Resistance Gene Database by Using Antimicrobial Resistance Genotype-Phenotype Correlations in a Collection of Isolates. *Antimicrob. Agents Chemother.* **2019**, *63*, e00483-19. [CrossRef]
38. Carattoli, A.; Zankari, E.; Garcia-Fernandez, A.; Larsen, M.V.; Lund, O.; Villa, L.; Aarestrup, F.M.; Hasman, H. In Silico Detection and Typing of Plasmids using PlasmidFinder and Plasmid Multilocus Sequence Typing. *Antimicrob. Agents Chemother.* **2014**, *58*, 3895–3903. [CrossRef]
39. Liu, B.; Zheng, D.D.; Zhou, S.Y.; Chen, L.H.; Yang, J. VFDB 2022: A general classification scheme for bacterial virulence factors. *Nucleic Acids Res.* **2022**, *50*, D912–D917. [CrossRef]
40. Li, X.B.; Xie, Y.Z.; Liu, M.; Tai, C.; Sung, J.Y.; Deng, Z.X.; Ou, H.Y. oriTfinder: A web-based tool for the identification of origin of transfers in DNA sequences of bacterial mobile genetic elements. *Nucleic Acids Res.* **2018**, *46*, W229–W234. [CrossRef]
41. Pezzicoli, A.; Ruggiero, P.; Amerighi, F.; Telford, J.L.; Soriani, M. Exogenous sialic acid transport contributes to group B streptococcus infection of mucosal surfaces. *J. Infect. Dis.* **2012**, *206*, 924–931. [CrossRef]
42. Puente-Polledo, L.; Reglero, A.; Gonzalez-Clemente, C.; Rodriguez-Aparicio, L.B.; Ferrero, M.A. Biochemical conditions for the production of polysialic acid by Pasteurella haemolytica A2. *Glycoconj. J.* **1998**, *15*, 855–861. [CrossRef] [PubMed]
43. Navasa, N.; Rodriguez-Aparicio, L.B.; Ferrero, M.A.; Monteagudo-Mera, A.; Martinez-Blanco, H. Transcriptional control of RfaH on polysialic and colanic acid synthesis by *Escherichia coli* K92. *FEBS Lett.* **2014**, *588*, 922–928. [CrossRef]
44. Lin, B.X.; Qiao, Y.; Shi, B.; Tao, Y. Polysialic acid biosynthesis and production in Escherichia coli: Current state and perspectives. *Appl. Microbiol. Biotechnol.* **2016**, *100*, 1–8. [CrossRef] [PubMed]

45. Cress, B.F.; Englaender, J.A.; He, W.; Kasper, D.; Linhardt, R.J.; Koffas, M.A. Masquerading microbial pathogens: Capsular polysaccharides mimic host-tissue molecules. *FEMS Microbiol. Rev.* **2014**, *38*, 660–697. [CrossRef] [PubMed]
46. Colley, K.J.; Kitajima, K.; Sato, C. Polysialic acid: Biosynthesis, novel functions and applications. *Crit. Rev. Biochem. Mol. Biol.* **2014**, *49*, 498–532. [CrossRef]
47. Bailey, M.J.; Hughes, C.; Koronakis, V. RfaH and the ops element, components of a novel system controlling bacterial transcription elongation. *Mol. Microbiol.* **1997**, *26*, 845–851. [CrossRef]
48. Lekota, K.E.; Bezuidt, O.K.I.; Mafofo, J.; Rees, J.; Muchadeyi, F.C.; Madoroba, E.; van Heerden, H. Whole genome sequencing and identification of *Bacillus endophyticus* and *B. anthracis* isolated from anthrax outbreaks in South Africa. *BMC Microbiol.* **2018**, *18*, 67. [CrossRef]
49. Vimr, E.R.; Kalivoda, K.A.; Deszo, E.L.; Steenbergen, S.M. Diversity of microbial sialic acid metabolism. *Microbiol. Mol. Biol. Rev.* **2004**, *68*, 132–153. [CrossRef]
50. Ferrero, M.A.; Aparicio, L.R. Biosynthesis and production of polysialic acids in bacteria. *Appl. Microbiol. Biotechnol.* **2010**, *86*, 1621–1635. [CrossRef]
51. Daines, D.A.; Wright, L.F.; Chaffin, D.O.; Rubens, C.E.; Silver, R.P. NeuD plays a role in the synthesis of sialic acid in *Escherichia coli* K1. *FEMS Microbiol. Lett.* **2000**, *189*, 281–284. [CrossRef]
52. Lubin, J.B.; Kingston, J.J.; Chowdhury, N.; Boyd, E.F. Sialic acid catabolism and transport gene clusters are lineage specific In Vibrio vulnificus. *Appl. Environ. Microbiol.* **2012**, *78*, 3407–3415. [CrossRef]
53. Rosa, L.T.; Bianconi, M.E.; Thomas, G.H.; Kelly, D.J. Tripartite ATP-Independent Periplasmic (TRAP) Transporters and Tripartite Tricarboxylate Transporters (TTT): From Uptake to Pathogenicity. *Front. Cell Infect. Microbiol.* **2018**, *8*, 33. [CrossRef]
54. Revilla-Nuin, B.; Rodriguez-Aparicio, L.B.; Ferrero, M.A.; Reglero, A. Regulation of capsular polysialic acid biosynthesis by N-acetyl-D-mannosamine, an intermediate of sialic acid metabolism. *FEBS Lett.* **1998**, *426*, 191–195. [CrossRef]
55. Horne, C.R.; Venugopal, H.; Panjikar, S.; Wood, D.M.; Henrickson, A.; Brookes, E.; North, R.A.; Murphy, J.M.; Friemann, R.; Griffin, M.D.W.; et al. Mechanism of NanR gene repression and allosteric induction of bacterial sialic acid metabolism. *Nat. Commun.* **2021**, *12*, 1988. [CrossRef]
56. Severi, E.; Hood, D.W.; Thomas, G.H. Sialic acid utilization by bacterial pathogens. *Microbiology* **2007**, *153*, 2817–2822. [CrossRef]
57. Brigham, C.; Caughlan, R.; Gallegos, R.; Dallas, M.B.; Godoy, V.G.; Malamy, M.H. Sialic acid (N-acetyl neuraminic acid) utilization by Bacteroides fragilis requires a novel N-acetyl mannosamine epimerase. *J. Bacteriol.* **2009**, *191*, 3629–3638. [CrossRef]
58. Pastorello, I.; Rossi Paccani, S.; Rosini, R.; Mattera, R.; Ferrer Navarro, M.; Urosev, D.; Nesta, B.; Lo Surdo, P.; Del Vecchio, M.; Rippa, V.; et al. EsiB, a novel pathogenic Escherichia coli secretory immunoglobulin A-binding protein impairing neutrophil activation. *mBio* **2013**, *4*, e00206-13. [CrossRef]
59. Piotrowska, M.; Przygodzinska, D.; Matyjewicz, K.; Popowska, M. Occurrence and Variety of beta-Lactamase Genes among *Aeromonas* spp. Isolated from Urban Wastewater Treatment Plant. *Front. Microbiol.* **2017**, *8*, 863. [CrossRef]
60. Vazquez-Lopez, R.; Solano-Galvez, S.; Alvarez-Hernandez, D.A.; Ascencio-Aragon, J.A.; Gomez-Conde, E.; Pina-Leyva, C.; Lara-Lozano, M.; Guerrero-Gonzalez, T.; Gonzalez-Barrios, J.A. The Beta-Lactam Resistome Expressed by Aerobic and Anaerobic Bacteria Isolated from Human Feces of Healthy Donors. *Pharmaceuticals* **2021**, *14*, 533. [CrossRef]
61. Tekedar, H.C.; Abdelhamed, H.; Kumru, S.; Blom, J.; Karsi, A.; Lawrence, M.L. Comparative Genomics of *Aeromonas hydrophila* Secretion Systems and Mutational Analysis of hcp1 and vgrG1 Genes From T6SS. *Front. Microbiol.* **2018**, *9*, 3216. [CrossRef]
62. Jacobs, L.; Chenia, H.Y. Characterization of integrons and tetracycline resistance determinants in *Aeromonas* spp. isolated from South African aquaculture systems. *Int. J. Food Microbiol.* **2007**, *114*, 295–306. [CrossRef]
63. Kirov, S.M.; Barnett, T.C.; Pepe, C.M.; Strom, M.S.; Albert, M.J. Investigation of the role of type IV *Aeromonas* pilus (Tap) in the pathogenesis of *Aeromonas* gastrointestinal infection. *Infect. Immun.* **2000**, *68*, 4040–4048. [CrossRef] [PubMed]
64. Oh, D.; Yu, Y.; Lee, H.; Jeon, J.H.; Wanner, B.L.; Ritchie, K. Asymmetric polar localization dynamics of the serine chemoreceptor protein Tsr in *Escherichia coli*. *PLoS ONE* **2018**, *13*, e0195887. [CrossRef]
65. Ortega, A.; Zhulin, I.B.; Krell, T. Sensory Repertoire of Bacterial Chemoreceptors. *Microbiol. Mol. Biol. R* **2017**, *81*, e00033-17. [CrossRef] [PubMed]
66. Lacal, J.; Garcia-Fontana, C.; Munoz-Martinez, F.; Ramos, J.L.; Krell, T. Sensing of environmental signals: Classification of chemoreceptors according to the size of their ligand binding regions. *Environ. Microbiol.* **2010**, *12*, 2873–2884. [CrossRef] [PubMed]

antibiotics

MDPI

Article

Antibiotic Resistance Mediated by *Escherichia coli* in Kuwait Marine Environment as Revealed through Genomic Analysis

Hanan A. Al-Sarawi [1,*], Nazima Habibi [2,*], Saif Uddin [2], Awadhesh N. Jha [3], Mohammed A. Al-Sarawi [4] and Brett P. Lyons [5]

[1] Environment Public Authority, Fourth Ring Road, Shuwaikh Industrial 70050, Kuwait
[2] Environment and Life Science Research Centre, Kuwait Institute for Scientific Research, Safat 13109, Kuwait; sdin@kisr.edu.kw
[3] School of Biological Sciences, Plymouth University, Drake Circus, Plymouth PL4 8AA, UK; a.jha@plymouth.ac.uk
[4] Department of Earth & Environmental Sciences, Kuwait University, Faculty of Science, P.O. Box 5969, Safat 13060, Kuwait; sarawi500@gmail.com
[5] Research & Monitoring Coordination Nature Conservation Department, Neom 49625, Saudi Arabia; brettlyons1@hotmail.com
* Correspondence: h.alsarawi@gmail.com (H.A.A.-S.); nhabibi@kisr.edu.kw (N.H.)

Abstract: Antibiotic-resistance gene elements (ARGEs) such as antibiotic-resistance genes (ARGs), integrons, and plasmids are key to the spread of antimicrobial resistance (AMR) in marine environments. Kuwait's marine area is vulnerable to sewage contaminants introduced by numerous storm outlets and indiscriminate waste disposal near recreational beaches. Therefore, it has become a significant public health issue and warrants immediate investigation. Coliforms, especially Gram-negative *Escherichia coli*, have been regarded as significant indicators of recent fecal pollution and carriers of ARGEs. In this study, we applied a genome-based approach to identify ARGs' prevalence in *E. coli* isolated from mollusks and coastal water samples collected in a previous study. In addition, we investigated the plasmids and *intI1* (class 1 integron) genes coupled with the ARGs, mediating their spread within the Kuwait marine area. Whole-genome sequencing (WGS) identified genes resistant to the drug classes of beta-lactams ($bla_{CMY\text{-}150}$, $bla_{CMY\text{-}42}$, $bla_{CTX\text{-}M\text{-}15}$, $bla_{DHA\text{-}1}$, $bla_{MIR\text{-}1}$, $bla_{OKP\text{-}B\text{-}15}$, $bla_{OXA\text{-}1}$, $bla_{OXA\text{-}48}$, $bla_{TEM\text{-}1B}$, $bla_{TEM\text{-}35}$), trimethoprim (*dfrA14, dfrA15, dfrA16, dfrA1, dfrA5, dfrA7*), fluroquinolone (*oqxA, oqxB, qnrB38, qnrB4, qnrS1*), aminoglycoside (*aadA2, ant(3")-Ia, aph(3")-Ib, aph(3')-Ia, aph(6)-Id*), fosfomycin (*fosA7, fosA_6, fosA, fosB1*), sulfonamide (*sul1, sul2, sul3*), tetracycline (*tet-A, tet-B*), and macrolide (*mph-A*). The MFS-type drug efflux gene *mdf-A* is also quite common in *E. coli* isolates (80%). The plasmid *ColRNAI* was also found to be prevalent in *E. coli*. The integron gene *intI1* and gene cassettes (GC) were reported to be in 36% and 33%, respectively, of total *E. coli* isolates. A positive and significant ($p < 0.001$) correlation was observed between phenotypic AMR-*intI1* (r = 0.311) and phenotypic AMR-GC (r = 0.188). These findings are useful for the surveillance of horizontal gene transfer of AMR in the marine environments of Kuwait.

Keywords: class 1 integrons; antibiotic resistance genes; horizontal gene transfer; gene cassette; plasmids; marine environment

Citation: Al-Sarawi, H.A.; Habibi, N.; Uddin, S.; Jha, A.N.; Al-Sarawi, M.A.; Lyons, B.P. Antibiotic Resistance Mediated by *Escherichia coli* in Kuwait Marine Environment as Revealed through Genomic Analysis. *Antibiotics* **2023**, *12*, 1366. https://doi.org/10.3390/antibiotics12091366

Academic Editor: Akebe Luther King Abia

Received: 12 July 2023
Revised: 19 August 2023
Accepted: 21 August 2023
Published: 25 August 2023

1. Introduction

The excessive use of antibiotics to treat infectious diseases has legated the world to the public health hazard of antibiotic resistance [1–3]. Aquatic environs have been identified as reservoirs of antibiotic resistancegenes (ARGs); however, little is known about their distribution, spread and migration [4,5]. Marine environments are also sinks for pharmaceuticals, disinfectants, heavy metals, organic compounds, microplastics, and atmospheric dust [6–11]. Among these, pollutants, pharmaceuticals, and heavy metals have been evidenced to impose selective pressure on inherent bacterial communities that often develop resistance genes against them [9,11–18]. In addition, genetic elements, for example, class 1 integrons, package ARGs into gene cassettes (GCs) and mediate their transfer to non-resistant bacterial communities via horizontal gene transfer (HGT) [19–22]. Although more consideration has been given to animal and human health with respect to antimicrobial resistance (AMR) monitoring, the environment often remains ignored. The World Health Organization propelled the One Health Concept, which calls for the evaluation of overall environmental health [23]. Immediate action is also warranted to monitor the threats of AMR in the Gulf Cooperation Council [24,25].

Emergency waste and unauthorized sewage discharge in Kuwait have introduced several antibiotic-resistant bacteria (ARBs) into Kuwait's marine environments [18,26]. Among these, *Escherichia coli* could become an infectious animal and human bacterium showing resistance to almost all clinically used antibiotics. A wide profile of AMR *E. coli* has been previously demonstrated through conventional phenotypic antibiotic susceptibility testing (AST) in Kuwait's marine environment [27–29]. However, data on the genes conferring resistance are lacking in these aquatic settings. In addition, class 1 integrons, GCs, and plasmids involved in their spread are unknown. Currently, microbiological methods of AMR surveillance are considered laborious, time-intensive, and provide limited phenotypic information. With the advent of molecular methods, a rapid and detailed genotypic assessment of all these components can be achieved [30–34]. These methods are now being embraced as a novel approach to map the whole genomes of bacterial isolates, ARGs, plasmids, integrons, and GCs simultaneously to complement the AMR phenotypic assays [32,35–37]. The goal of this research was to examine the genomic profiles of *E. coli* through whole-genome sequencing and to study the prevalence of ARGs, plasmids, integrons (*intI1*), and GCs.

2. Results

For the present investigation, selected *E. coli* isolates (n = 23) were subjected to whole-genome sequencing. All sequences ranged between 4,577,350 and 5,103,695 bases, with a Phred quality score above 20.

2.1. MLST and Phylogenetic Analysis

The open reading frames corresponding to seven sequence tags (STs), namely, *adk-fumC-gyrB-icd-mdh-purA-recA*, were identified in the assembled genomes of 23 *E. coli* isolates. Alignment of sequences against these STs established the *Enterobacteriaceae* origin of the strains. Further treatment with the mafft software and UGENE software confirmed 20 isolates as *E. coli*, and three of these closely matched with *Enterobacter cloacae* (SE111, SE181, and SE158). Molecular data analyses helped to correctly identify the species of *E. cloacae*; hence, we found the molecular tests to be technically superior for discriminating between closely related *E. coli* and *E. cloaca* strains. Further analysis was performed on the 20 *E. coli* isolates. The phylogenetic relationships of the selected *E. coli* were distributed into two clusters (Figure 1). A close relationship was observed between the isolates from spatially distant locations, different seasons, and varied matrices (marine waters or mollusks). For example, SE25 and KHE11 isolated from Al-Salam and Khiran were closely related. Strains SE19 and SC118 were isolated from different matrices, i.e., marine water during winter and mollusks collected during summer; however, they were positioned on the same branch of the phylogenetic tree for their similarity. Similarly, SC59 and 756E0 were also analogous. It was noticed that the three isolates of *E. cloacae*, namely, SE111, SE181, and SE158, exist separately as a group.

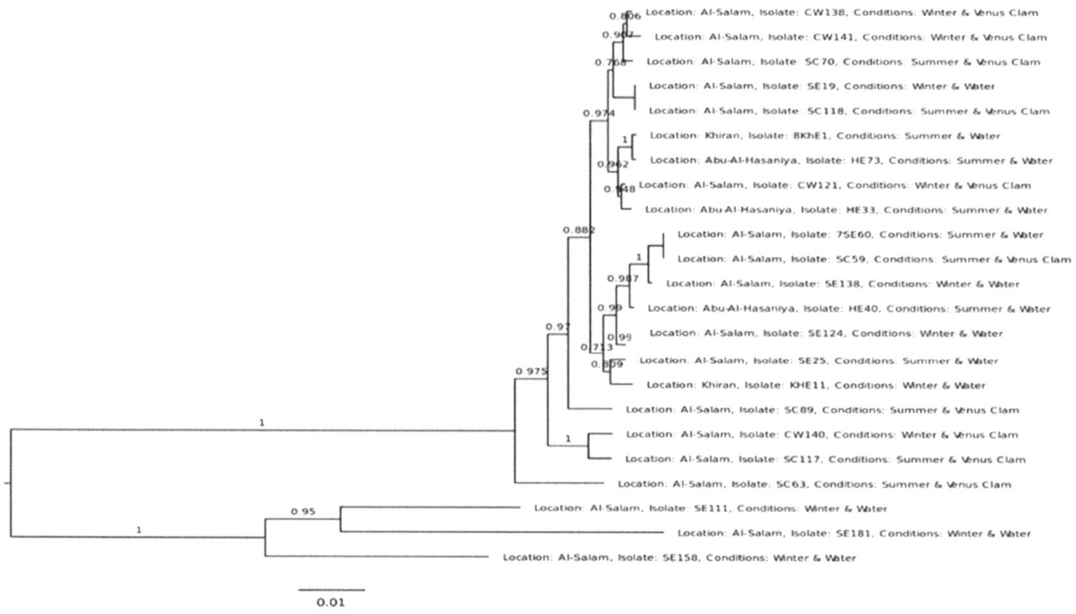

Figure 1. Phylogeny of the strains isolated from Kuwait. A maximum-likelihood tree was plotted on the distances between the MLST sequences of the selected strains.

2.2. Antibiotic-Resistance Gene Elements

We submitted the assembled *E. coli* sequences to the ResFinder database and found matches against 33 ARGs (Figure 2; Table S1). The percentage identity of the sequences ranged between 80 and 100%. The highest frequency (80%) was that of the *mdf (A)* gene found in at least 16 isolates. This was followed by bla_{Tem-1B}, present in 45% of *E. coli* strains.

The highest number of genes (10/33) originated from beta-lactam family ($bla_{CMY-150}$, bla_{CMY-42}, $bla_{CTX-M-15}$, bla_{DHA-1}, bla_{MIR-1}, $bla_{OKP-B-15}$, bla_{OXA-1}, bla_{OXA-48}, bla_{TEM-1B}, bla_{TEM-35}). This was followed by trimethoprim (6/33),-(*dfrA14, dfrA15, dfrA16, dfrA1, dfrA5, dfrA7*), fluoroquinolone (5/33) (*oqxA, oqxB, QnrB38, QnrB4, QnrS1*),aminoglycoside (5/33) (*aadA2, ANT (3″)-Ia, APH (3″)-Ib, APH (3′)-Ia, APH(6)-Id*), fosfomycin (4/33) (*FosA7, FosA6, FosA, FosB1*), sulfonamide (2/33) (*sul1, sul2*), and tetracycline (2/33) resistance genes (*tetA, tetB*). Single genes belonged to the drug class macrolide (*mphA*) and MFS-type drug efflux (*mdfA*).

We compared the ARG summaries of these 20 strains with their AMR phenotypes (tested against a panel of 23 antibiotics). According to the genotypic assay, all these strains possessed ARGs; therefore, they were considered as potentially resistant to at least one of the drug classes. Phenotypically, the strains SC59, HE33, 7SE60, SE124, and CW140 were sensitive to all the antibiotics (Figure 3).

Resistance to beta-lactams was confirmed both genotypically and phenotypically in 40% of the isolates, namely, HE40 (bla_{TEM-1B}), SC63 (bla_{TEM-1B}), SC70 (bla_{OXA-1}, bla_{OXA-48}, bla_{TEM-35}), SC118 (bla_{CMY-42}, bla_{TEM-1B}), SE25 ($bla_{CTX-M-15}$), SE19 (bla_{TEM-1B}), KHE11 ($bla_{CMY-150}$, bla_{TEM-1B}), and CW138 (bla_{TEM-1B}). Strain SE138 bearing beta-lactamase genes (bla_{DHA-1}, bla_{MIR-1}, bla_{TEM-1B}) depicted an intermediate phenotype against this drug class. Strain 8KHE1 was phenotypically resistant to beta-lactams + beta-lactamase inhibitors and cephalosporins. None of the genes were resistant to the above drug classes; rather, the *mdfA* (MFS-type drug efflux) resistant against tetracycline, disinfectants, and antiseptics was found in the genotype. Similar was the case with strains SC117 and SC89. Within the beta-lactamase, genes resistant to CMY-beta lactamase (cephamycin), CTX-M-beta lactamase (penam, cephalosporin), DHA-beta lactamase (cephalosporin, cephamycin), MIR-beta lactamase (monobactam, cephalosporin), OKP-beta lactamase (penam, cephalosporin), OXA-beta lactamase (penam, cephalosporin, carbapenem), and TEM-beta lactamase (penam, monobactam, penem, cephalosporin) were observed in strains SC118; SE25, SE138; SE138; SE124; SC70; and SC59, HE40, SC63, SC70, SC118, SE19, KHE11, SE138, CW138, and CW140, respectively. Cephalosporin was one of the drugs in the antibiotic panel. As evident from the above statements, this first-generation beta-lactamase confers resistance against all the sub-categories of beta-lactams. TEM-beta lactamase was one of the most common genes detected in the tested isolates (45%). Among the carbapenems, the SE19 isolate expressed a meropenem (carbapenem)-resistant phenotype and also possessed bla_{TEM} (TEM-beta lactamase) gene. All the remaining strains were susceptible to meropenem. In addition to this, susceptibility to imipenem (carbapenem) was observed in all the strains (Figure 3). None of the genotypes were positive for the bla_{IMP} group of genes. Strain CW141, phenotypically resistant to piperacillin (beta-lactams), was devoid of relevant genes.

Gene ID	*E. coli* isolates																			
	SC59	8KhE1	HE40	SC63	SC70	SC117	SC118	HE73	HE33	SC89	SE25	7SE60	SE19	KHE11	SE124	SE138	CW138	CW140	CW121	CW141
ant(3")-Ia	.	.	.	.	82.3	.	.	.	.	.	.	.	.	95.1	.	.	.	.	.	.
aph(3")-Ib	100	.	.	100	.	.	.	100	.	.	.	.	.	.	.	100	100	100	.	.
aph(6)-Id	100	.	100	100	.	.	.	100	.	.	.	.	.	.	.	100	100	100	.	.
blaCMY-150	.	.	.	.	.	.	.	.	.	.	.	.	.	100	.	.	.	.	.	.
blaCMY-42	.	.	.	.	.	.	100	.	.	.	.	.	.	.	.	.	.	.	.	.
blaCTX-M-15	.	.	.	.	.	.	.	.	.	.	100	.	.	.	.	.	.	.	.	.
blaDHA-1	.	.	.	.	.	.	.	.	.	.	.	.	.	.	.	100	.	.	.	.
blaMIR-1	.	.	.	.	.	.	.	.	.	.	.	.	.	.	.	100	.	.	.	.
blaOKP-B-15	.	.	.	.	.	.	.	.	.	.	.	.	.	.	99.9	.	.	.	.	.
blaOXA-1	.	.	.	.	99.0	.	.	.	.	.	.	.	.	.	.	.	.	.	.	.
blaOXA-48	.	.	.	.	100	.	.	.	.	.	.	.	.	.	.	.	.	.	.	.
blaTEM-1B	100	.	100	100	.	.	100	.	.	.	.	.	100	100	.	100	100	100	.	.
blaTEM-35	.	.	.	.	100	.	.	.	.	.	.	.	.	.	.	.	.	.	.	.
dfrA14	100	.	100	.	.	.	.	.	.	.	.	.	.	.	.	.	.	.	.	.
dfrA15	.	.	.	.	.	.	.	.	.	.	.	.	.	.	.	100	.	.	.	.
dfrA16	.	.	.	.	.	.	.	.	.	.	.	.	.	100	.	.	.	.	.	.
dfrA1	.	.	.	.	100	.	.	.	.	.	.	.	.	.	.	.	.	.	.	.
dfrA7	.	.	.	.	.	.	.	.	.	.	.	.	.	.	.	.	100	100	.	.
fosA7	.	.	.	.	.	.	.	.	.	.	100	.	.	.	.	.	.	.	.	.
fosA_6	.	.	.	.	.	.	.	.	.	.	.	.	.	.	100	.	.	.	.	.
fosA	.	.	.	.	.	.	.	.	.	.	.	.	.	.	.	100	.	.	.	.
fosB1	.	.	.	.	.	.	.	.	.	.	.	.	.	.	.	.	.	.	.	99.8
mdf(A)	100	100	100	100	100	100	100	100	100	100	100	100	100	.	.	.	100	100	100	.
mph(A)	.	.	100	.	100	.	.	.	.	.	.	.	.	.	.	.	.	.	.	.
oqxA	.	.	.	.	.	.	.	.	.	.	.	.	.	.	100	100	.	.	.	.
oqxB	.	.	.	.	.	.	.	.	.	.	.	.	.	.	100	99.0	.	.	.	.
qnrB38	.	.	.	.	.	.	.	.	.	.	.	.	.	100	.	.	.	.	.	.
qnrB4	.	.	.	.	.	.	.	.	.	.	.	.	.	.	.	100	.	.	.	.
qnrS1	100	.	100	.	100	.	.	.	.	.	100	.	.	.	.	.	.	.	.	.
sul1	.	.	.	.	.	.	.	.	.	.	.	.	.	100	.	100	.	.	.	.
sul2_2	100	.	100	100	.	.	.	100	.	.	.	.	.	.	.	100	100	100	.	.
tet(A)	97.8	.	97.8	97.8	.	.	.	100	.	.	.	.	.	.	.	.	97.8	97.8	.	.
tet(B)	.	.	.	.	100	.	.	.	.	.	.	.	100	.	.	.	.	.	.	.

Figure 2. ARGs distributed in the *E. coli* genomes. Colored boxes are positive for the respective ARG listed on the left-hand side panel. The values in each box show the percentage identity in the ResFinder database v4.0.0 (red > 80%; yellow > 90%; green > 100%; white < 0.0%).

Matching genotypes and phenotypes (20%) for aminoglycoside resistance were recorded in HE40 (*aph(6)-Id*), HE73 (*aph(3″)-Ib*, *aph(6)-Id*), KHE11 (*ant(3″)-Ia*), and SE138 (*aph(3″)-Ib*, *aph(6)-Id*), whereas genes without any phenotypic expression for this drug class were observed in SC59 (*aph(3″)-Ib*, *aph(3″)-Ib*), SC70 (*ant(3″)-Ia*), CW138 (*aph(3″)-Ib*, *aph(6)-Id*), and CW140 (*aph(3″)-Ib*, *aph(6)-Id*). Strains 8KHE1, SC117, and SC89 depicted an aminoglycoside-resistant profile but were devoid of related genes. Contrastingly, its genotype possessed *mdfA* (MFS-type drug efflux) resistance against tetracycline, disinfectants, and antiseptics.

Isolate id	Phenotypic Resistance: Aminoglycoside			Beta-lactams				Aminoglycoside + Beta-lactams	beta-lactam/beta-lactamase inhibitor		Cephalosporin								Fluoroquinolones		Imipenem	Quinolone	Dihydrofolate reductase/Sulfonamide	Genotypic Resistance	
	AMI	GEN	TOB	AMP	AZT	MERO	PIP	A/S2	P/T4	TM2	FAZ	FEP	TANS	AXO	TAZ	FOX	POD	FUR	CIP	GAT	IMI	NIT	SXT	ARGs	Drug class
SC59	0	0	0	0	0	0	0	0	0	0	0	0	0	0	0	4	0	0	0	0	0	0	0	aph(3'')-Ib, aph(3'')-Ib, blaTEM-1B, dfrA14, mdf(A), qnrS1, sul2, tet(A)	aminoglycoside, TEM beta-lactamase (penam, monobactam, penem, cephalosporin), trimethoprim, MFS type drug efflux, quinolone, Sulfonamide, tetracycline
8KHE1	0	2	0	16	8	0	32	32	0	64	32	0	0	16	2	4	0	32	0	0	0	0	4	mdf(A)	MFS type drug efflux
HE40	0	8	4	32	32	0	128	32	128	64	32	8	32	64	32	32	16	32	4	8	0	0	4	aph(6)-Id, blaTEM-1B, dfrA14, mdf (A), mph(A), qnrS1, sul2, tet (A)	aminoglycoside, TEM beta-lactamase (penam, monobactam, penem, cephalosporin), trimethoprim, MFS type drug efflux, quinolone, sulfonamide, tetracycline
SC63	0	0	0	32	0	0	128	8	0	16	0	0	0	0	0	4	0	0	4	8	0	0	4	aph(3'')-Ib, aph(6)-Id, blaTEM-1B, mdf(A), sul2, tet(A)	aminoglycoside, TEM beta-lactamase (penam, monobactam, penem, cephalosporin), trimethoprim, MFS type drug efflux, sulfonamide, tetracycline
SC70	0	0	0	32	0	0	128	4	0	0	8	0	0	0	0	4	0	0	1	1	0	0	4	ant(3'')-Ia, blaOXA-1, blaOXA-48, blaTEM-35, dfrA1, mdf(A), mph(A), qnrS1, tet(B)	aminoglycoside, OXA beta-lactamase (penam, cephalosporin), TEM beta-lactamase (penam, monobactam, penem, cephalosporin), trimethoprim, MFS type drug efflux, macrolide, sulfonamide, tetracycline
SC117	0	2	0	32	16	0	32	16	0	64	32	0	16	64	32	32	16	32	4	4	0	0	0	mdf(A)	MFS type drug efflux
SC118	0	0	0	32	32	0	128	16	0	64	32	0	32	64	32	32	16	32	4	4	0	0	0	blaCMY-42, blaTEM-1B, mdf(A),	CMY beta lactamase (cephalosporin, cephamycin), TEM beta-lactamase (penam, monobactam, penem, cephalosporin), MFS type drug efflux
HE73	0	8	0	32	32	0	128	32	0	64	32	4	0	32	8	16	16	32	4	8	0	0	4	aph(3'')-Ib, aph(6)-Id, mdf(A), sul 2, tet(A),	aminoglycoside, MFS type drug efflux, sulfonamide, tetracycline
HE33	0	0	0	0	0	0	0	0	0	0	0	0	0	0	0	0	0	0	0	0	0	0	0	mdf(A)	MFS type drug efflux
SC89	0	0	0	32	0	0	64	4	0	0	4	0	0	0	0	4	0	0	0	0	0	0	4	mdf(A)	MFS type drug efflux
SE25	0	0	0	32	32	0	128	8	0	0	32	32	0	64	4	4	16	32	0	0	0	0	0	blaCTX-M-15, fosA7, mdf(A), qnrS1,	CTX-M beta-lactamase (cephalosporin, penam), MFS type drug efflux, tetracycline
7SE60	0	0	0	0	0	0	0	0	0	0	0	0	0	0	0	0	0	0	0	0	0	0	0	mdf(A)	MFS type drug efflux
SE19	8	16	8	32	32	8	128	32	0	64	32	16	32	4	32	32	16	32	4	8	0	32	0	blaTEM-1B, mdf(A), tet(B)	TEM beta-lactamase (penam, monobactam, penem, cephalosporin), MFS type drug efflux, tetracycline
KHE11	64	16	8	32	32	1	128	32	128	64	32	4	32	64	32	4	16	32	4	8	0	128	8	ant(3'')-Ia, blaCMY-150, blaTEM-1B, dfrA16, qnrB38, sul1,	aminoglycoside, TEM beta-lactamase (penam, monobactam, penem, cephalosporin), trimethoprim, quinolone, sulfonamide, tetracycline
SE124	0	0	0	0	0	0	0	0	0	0	0	0	0	0	0	4	0	4	0	0	0	0	0	blaOKP-B-15, fosA_6, oqxA, oqxB,	OKP beta-lactamase (penam, cephalosporin), fosfomycin, quinolone
SE138	0	16	4	16	8	0	64	4	0	0	32	0	0	32	2	4	16	8	4	1	0	0	4	aph(3'')-Ib, aph(6)-Id, blaDHA-1, blaMIR-1, blaTEM-1B, dfrA15, fosA, oqxA, oqxB, qnrB4, sul1, sul2,	aminoglycoside, CTX-M beta-lactamase (cephalosporin, penam), TEM beta-lactamase (penam, monobactam, penem, cephalosporin), DHA beta-lactamase (cephamycin, cephalosporin), trimethoprim, fosfomycin, quinolone, sulfonamide, tetracycline
CW138	0	0	0	32	0	0	128	8	0	0	32	0	0	0	0	32	0	0	4	2	0	0	8	aph(3'')-Ib, aph(6)-Id, blaTEM-1B, dfrA7, mdf(A), sul2, tet(A)	aminoglycoside, TEM beta-lactamase (penam, monobactam, penem, cephalosporin), trimethoprim, MFS type drug efflux, sulfonamide, tetracycline
CW140	0	0	0	0	0	0	0	0	0	0	0	0	0	0	0	4	0	0	0	0	0	0	0	aph(3'')-Ib, aph(6)-Id, blaTEM-1B, dfrA7, mdf(A), sul2, tet(A)	aminoglycoside, TEM beta-lactamase (penam, monobactam, penem, cephalosporin), trimethoprim, MFS type drug efflux, sulfonamide, tetracycline
CW121	0	0	0	0	0	0	0	0	0	0	0	0	0	0	0	0	0	0	0	0	0	0	8	mdf(A)	MFS type drug efflux
CW141	0	0	0	16	0	0	128	16	0	16	4	0	0	0	0	4	0	0	0	0	0	0	8	fosB1	Fosfomycin
	Amikacin	Gentamycin	Tobramycin	Ampicillin	Aztreonam	Meropenem	Piperacillin	Ampicillin/sulbactam	Piperacillin/tazobactam	Ticercillin/clavulanic acid	Cefazolin	Cefepime	Cefotetan Na	Ceftriaxone	Ceftazidime	Cefoxitin	Cefpodoxime	Cefuroxime	Ciprofloxacin	Gatifloxacin	Imipenem	Nitrofurantoin	Trimethorprim/sulfamethoxazole		

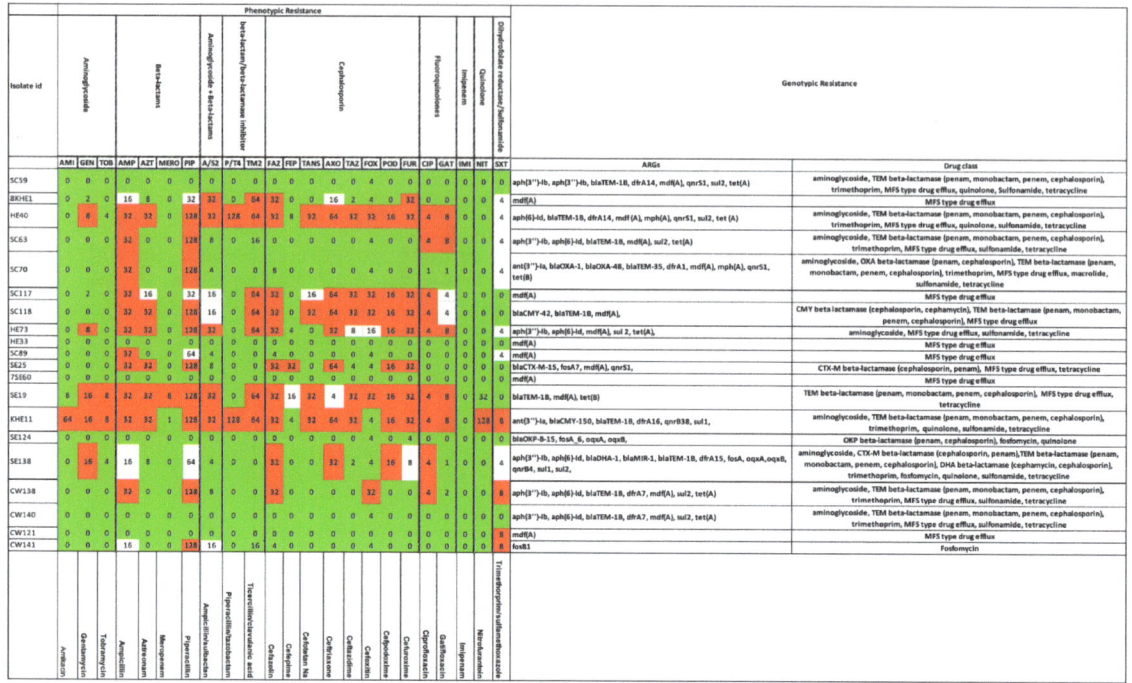

Figure 3. Genotypic versus phenotypic resistance in selected isolates of *E. coli*. Phenotypes are presented on the left-hand side panel. The color codes represent Red—Resistant, Green—Susceptible, and White—Intermediate. Corresponding genotypes are shown on the right-hand side.

In the case of fluroquinolones, phenotypic resistance was expressed in 45% of isolates (HE40, SC63, SC117, SC118, HE733, SE19, KHE11, SE138, and CW138). Among these, only 15% (3/20) of the isolates, i.e., HE40, KHE11, and SE138, possessed resistance genes (*qnrS1*). Phenotypic sensitivity against quinolone (used interchangeably with fluroquinolone) was demonstrated by all the strains except KHE11. ARGs against this drug class were located in strains SC59 (*qnrS1*), HE40 (*qnrS1*), SC70 (*qnrS1*), SE25 (*qnrS1*), and SE138 (*oqxA*, *oqxB*, *qnrB4*).

Trimethoprim- or sulfonamide-resistant phenotypes were observed in KHE11, CW138, CW121, and CW141, of which only the first two strains (10%) possessed ARGs (KHE11—*dfrA15*, *sul1*; CW138—*dfrA7*, *sul2*). Four strains with intermediate phenotypes were positive for corresponding ARGs (HE40—*dfrA14*, *sul2*; SC63—*sul2*; HE73—*sul2*; and SE138—*dfrA15*, *sul1*, *sul2*).

Moreover, SC59, HE40, SC63, SC70, HE73, SE25, SE19, KHE11, SE138, CW138, and CW140 all possessed tetracycline-resistant genotypes (ARG—*tetA*, *tetB*), which was not captured by the AST as the chosen panel lacked tetracycline. Similarly, macrolide-resistant genes (*mphA*) were recorded in SC70 and fosfomycin-resistant genes (*fosB1*) in CW141 that were not tested phenotypically.

The alignment of sequences against the plasmid finder database revealed 13 isolates as hosts to 22 plasmids (Table S2). The most prevalent was the *ColRNAI* plasmid found in 11 isolates (42.3%) (Figure 4). Sequences were then concomitantly mined for integrons, recombination sites, and promoters. The genetic elements identified were *attC* (gene cassette recombination sites), *intI* (intersection tyr-integrase), *Pc_1* (gene cassette promoter class), *Pint_1* (integron promoter), and *attI_1* (integron recombination site). The elements *attC* and *intI* were reported in 20% (4/20) of the strains, whereas *Pc_1* and *attI_1* were detected in 10% (2/20) of the isolates. *Pint_1* was found in 15% (3/20) of the tested samples. Isolates

CW138, CW121, and CW141 were positive for integron with the integron integrase (*intI*) and *attC* site nearby, whereas HE70 was positive for the latter only, lacking recombination sites (Table 1). These elements aid the mobilization of ARGs in other strains. The *intI1* gene encodes the integrase enzyme, the promoter Pc ensures its expression, and the site-specific recombination takes place between the *attI* and *attC* sites. The GC is an open reading frame (ORF) without a promoter but with a recombination site. These GCs can integrate novel genes and support the bacterial strains to adapt. On the other hand, strain SC70 possessed only a cluster of *attC* sites without any integrase in its vicinity (Table S3). Classification of integrons and gene cassettes revealed the presence of class 1 integron (*intI1*) and GC1. All the genetic elements within strain CW141 are shown in Figure 5. Intriguingly, this strain possessed the fosfomycin-resistant gene (*fosB1*) and expressed phenotypic AMR against piperacillin (an extended spectrum beta-lactam) and trimethoprim, as well as harbored the incX1 plasmid.

PLASMIDS	***E. coli* isolates**												
	SC59	**HE40**	**SC70**	**HE73**	**HE33**	**SE25**	**7SE60**	**SE19**	**SE138**	**CW138**	**CW140**	**CW121**	**CW141**
Col(KPHS6)	.	.	.	.	.	.	.	.	.	.	.	100	.
Col(MG828)	.	.	.	.	.	.	.	.	.	.	.	.	.
Col156	.	.	100	.	.	.	.	.	.	98.7	.	100	100
Col440I	100	.	.	.	.	.	.	.	.	97.4	.	.	.
Col8282	.	.	.	.	.	97.6	.	.	.	.	.	.	.
ColE10	.	.	100	.	.	.	.	.	.	.	.	.	.
ColRNAI	.	.	99.2	100	100	.	100	.	100	98.5	98.5	.	100
IncB/O/K/Z	.	.	.	.	.	.	.	.	.	.	.	.	.
IncFIA(HI1)_1_HI1	99.7	.	.	.	.	.	99.7	.	.	.	.	.	.
IncFIA	.	.	.	.	.	.	.	100	.	.	.	.	.
IncFIB(AP001918)	.	.	.	.	.	.	.	.	.	.	.	.	.
IncFIB(K)_1_Kpn3	100	100	.	.	.	.	100	.	.	.	.	.	.
IncFIC(FII)	.	.	.	.	.	.	.	.	.	.	.	.	.
IncFII(29)_1_pUTI89	.	.	.	.	.	.	.	.	.	.	.	100	.
IncFII(pRSB107)_1_pRSB107	.	.	.	.	.	.	.	.	.	.	.	.	.
IncI1_1_Alpha	.	.	.	.	.	.	.	.	.	.	.	.	.
IncI2_1_Delta	.	.	.	.	100	.	.	.	.	.	.	.	.
IncI_Gamma	.	.	.	.	.	.	.	97.2	.	.	.	.	97.2
IncN	.	100	.	.	.	.	.	.	.	.	.	.	.
IncX1	.	.	.	.	.	.	.	.	.	.	.	100	100
IncX4_1	.	.	.	100	.	.	.	.	.	.	.	.	.
IncX4_2	.	.	.	.	100	.	.	.	.	.	.	.	.

Figure 4. The plasmids found in selected isolates of *E. coli* revealed by whole-genome sequencing. Colored boxes mark the presence of the plasmids and their percentage identity in the database (red > 80%; yellow > 90%; green > 100%; white < 0.0%). Plasmids were fetched from the PlasmidFinder database.

Table 1. Integrons in *E. coli* isolates.

Sample	Elements Identified by Integron Finder					Integron Class	
	attC	intI	*Pc_1*	*Pint_1*	*attI_1*	*intI1*	GC
HE40	-	Yes	Yes	-	Yes	-	-
CW138	Yes	Yes	-	Yes	-	Yes	Yes
CW121	Yes	Yes	-	Yes	-	Yes	Yes
CW141	Yes	Yes	Yes	Yes	Yes	Yes	-
SC70	Yes	-	-	-	-	-	-

attC—GC recombination site; intI—intersection tyr-integrase; *Pc-1*—gene cassette promoter int1; *Pint_1*—promoter intI1; *attI_1*—integron recombination site; *intI1*—integrase gene; GC—gene cassette.

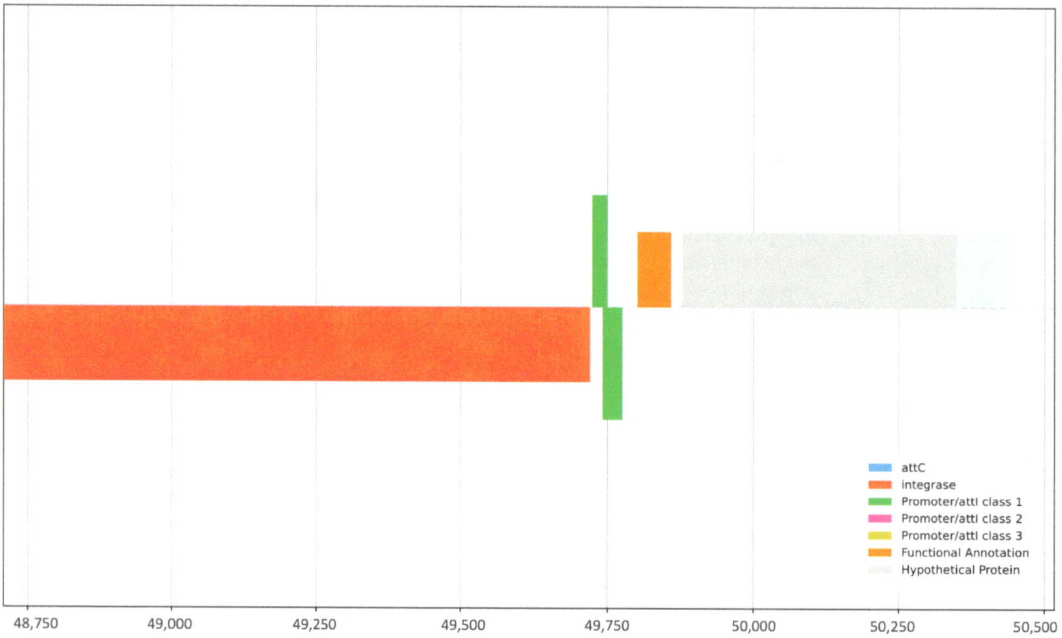

Figure 5. Graphical representation of integrons, recombination sites, and promoters present in *E. coli* strain CW141.

2.3. PCR-Based Identification of IntI1 and GCs

Among all the isolated strains (n = 598 from both mollusks and seawater), 216 were positive for the *intI1* (36%) gene, exhibiting a band of 400 bp in size on the agarose gel. These were associated with 198 GCs (36%) (Figure 6A). We looked at the AMR phenotypes of *intI1*-positive isolates (n = 216); interestingly, 95% of them were phenotypically resistant to at least one antibiotic among the panel (aminoglycoside, beta-lactams, aminoglycoside + beta-lactam inhibitors, beta-lactams/beta-lactamase inhibitors, cephalosporins, fluroquinolones, quinolones, imipenem, and dihydrofolate-reductase/trimethoprim) and the remaining 5% were susceptible (Figure 6C) to all the tested antibiotics. Considering the total AMR phenotypes of *E. coli* (n = 420), approximately 49% were negative for *intI1* (Figure 6B). Spearman's correlation model established a positive correlation between phenotypic AMR-*intI1*-GC. Overall, the coefficients were statistically significant (*intI1* ß–0.230, $p < 0.001$; GC ß–0.121, $p < 0.001$). There was 7.5% variance between *intI1*-GC resistance (F—24.28, $p < 0.001$). Positive correlations were observed between phenotypic AMR-*intI1* (0.310; $p < 0.001$) and phenotypic AMR-GC (0.190; $p < 0.001$). The *intI1* and GC were also significantly correlated (0.120; $p < 0.003$).

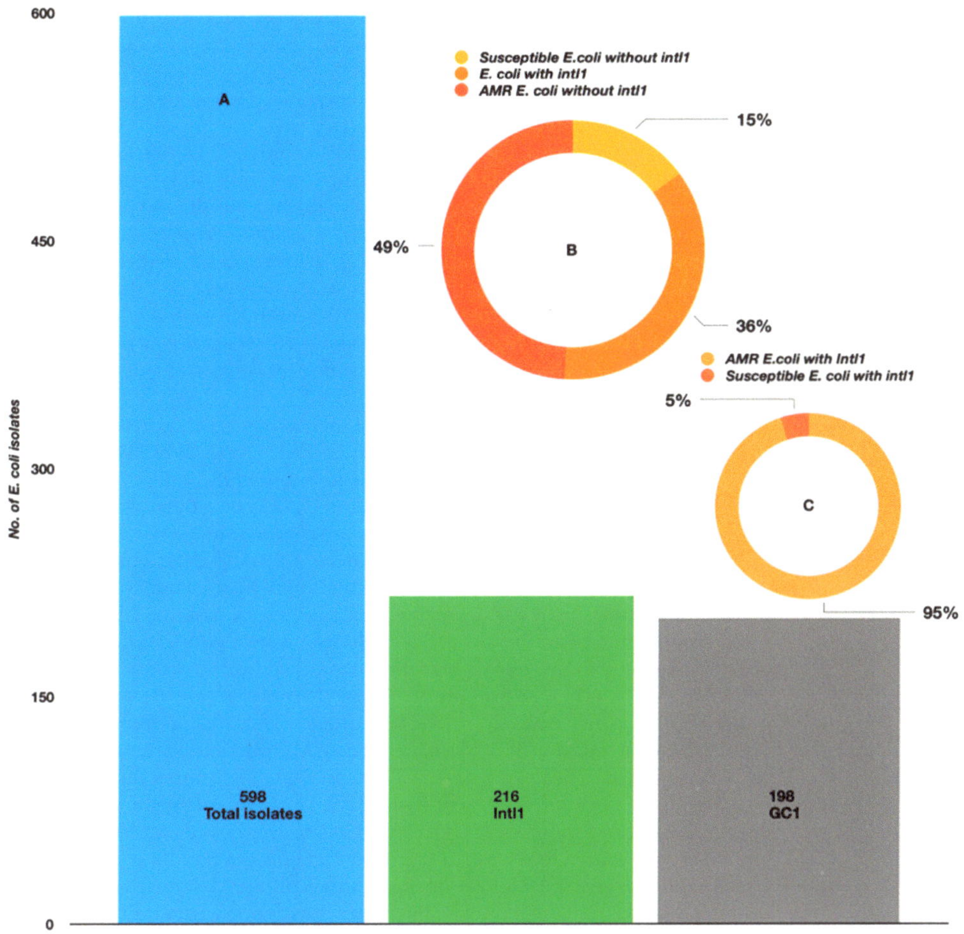

Figure 6. (**A**) Prevalence of class 1 integrons and gene cassettes in *E. coli* isolated from the Kuwait marine waters and molluscans. (**B**) The occurrence of class 1 integrons in *E. coli* isolated during summer and winter seasons. (**C**) AMR-susceptible *E. coli* with *intI1*.

3. Discussion

WGS has become the most preferred method to identify ARGs and associated genetic elements [38]. Recently, it identified ARGs in both highly resistant and susceptible isolates in the order of Enterobacterales [38]. This indicates that a population of resistant *E.coli* is floating in the coastal waters of Kuwait [36,39]. In addition to resistance profiling, WGS was also used presently for the identification of *Enterobacteriaceae* species. Interestingly, three of the isolates (13.0%) were identified as *Enterobacter cloacae*. A study from the Norwegian coast demonstrated that MALDI-TOF-MS (Matrix-assisted laser desorption ionization–Time of flight mass spectrometry) identified 90% of isolated strains as *E. coli*, whereas the remaining 10% were *Klebsiella*, *Citrobacter*, and *Enterobacter* [40]. More robust and precise identification approaches such as molecular methods are preferred over conventional microbiological assays, especially in mollusks and other filter feeders in the marine environment that are prone to pathogenic exposure, in addition to *E. coli*, for accurate discrimination between closely related species [41]. Further, the MLST-based phylogeny established a close relationship between the 20 isolates. This indicates a common origin of *E. coli*, most probably one of the point sources of emergency outfalls. The genetic similarity between the *E. coli* isolates of seawater and mollusks is most probably due to the filter feeding mechanism of the latter [42]. A comprehensive analysis might assist in contact tracing of these AMR strains.

Intriguingly, the *E. coli* isolates (n = 20) possessed genes resistant against seven drug classes. This is most likely due to the selective pressure imposed by antibiotics such as Azithromycin, Cefalexin, Ciprofloxacin, Clarithromycin, Dimetridazole, Erythromycin, Metronidazole, Metronidazole-OH, Ofloxacin, Ronidazole, Sulfamethoxazole, Tetracycline, and Trimethoprim found in seawater samples [8] and the effluent streams of waste-water treatment plants in Kuwait [43]. Moreover, the presence of conjugative plasmids and integrons in these strains is indicative of ARG transmission through horizontal gene transfer [19,20,22,44,45]. Nevertheless, this study only targeted the fecal coliforms, and the likelihood of other microbial communities with diverse ARG profiles is expected. The advanced method of high-throughput shotgun metagenomic sequencing would be a more valuable tool in the assessment of resistomes at contaminated and non-contaminated sites [26,38].

The presence of beta-lactam genes and their phenotypic expression in strains such as HE40, SC63, SC70, SC118, SE25, SE19, KHE11, SE138, and CW138 draws our immediate attention. Moreover, plasmid vectors were also recorded in HE40, SC70, SE25, SE19, SE138, and CW138. In addition, the strains HE40 and CW138 also possessed integrons and gene cassettes, indicating the possibility of horizontal gene transfer of beta-lactamase genes in the region. Extended spectrum beta-lactams are the last-choice drugs to treat hardcore bacterial infections [46,47]. Worldwide circulation of beta-lactamases have been reported recently with more than 40% in Asian countries [48]. A baseline study also documented the presence of beta-lactams in aerosols collected from a public building situated near the coast of Kuwait [49]. Moreover, trimethoprim resistance was confirmed in strains KHE11 and CW138. The dominance of the MFS-type drug efflux gene (tetracycline, disinfectants, antiseptics) was also noticed in 75% of sequenced isolates. Tetracycline-resistant genes (*tetA/tetB)* were found in 55% of isolates. The AMR phenotypes for these antibiotics were missing and need to be taken into consideration while performing future phenotypic assays.

We also report that 35.99% of AMR *E.coli* held the *intI1* gene, in parallel with *Enterobacteriaceae* found in Korea (41.4%) [50]. Contrastingly, only 12.1% of *Enterobacteriaceae* strains were positive for class 1 integrons in an effluent handling system in Poland [51]. *IntI1* positive strains were maximum in locations proximal to the coastal emergency waste outfalls. Numerous storm outlets discharge emergency waste into the country's marina, leading to deteriorated water quality [24,27,52,53]. These findings are in congruence with our earlier reports on the presence of AMR microbes, ARGs, integrons, plasmids, and insertion sequences near the outfalls [18,26]. We attribute this to the antibiotics, pharmaceuticals, and other contaminants introduced into the seawater [8,43]. A constant selection pressure is thought to elevate the horizontal gene transfer frequency within these aquatic milieus [25,33,36,45,54,55]. Regression analysis predicted a relationship (7.5% variance) between *intI1*-GC resistance. This suggests that the class 1 integron could potentially play a role in the transmission of AMR in *Enterobacteriaceae* [45]; however, other contaminants, such as metals, cannot be ignored [5,56–58].

In the present investigation, WGS identified ARGs in both resistant and susceptible *E. coli* phenotypes. The presence of *intI1* and GCs indicates the HGT of AMR in the region. WGS is recommended as an accurate and precise monitoring tool for individual AMR strains perpetrating in marine ecosystems.

4. Materials and Methods

4.1. Sampling Locations, Collection and Isolation of Strains

A detailed overview of the sampling task is provided elsewhere [28] as they were previously collected and tested for AMR through standard microbiological methods. However, for ease of readership, a succinct description is provided in Sections 4.1.1–4.1.3. A detailed description of the genomic analysis performed in the current study has been described in Sections 4.2–4.5.

4.1.1. Marine Waters

Seawater was collected from Al-Ghazali (29°347784 N, 47°911974 E), Al-Salam (29°357207 N, 47°946784 E), Abu Al-Hasaniya (29°125652 N, 48°633155 E), and Al-Khairan (28°665070 N, 48°387640 E) in an earlier campaign [28]. Six replicates were sampled in 200 ml sterile bottles from each site in both summer (Jul–Aug 2015; 34.0 °C ± 2.0) and winter (Dec–Feb 2016; 17.2 °C ± 2.0) seasons (Table S4). In situ measurements of pH (8.2 ± 0.2), salinity (42 ± 2.0), and temperature were made employing a hand-held, multi-probe water quality meter (Hanna instruments, Smithfield, RI, USA). Samples were transported on ice to the Environment Public Authority (EPA) Kuwait laboratories. Samples were processed at EPA laboratories following an established protocol [36]. Briefly, 10 mL of seawater was pipetted into 1/4 strength Ringer's solution and serially diluted (10 to 10^5). Serial dilutions were passed through 0.45 µm Merck filters (Merck Life Sciences Limited, Dorset, UK). The filters were placed on Tryptone Bile X-Glucuronide chromogenic media (TBX) selective for *E. coli*. The Petri dishes were placed inverted at 30 °C for 4 h and 44 °C for 21 h. The plates were examined for the growth of blue–green colonies marking the presence of *E. coli*. A total of 351 strains were isolated from the collected water samples.

4.1.2. Mollusk Samples

Concurrent to the seawater sampling, mollusk samples were gathered in the summer (Jul–Aug 2015; 34.0 °C ± 2.0) and winter seasons (Dec–Feb 2016; 17.2 °C ± 2.0). Shells (n = 55–60) were hand-picked, sorted in autoclaved bags (4 °C), and transported to the College of Science, Kuwait University laboratories for further processing [28]. The mollusc shells were removed to collect the flesh and fluid in a pre-autoclaved beaker (Borosil, Poole, UK). Approximately 20 g was macerated with 0.1% peptone water (Sigma, Plymouth, UK) and serially diluted [28]. The dilutions were passed through the 0.45 µm nitrocellulose membrane filters and placed on TBX-agar for *E. coli*, as mentioned previously. In total, 247 mollusc strains were isolated.

4.1.3. Antimicrobial Susceptibility Testing

Antibiotic susceptibility assays for all these isolates were performed, and minimum inhibitory concentration (MIC) was recorded and presented in Al-Sarawi et al. [28]. Briefly, the isolates were tested for susceptibility and resistance against a panel of 23 antibiotics as per the guidelines of Clinical and Laboratory Standards Institutes [59]. The micro-dilution method was employed to determine the MIC by inoculating a loopful of isolate into 10 mL of Cation-Adjusted Muller Hinton (CAMBH) broth (incubated on shaker incubator for 24 h at 37 °C). Turbidity was adjusted with 0.5 M MacFarland solution and loaded to custom, dehydrated, 96-well Sensititre™ plates (GN2F, Thermo Scientific, Paisley, UK), which were further incubated at 25 °C for 24 h. Strains were classified as resistant, intermediate, or susceptible based on the MIC breakpoints standardized by CEFAS [27].

4.2. Whole-Genome Sequencing (WGS) and Filtering of ARGEs

From the 598 isolates, selected strains (n = 23, Table S5) with interesting AMR phenotypes, i.e., resistant to 2 or more antibiotics Al- Sarawi et al. [28] or susceptible to all, were subjected to WGS. These isolates were also chosen to represent varied spatiotemporal variability (three sites and two seasons). Whole-genome DNA was isolated from an over-nightly activated broth. Approximately 15 mL of Tryptic Soy Broth was seeded with a loopful of *E. coli* and incubated at 37 °C. The culture tube was centrifuged at 13,000× *g* to pellet the organisms and subjected to DNA purification as per the standard protocol of Promega Wizard ®Genomic DNA extraction Kit (Promega, Chilworth Southampton, Hampshire, UK) [60]. Fluorometric quantification of DNA was conducted on a Quantus fluorometer (Promega, Chilworth Southampton, Hampshire, UK). Sequencing libraries were prepared following the Nextera XT kit (Illumina, USA). The libraries were purified using AMPure® XP (Beckman Coulter, Brea, CA, USA) magnetic beads. Libraries were normalized and pooled before loading on a MiSeq V3 sequencing cartridge. Sequencing was performed on an Illumina MiSeq platform available at the Centre for Environment Fisheries and Aquaculture Science (CEFAS), Weymouth laboratories through paired-end (2 × 300 bp) chemistry [36]. Post-sequencing, the Illumina adapters were removed by Trimmomatic v 0.36 [61] and a quality check was performed on the web version of FastQC v 0.11.5 [62]. Raw reads were thereafter aligned in Spades v 3.10.1 for prokaryotic assembly [63] and annotated via Prokka v1.11 [64]. The ABRicate tool [65] was used to screen the 'assembled fasta' for antibiotic-resistant genes (ARGs), employing the ResFinder v 4.0.0 [66] database (accessed on 2 April 2023). The sequences were also mined for plasmids through the plasmid finder database [67]. The integron finder database v 2.0.2 was used to annotate the complete integron with integron integrase, *attC* recombination sites, promoters, and nearby gene cassettes [68].

4.3. MLST (Muti-Locus Sequence Typing) and Phylogenetic Analysis

Seven MLST genes, namely, *adk-fumC-gyrB-icd-mdh-purA-recA* were retrieved from the Pfam archive. The respective ids of the gene sets were PF00406, PF05683, PF00204, PF00180, PF00056, PF00709, and PF00154, respectively [69]. The hmmscan v 3.1, [70] was then used to align the assembled *E. coli* genomes with the abovementioned MLSTs. The identified MLSTs were aligned in mafft v 7.305 using the default settings [71]. UGENE v 1.98 was employed to remove and concatenate the unaligned sequences from the 5′ and 3′ ends [72]. A maximum likelihood tree analysis was performed on the aligned MLSTs through FastTree v 2.1.8 [73]. A phylogenetic tree was plotted in FigTree v 1.4.2 [74].

4.4. Screening for Class 1 Integrons and Associated Gene Cassettes

A total of 598 *E. coli* pure cultures isolated from marine waters (n = 351) and marine organisms/mollusks (n = 247) were used for *intI1* gene screening [28,75] and associated gene cassettes (GC). DNA was isolated as per the protocol described elsewhere [76]. Primers int1.F/R (F-5′GGGTCAAGGATCTGGATTTCG 3′; R-5′ACATGCGTGTAAATCATCGTCG3′) and HS286 (F-5′ GGGATCCTCSGCTKGARCGAMTTGTTAGVC) HS287 (R-5′GGGATCCG-CSGCTKANCTCVRRCGTTAGSC3′) were used to amplify the *intI1* and GCs, respectively [33,77]. A PCR mix (25 μL) was prepared by combining 2 μL (4 μM) each of forward and reverse primers, 6.5 μL of PCR grade water, 12.5 μL of buffer (MangoMix™, Bioline, London, UK), and 2 μL of template DNA. The reaction was run for initial denaturation (94 °C for 60 s) followed by 35 repetitions (denaturation—94 °C, 60 s; annealing—58 °C for 30 s; extension—72 °C for 150 s) and final extension at 72 °C on a Gene Amp PCR system 9700 (Applied Biosystem, Cheshire, UK). PCR products were passed through a 1.5% agarose gel (Fisher, NJ, USA) and visualized on a GelDoc XR gel imaging system (Bio-Rad, Hertfordshire, UK).

4.5. Statistical Analysis

Statistical analysis was performed in SPSS 23.0 (IBM, SPSS, Hampshire, UK). The normality of data was tested through the Shapiro–Wilk test. A *t*-test was run to check for the no-normality violation and homogeneity assumptions. Data were considered significant at a confidence interval of 99.95% ($p < 0.05$). Regression tests applying rectilinear models were employed to establish the correlation between *intI1*-GC resistance. Homogeneity of variance, data normality, and dimensions of linearity were also explored.

Supplementary Materials: The following supporting information can be downloaded at: https://www.mdpi.com/article/10.3390/antibiotics12091366/s1. Table S1: Antibiotic resistance genes filtered through ResFinder; Table S2: Plasmids found in selected isolates of *E. coli*; Table S3: Integrons and associated elements filtered from the integrall database.; Table S4: GPS coordinates and physicochemical parameters of sampling sites; Table S5: Metadata of *E. coli* isolates used for sequencing.

Author Contributions: H.A.A.-S.: conceptualization, methodology, validation, resources; N.H.: software, data curation, writing—original draft, writing—review and editing, visualization; S.U.: investigation, writing—review and editing; A.N.J.: investigation, methodology; M.A.A.-S.: investigation, methodology; B.P.L.: conceptualization, supervision, project administration. All authors have read and agreed to the published version of the manuscript.

Funding: This research received no external funding.

Institutional Review Board Statement: Not Applicable.

Informed Consent Statement: Not Applicable.

Data Availability Statement: Raw Sequences are hosted on the web portal of the National Centre for Biotechnology Information (NCBI) under accession no. PRJNA955288 (SRR24162651 to SRR24162673) https://dataview.ncbi.nlm.nih.gov/object/PRJNA955288?reviewer=gfeu7sag3l3hgq6o8k49nk974 (accessed on 15 June 2023).

Acknowledgments: We are thankful to Plymouth University for providing the facilities for whole-genome sequencing.

Conflicts of Interest: The authors declare no conflict of interest.

References

1. Bungau, S.; Tit, D.M.; Behl, T.; Aleya, L.; Zaha, D.C. Aspects of excessive antibiotic consumption and environmental influences correlated with the occurrence of resistance to antimicrobial agents. *Curr. Opin. Environ. Sci. Health* **2021**, *19*, 100224.
2. Kraemer, S.A.; Ramachandran, A.; Perron, G.G. Antibiotic pollution in the environment: From microbial ecology to public policy. *Microorganisms* **2019**, *7*, 180.
3. Thompson, T. The staggering death toll of drug-resistant bacteria. *Nature* **2022**, *Online ahead of print*.
4. Marti, E.; Variatza, E.; Balcazar, J.L. The role of aquatic ecosystems as reservoirs of antibiotic resistance. *Trends Microbiol.* **2014**, *22*, 36–41. [CrossRef]
5. Baquero, F.; Alvarez-Ortega, C.; Martinez, J.L. Ecology and evolution of antibiotic resistance. *Environ. Microbiol. Rep.* **2009**, *1*, 469–476.
6. Al-Ghadban, A.; Uddin, S.; Aba, A.; Ali, L.N.; Al-Sharmoukh, D.; Al-Khabbaz, A.; Al-Mutairi, A. *Measurement and Assessment of Radionuclide Concentrations in the Coastal Marine Environment*; Kuwait Institute for Scientific Research: Kuwait City, Kuwait, 2011; p. 128.
7. Gevao, B.; Jaward, F.M.; Uddin, S.; Al-Ghadban, A.N. Occurrence and concentrations of polychlorinated dibenzo-p-dioxins (PCDDs) and polychlorinated dibenzofurans (PCDFs) in coastal marine sediments in Kuwait. *Mar. Pollut. Bull.* **2009**, *58*, 452–455.
8. Gevao, B.; Uddin, S.; Dupont, S. Baseline concentrations of pharmaceuticals in Kuwait's coastal marine environment. *Mar. Pollut. Bull.* **2021**, *173*, 113040.
9. Uddin, S.; Aba, A.; Fowler, S.; Behbehani, M.; Ismaeel, A.; Al-Shammari, H.; Alboloushi, A.; Mietelski, J.; Al-Ghadban, A.; Al-Ghunaim, A. Radioactivity in the Kuwait marine environment—Baseline measurements and review. *Mar. Pollut. Bull.* **2015**, *100*, 651–661.
10. Uddin, S.; Fowler, S.W.; Saeed, T. Microplastic particles in the Persian/Arabian Gulf–a review on sampling and identification. *Mar. Pollut. Bull.* **2020**, *154*, 111100.
11. Uddin, S.; Fowler, S.W.; Habibi, N.; Behbehani, M. Micro-Nano Plastic in the Aquatic Environment: Methodological Problems and Challenges. *Animals* **2022**, *12*, 297.
12. Hernando-Amado, S.; Coque, T.M.; Baquero, F.; Martínez, J.L. Defining and combating antibiotic resistance from One Health and Global Health perspectives. *Nat. Microbiol.* **2019**, *4*, 1432–1442.
13. Chen, J.; McIlroy, S.E.; Archana, A.; Baker, D.M.; Panagiotou, G. A pollution gradient contributes to the taxonomic, functional, and resistome diversity of microbial communities in marine sediments. *Microbiome* **2019**, *7*, 1–12.
14. Amarasiri, M.; Sano, D.; Suzuki, S. Understanding human health risks caused by antibiotic resistant bacteria (ARB) and antibiotic resistance genes (ARG) in water environments: Current knowledge and questions to be answered. *Crit. Rev. Environ. Sci. Technol.* **2020**, *50*, 2016–2059.
15. Uddin, S.; Fowler, S.W.; Uddin, M.F.; Behbehani, M.; Naji, A. A review of microplastic distribution in sediment profiles. *Mar. Pollut. Bull.* **2021**, *163*, 111973.
16. Habibi, N.; Uddin, S.; Bottein, M.Y.D.; Faizuddin, M. Ciguatera in the Indian Ocean with Special Insights on the Arabian Sea and Adjacent Gulf and Seas: A Review. *Toxins* **2021**, *13*, 525.
17. Uddin, S.; Al-Ghadban, A.; Gevao, B.; Al-Shamroukh, D.; Al-Khabbaz, A. Estimation of suspended particulate matter in Gulf using MODIS data. *Aquat. Ecosyst. Health Manag.* **2012**, *15*, 41–44. [CrossRef]
18. Habibi, N.; Uddin, S.; Al-Sarawi, H.; Aldhameer, A.; Shajan, A.; Zakir, F.; Abdul Razzack, N.; Alam, F. Metagenomes from Coastal Sediments of Kuwait: Insights into the Microbiome, Metabolic Functions and Resistome. *Microorganisms* **2023**, *11*, 531.
19. Wright, G.D. Antibiotic resistance in the environment: A link to the clinic? *Curr. Opin. Microbiol.* **2010**, *13*, 589–594.

20. Perry, J.A.; Wright, G.D. The antibiotic resistance "mobilome": Searching for the link between environment and clinic. *Front. Microbiol.* **2013**, *4*, 138.
21. Von Wintersdorff, C.J.; Penders, J.; Van Niekerk, J.M.; Mills, N.D.; Majumder, S.; Van Alphen, L.B.; Savelkoul, P.H.; Wolffs, P.F. Dissemination of antimicrobial resistance in microbial ecosystems through horizontal gene transfer. *Front. Microbiol.* **2016**, *7*, 173.
22. Perry, J.A.; Wright, G.D. Forces shaping the antibiotic resistome. *BioEssays* **2014**, *36*, 1179–1184.
23. Anonymous. *Antimicrobial Resistance: Global Report on Surveillance*; World Health Organization: Geneva, Switzerland, 2014.
24. Devlin, M.; Le Quesne, W.J.; Lyons, B.P. The marine environment of Kuwait—Emerging issues in a rapidly changing environment. *Mar. Pollut. Bull.* **2015**, *100*, 593–596.
25. Le Quesne, W.J.; Baker-Austin, C.; Verner-Jeffreys, D.W.; Al-Sarawi, H.A.; Balkhy, H.H.; Lyons, B.P. Antimicrobial resistance in the Gulf Cooperation Council region: A proposed framework to assess threats, impacts and mitigation measures associated with AMR in the marine and aquatic environment. *Environ. Int.* **2018**, *121*, 1003–1010.
26. Habibi, N.; Uddin, S.; Lyons, B.; Al-Sarawi, H.A.; Behbehani, M.; Shajan, A.; Razzack, N.A.; Zakir, F.; Alam, F. Antibiotic Resistance Genes Associated with Marine Surface Sediments: A Baseline from the Shores of Kuwait. *Sustainability* **2022**, *14*, 8029.
27. Al-Sarawi, H.A.; Jha, A.N.; Al-Sarawi, M.A.; Lyons, B.P. Historic and contemporary contamination in the marine environment of Kuwait: An overview. *Mar. Pollut. Bull.* **2015**, *100*, 621–628.
28. Al-Sarawi, H.A.; Jha, A.N.; Baker-Austin, C.; Al-Sarawi, M.A.; Lyons, B.P. Baseline screening for the presence of antimicrobial resistance in E. coli isolated from Kuwait's marine environment. *Mar. Pollut. Bull.* **2018**, *129*, 893–898.
29. Al-Sarawi, H.A.; Najem, A.B.; Lyons, B.P.; Uddin, S.; Al-Sarawi, M.A. Antimicrobial Resistance in Escherichia coli Isolated from Marine Sediment Samples from Kuwait Bay. *Sustainability* **2022**, *14*, 11325. [CrossRef]
30. Zhu, L.-X.; Zhang, Z.-W.; Liang, D.; Jiang, D.; Wang, C.; Du, N.; Zhang, Q.; Mitchelson, K.; Cheng, J. Multiplex asymmetric PCR-based oligonucleotide microarray for detection of drug resistance genes containing single mutations in Enterobacteriaceae. *Antimicrob. Agents Chemother.* **2007**, *51*, 3707–3713.
31. Papan, C.; Meyer-Buehn, M.; Laniado, G.; Nicolai, T.; Griese, M.; Huebner, J. Assessment of the multiplex PCR-based assay Unyvero pneumonia application for detection of bacterial pathogens and antibiotic resistance genes in children and neonates. *Infection* **2018**, *46*, 189–196.
32. Burakoff, A.; Brown, K.; Knutsen, J.; Hopewell, C.; Rowe, S.; Bennett, C.; Cronquist, A. Outbreak of fluoroquinolone-resistant Campylobacter jejuni infections associated with raw milk consumption from a herdshare dairy—Colorado, 2016. *Morb. Mortal. Wkly. Rep.* **2018**, *67*, 146.
33. Nemergut, D.; Martin, A.; Schmidt, S. Integron diversity in heavy-metal-contaminated mine tailings and inferences about integron evolution. *Appl. Environ. Microbiol.* **2004**, *70*, 1160–1168.
34. Pournajaf, A.; Ardebili, A.; Goudarzi, L.; Khodabandeh, M.; Narimani, T.; Abbaszadeh, H. PCR-based identification of methicillin–resistant Staphylococcus aureus strains and their antibiotic resistance profiles. *Asian Pac. J. Trop. Biomed.* **2014**, *4*, S293–S297.
35. Khan, M.W.; Habibi, N.; Shaheed, F.; Mustafa, A.S. Draft genome sequences of five clinical strains of Brucella melitensis isolated from patients residing in Kuwait. *Genome Announc.* **2016**, *4*, e01144-16. [CrossRef]
36. Light, E.; Baker-Austin, C.; Card, R.M.; Ryder, D.; Alves, M.T.; Al-Sarawi, H.A.; Abdulla, K.H.; Stahl, H.; Aliya, A.-G.; Al Ghoribi, M. Establishing a marine monitoring programme to assess antibiotic resistance: A case study from the Gulf Cooperation Council (GCC) region. *medRxiv* **2022**, *9*, 100268.
37. Cabello-Yeves, P.J.; Callieri, C.; Picazo, A.; Mehrshad, M.; Haro-Moreno, J.M.; Roda-Garcia, J.J.; Dzhembekova, N.; Slabakova, V.; Slabakova, N.; Moncheva, S. The microbiome of the Black Sea water column analyzed by shotgun and genome centric metagenomics. *Environ. Microbiome* **2021**, *16*, 1–15.
38. Ruppé, E.; Cherkaoui, A.; Charretier, Y.; Girard, M.; Schicklin, S.; Lazarevic, V.; Schrenzel, J. From genotype to antibiotic susceptibility phenotype in the order Enterobacterales: A clinical perspective. *Clin. Microbiol. Infect.* **2020**, *26*, 643.e641–643.e647.
39. Zhang, X.-X.; Zhang, T.; Zhang, M.; Fang, H.H.; Cheng, S.-P. Characterization and quantification of class 1 integrons and associated gene cassettes in sewage treatment plants. *Appl. Microbiol. Biotechnol.* **2009**, *82*, 1169–1177.
40. Grevskott, D.H.; Svanevik, C.S.; Sunde, M.; Wester, A.L.; Lunestad, B.T. Marine bivalve mollusks as possible indicators of multidrug-resistant Escherichia coli and other species of the Enterobacteriaceae family. *Front. Microbiol.* **2017**, *8*, 24. [CrossRef]
41. Beaz-Hidalgo, R.; Balboa, S.; Romalde, J.L.; Figueras, M.J. Diversity and pathogenecity of Vibrio species in cultured bivalve molluscs. *Environ. Microbiol. Rep.* **2010**, *2*, 34–43.
42. Giacometti, F.; Pezzi, A.; Galletti, G.; Tamba, M.; Merialdi, G.; Piva, S.; Serraino, A.; Rubini, S. Antimicrobial resistance patterns in Salmonella enterica subsp. enterica and Escherichia coli isolated from bivalve molluscs and marine environment. *Food Control* **2021**, *121*, 107590.
43. Gevao, B.; Uddin, S.; Krishnan, D.; Rajagopalan, S.; Habibi, N. Antibiotics in Wastewater: Baseline of the Influent and Effluent Streams in Kuwait. *Toxics* **2022**, *10*, 174. [CrossRef] [PubMed]
44. Wright, G.D. The antibiotic resistome: The nexus of chemical and genetic diversity. *Nat. Rev. Microbiol.* **2007**, *5*, 175–186. [CrossRef] [PubMed]
45. Wright, M.S.; Baker-Austin, C.; Lindell, A.H.; Stepanauskas, R.; Stokes, H.W.; McArthur, J.V. Influence of industrial contamination on mobile genetic elements: Class 1 integron abundance and gene cassette structure in aquatic bacterial communities. *ISME J.* **2008**, *2*, 417–428. [CrossRef]

46. Waśko, I.; Kozińska, A.; Kotlarska, E.; Baraniak, A. Clinically Relevant β-Lactam Resistance Genes in Wastewater Treatment Plants. *Int. J. Environ. Res. Public Health* **2022**, *19*, 13829. [CrossRef]
47. Tooke, C.L.; Hinchliffe, P.; Bragginton, E.C.; Colenso, C.K.; Hirvonen, V.H.; Takebayashi, Y.; Spencer, J. β-Lactamases and β-Lactamase Inhibitors in the 21st Century. *J. Mol. Biol.* **2019**, *431*, 3472–3500. [CrossRef] [PubMed]
48. Pongchaikul, P.; Mongkolsuk, P. Comprehensive Analysis of Imipenemase (IMP)-Type Metallo-β-Lactamase: A Global Distribution Threatening Asia. *Antibiotics* **2022**, *11*, 236. [CrossRef] [PubMed]
49. Habibi, N.; Uddin, S.; Behbehani, M.; Kishk, M.; Abdul Razzack, N.; Zakir, F.; Shajan, A. Antibiotic Resistance Genes in Aerosols: Baseline from Kuwait. *Int. J. Mol. Sci.* **2023**, *24*, 6756. [CrossRef] [PubMed]
50. Ryu, S.-H.; Park, S.-G.; Choi, S.-M.; Hwang, Y.-O.; Ham, H.-J.; Kim, S.-U.; Lee, Y.-K.; Kim, M.-S.; Park, G.-Y.; Kim, K.-S. Antimicrobial resistance and resistance genes in Escherichia coli strains isolated from commercial fish and seafood. *Int. J. Food Microbiol.* **2012**, *152*, 14–18. [CrossRef]
51. Koczura, R.; Mokracka, J.; Jabłońska, L.; Gozdecka, E.; Kubek, M.; Kaznowski, A. Antimicrobial resistance of integron-harboring Escherichia coli isolates from clinical samples, wastewater treatment plant and river water. *Sci. Total Environ.* **2012**, *414*, 680–685. [CrossRef]
52. Lyons, B.; Devlin, M.; Hamid, S.A.; Al-Otiabi, A.; Al-Enezi, M.; Massoud, M.; Al-Zaidan, A.; Smith, A.; Morris, S.; Bersuder, P. Microbial water quality and sedimentary faecal sterols as markers of sewage contamination in Kuwait. *Mar. Pollut. Bull.* **2015**, *100*, 689–698. [CrossRef]
53. Lyons, B.; Barber, J.; Rumney, H.; Bolam, T.; Bersuder, P.; Law, R.; Mason, C.; Smith, A.; Morris, S.; Devlin, M. Baseline survey of marine sediments collected from the State of Kuwait: PAHs, PCBs, brominated flame retardants and metal contamination. *Mar. Pollut. Bull.* **2015**, *100*, 629–636. [CrossRef]
54. Gaze, W.H.; Zhang, L.; Abdouslam, N.A.; Hawkey, P.M.; Calvo-Bado, L.; Royle, J.; Brown, H.; Davis, S.; Kay, P.; Boxall, A. Impacts of anthropogenic activity on the ecology of class 1 integrons and integron-associated genes in the environment. *ISME J.* **2011**, *5*, 1253–1261. [CrossRef]
55. Stalder, T.; Barraud, O.; Casellas, M.; Dagot, C.; Ploy, M.-C. Integron involvement in environmental spread of antibiotic resistance. *Front. Microbiol.* **2012**, *3*, 119. [CrossRef]
56. Zhang, H.; Wang, Y.; Liu, P.; Sun, Y.; Dong, X.; Hu, X. Unveiling the occurrence, hosts and mobility potential of antibiotic resistance genes in the deep ocean. *Sci. Total Environ.* **2022**, *816*, 151539. [CrossRef] [PubMed]
57. Yang, H.; Liu, R.; Liu, H.; Wang, C.; Yin, X.; Zhang, M.; Fang, J.; Zhang, T.; Ma, L. Evidence for Long-Term Anthropogenic Pollution: The Hadal Trench as a Depository and Indicator for Dissemination of Antibiotic Resistance Genes. *Environ. Sci. Technol.* **2021**, *55*, 15136–15148. [CrossRef] [PubMed]
58. Domingues, S.; Da Silva, G.J.; Nielsen, K.M. Global dissemination patterns of common gene cassette arrays in class 1 integrons. *Microbiology* **2015**, *161*, 1313–1337. [CrossRef] [PubMed]
59. Hastey, C.J.; Boyd, H.; Schuetz, A.N.; Anderson, K.; Citron, D.M.; Dzink-Fox, J.; Hackel, M.; Hecht, D.W.; Jacobus, N.V.; Jenkins, S.G. Changes in the antibiotic susceptibility of anaerobic bacteria from 2007–2009 to 2010–2012 based on the CLSI methodology. *Anaerobe* **2016**, *42*, 27–30. [CrossRef] [PubMed]
60. Al Salameen, F.; Habibi, N.; Uddin, S.; Al Mataqi, K.; Kumar, V.; Al Doaij, B.; Al Amad, S.; Al Ali, E.; Shirshikhar, F. Spatio-temporal variations in bacterial and fungal community associated with dust aerosol in Kuwait. *PLoS ONE* **2020**, *15*, e0241283. [CrossRef]
61. Bolger, A.M.; Lohse, M.; Usadel, B. Trimmomatic: A flexible trimmer for Illumina sequence data. *Bioinformatics* **2014**, *30*, 2114–2120. [CrossRef]
62. Andrews, S. FastQC: A quality control tool for high throughput sequence data. *Retrieved May* **2010**, *17*, 2018.
63. Bankevich, A.; Nurk, S.; Antipov, D.; Gurevich, A.A.; Dvorkin, M.; Kulikov, A.S.; Lesin, V.M.; Nikolenko, S.I.; Pham, S.; Prjibelski, A.D. SPAdes: A new genome assembly algorithm and its applications to single-cell sequencing. *J. Comput. Biol.* **2012**, *19*, 455–477. [CrossRef]
64. Seemann, T. Prokka: Rapid prokaryotic genome annotation. *Bioinformatics* **2014**, *30*, 2068–2069. [CrossRef]
65. Seemann, T. *ABRicate: Mass Screening of Contigs for Antibiotic Resistance Genes*; GitHub: San Francisco, CA, USA, 2016.
66. Bortolaia, V.; Kaas, R.S.; Ruppe, E.; Roberts, M.C.; Schwarz, S.; Cattoir, V.; Philippon, A.; Allesoe, R.L.; Rebelo, A.R.; Florensa, A.F. ResFinder 4.0 for predictions of phenotypes from genotypes. *J. Antimicrob. Chemother.* **2020**, *75*, 3491–3500. [CrossRef]
67. Carattoli, A.; Hasman, H. PlasmidFinder and In Silico pMLST: Identification and Typing of Plasmid Replicons in Whole-Genome Sequencing (WGS). In *Horizontal Gene Transfer. Methods in Molecular Biology*; de la Cruz, F., Ed.; Humana: New York, NY, USA, 2020; Volume 2075, pp. 285–294. [CrossRef]
68. Néron, B.; Littner, E.; Haudiquet, M.; Perrin, A.; Cury, J.; Rocha, E.P. IntegronFinder 2.0: Identification and analysis of integrons across bacteria, with a focus on antibiotic resistance in Klebsiella. *Microorganisms* **2022**, *10*, 700. [CrossRef] [PubMed]
69. Finn, R.D.; Tate, J.; Mistry, J.; Coggill, P.C.; Sammut, S.J.; Hotz, H.-R.; Ceric, G.; Forslund, K.; Eddy, S.R.; Sonnhammer, E.L. The Pfam protein families database. *Nucleic Acids Res.* **2007**, *36*, D281–D288. [CrossRef] [PubMed]
70. Finn, R.D.; Clements, J.; Eddy, S.R. HMMER web server: Interactive sequence similarity searching. *Nucleic Acids Res.* **2011**, *39*, W29–W37. [CrossRef] [PubMed]
71. Katoh, K.; Misawa, K.; Kuma, K.i.; Miyata, T. MAFFT: A novel method for rapid multiple sequence alignment based on fast Fourier transform. *Nucleic Acids Res.* **2002**, *30*, 3059–3066. [CrossRef]

72. Okonechnikov, K.; Golosova, O.; Fursov, M.; Team, U. Unipro UGENE: A unified bioinformatics toolkit. *Bioinformatics* **2012**, *28*, 1166–1167. [CrossRef]
73. Price, M.N.; Dehal, P.S.; Arkin, A.P. FastTree 2–approximately maximum-likelihood trees for large alignments. *PLoS ONE* **2010**, *5*, e9490. [CrossRef]
74. FigTree. Molecular, Evolution, Phylogenetic and Epidemiology v1.4.2. Available online: http://tree.bio.ed.ac.uk/software/figtree/ (accessed on 17 May 2017).
75. Alsarawi, H.A. *Developing an Integrated Strategy for the Assessment of Hazardous Substances in Kuwait's Marine Environment*; University of Plymouth: Plymouth, UK, 2017.
76. Mustafa, A.S.; Habibi, N.; Osman, A.; Shaheed, F.; Khan, M.W. Species identification and molecular typing of human *Brucella* isolates from Kuwait. *PLoS ONE* **2017**, *12*, e0182111. [CrossRef]
77. Mazel, D.; Dychinco, B.; Webb, V.A.; Davies, J. Antibiotic resistance in the ECOR collection: Integrons and identification of a novel aad gene. *Antimicrob. Agents Chemother.* **2000**, *44*, 1568–1574. [CrossRef] [PubMed]

antibiotics

MDPI

Review

The African Wastewater Resistome: Identifying Knowledge Gaps to Inform Future Research Directions

Akebe Luther King Abia [1,2,*], Themba Baloyi [1], Afsatou N. Traore [1] and Natasha Potgieter [1,*]

1 One Health Research Group, Biochemistry & Microbiology Department, University of Venda, Private Bag X5050, Thohoyandou 0950, South Africa; thembabaloyi17@gmail.com (T.B.); afsatou.traore@univen.ac.za (A.N.T.)

2 Environmental Research Foundation, Westville 3630, South Africa

* Correspondence: lutherkinga@yahoo.fr (A.L.K.A.); natasha.potgieter@univen.ac.za (N.P.)

Abstract: Antimicrobial resistance (AMR) is a growing global public health threat. Furthermore, wastewater is increasingly recognized as a significant environmental reservoir for AMR. Wastewater is a complex mixture of organic and inorganic compounds, including antibiotics and other antimicrobial agents, discharged from hospitals, pharmaceutical industries, and households. Therefore, wastewater treatment plants (WWTPs) are critical components of urban infrastructure that play a vital role in protecting public health and the environment. However, they can also be a source of AMR. WWTPs serve as a point of convergence for antibiotics and resistant bacteria from various sources, creating an environment that favours the selection and spread of AMR. The effluent from WWTPs can also contaminate surface freshwater and groundwater resources, which can subsequently spread resistant bacteria to the wider environment. In Africa, the prevalence of AMR in wastewater is of particular concern due to the inadequate sanitation and wastewater treatment facilities, coupled with the overuse and misuse of antibiotics in healthcare and agriculture. Therefore, the present review evaluated studies that reported on wastewater in Africa between 2012 and 2022 to identify knowledge gaps and propose future perspectives, informing the use of wastewater-based epidemiology as a proxy for determining the resistome circulating within the continent. The study found that although wastewater resistome studies have increased over time in Africa, this is not the case in every country, with most studies conducted in South Africa. Furthermore, the study identified, among others, methodology and reporting gaps, driven by a lack of skills. Finally, the review suggests solutions including standardisation of protocols in wastewater resistome works and an urgent need to build genomic skills within the continent to handle the big data generated from these studies.

Keywords: low- and middle-income countries; environmental health; public health; wastewater monitoring; antimicrobial resistance; antibiotic-resistant bacteria; antibiotic resistance genes; wastewater-based epidemiology

Citation: Abia, A.L.K.; Baloyi, T.; Traore, A.N.; Potgieter, N. The African Wastewater Resistome: Identifying Knowledge Gaps to Inform Future Research Directions. *Antibiotics* **2023**, *12*, 805. https://doi.org/10.3390/antibiotics12050805

Academic Editor: Jie Fu

Received: 16 March 2023
Revised: 20 April 2023
Accepted: 21 April 2023
Published: 24 April 2023

1. Introduction

Antimicrobial resistance (AMR) has been recognised by countries and organisations worldwide as one of the biggest threats to public health in recent times [1–3]. It is estimated that without appropriate preventive or remedial measures, the world may experience approximately 10 million losses of lives and over USD 100 trillion annually in the global economy by 2050 [4].

Although micro-organisms possess intrinsic resistance to naturally occurring stressors, the indiscriminate use of pharmaceuticals has been recognised as the most significant contributor to acquired resistance in these organisms, thus escalating the threat to human health [5,6]. For example, the massive and increasing demand for animal protein has engendered an unparalleled use of antibiotics in food animal production, which in 2017 was estimated at 93,309 tons per year globally, with an expected 11.5% increase by 2030 [7].

Furthermore, in humans, misdiagnosis of infections results in the inappropriate prescription of many antibiotics [8]. Therefore, to curb this ill, the World Health Organization (WHO) has identified critical factors driving AMR, including the abusive use of these pharmaceuticals, nonavailability of clean water, sanitation and hygiene (WASH) for human and animal use, inadequate measures to control and prevent infections and diseases in health and animal production settings, inaccessibility to good, and cost-effective medications, vaccines and test procedures, unawareness and lack of knowledge regarding the problem, and nonenforcement of legislation [9].

However, a considerable proportion of the antibiotics consumed by humans and animals are mostly excreted in partially or completely unmetabolised forms, usually containing active ingredients [10,11]. This results in the inevitable discharge of these pharmaceutically active compounds into the environment, especially water bodies, with the major consequence being the potential selection for the survival of resistant micro-organisms. With this, wastewater treatment plants (WWTPs) have been recognised as being among the hotspots for the discharge of antibiotics, their residues and antibiotic-resistant bacteria into the environment [12–17].

Despite the perceived role of these WWTPs on the spread of AMR, studies evaluating their impact are limited, especially in low- and middle-income countries (LMICs) such as South Africa, where such facilities are usually nonfunctional or function sub-optimally. Furthermore, where such studies are available, the link between environmental and clinical isolates is not apparent, probably because of the basic analyses performed that usually have low discriminating powers to establish such associations. Moreover, the lack of proper reporting of findings influences the acquisition of such data in the public domain. Thus, the present review evaluated the existing literature on AMR in Africa between 2012 and 2022, emphasising South Africa as a case study, to identify gaps that need to be filled to inform future preventive and mitigation measures towards AMR.

2. Overview of African Studies between 2012 and 2022

In Africa, the prevalence of AMR in wastewater is of particular concern due to the inadequate sanitation and wastewater treatment facilities, coupled with the overuse and misuse of antibiotics in healthcare and agriculture. African countries, especially in the sub-Saharan region, have the highest disease burdens in the world, with infectious diseases accounting for over 227 million healthy life years and over USD 800 billion yearly productivity loss globally [18]. The ripple effect of this health situation has been identified as the primary factor driving the excessive rate of antimicrobial prescriptions within the continent [19]. For example, consumption of antibiotics in the WHO Watch list increased by 165% in LMIC (including African countries) compared to approximately 28% in their high-income counterparts between 2000 and 2015 [19].

This high antibiotic use implies that wastewater in these countries would be rich in antibiotic residues, antibiotic-resistant bacteria (ARB) and their associated antibiotic-resistance genes (ARGs). For example, a study in Ghana investigated resistance genes, mobile genetic elements (MGEs), from drainage and canalizations before and after three hospitals and an urban waste treatment plant [20]. The main idea was to establish the relationship between the hospital and the wastewater resistome. The authors used a combination of culture-dependent and independent methods, including high-throughput whole-genome sequencing on two sequencing platforms, Nanopore (long reads) and Illumina (short reads). The authors recorded higher resistance rates to carbapenems in the canalization after the hospitals, indicating that the hospital wastewater contributed significantly to the dissemination of resistant bacteria in the environment. Furthermore, the study identified several carbapenemase/β-lactamase genes, including novel variants, such as $bla_{\text{DIM-1}}$, $bla_{\text{VIM-71}}$, $bla_{\text{CARB-53}}$, and $bla_{\text{CMY-172}}$, with some of these genes associated with MGEs, meaning that these could easily be transferred within and between bacterial communities.

In Nigeria, Akpan et al. [21] isolated Gram-negative bacteria from an abattoir's wastewater and tested them for antibiotic resistance against five antibiotics, to determine the impact of the abattoir on the environmental resistome. The organisms isolated included *Salmonella* spp., *E. coli*, *Klebsiella* spp., *Shigella* spp., *Pseudomonas* spp. and *Enterobacter* spp. The authors observed that a significant proportion of the isolates (~67%) were resistant to all antibiotics tested, with a 77% multidrug resistance recorded across the samples. However, no extended-spectrum β-lactamase (ESBL)-producing traits were observed in any of the isolates. This study demonstrated that abattoirs contributed considerably to AMR in the aquatic environment.

Tesfaye et al. [22] investigated antimicrobial resistance in *Enterobacteriaceae* in wastewater collected from health settings, an abattoir, and a WWTP, including downstream of a river in Addis Ababa, Ethiopia. The authors obtained 54 isolates, including *E. coli*, *Salmonella* spp., *Klebsiella pneumoniae*, *Enterobacter aerogenes*, *Citrobacter* spp., *Klebsiella oxytoca* and *Enterobacter cloacae*. Antibiotic susceptibility testing revealed that all the isolates were multidrug resistant, while 2 isolates were resistant to all the 12 antibiotics tested. ESBL production was also recorded in 27.3% of the resistant isolates. Furthermore, the hospital wastewater had a higher percentage of resistance than all the other sites, again identifying hospital wastewater as a hotspot for AMR dissemination.

A major shortcoming in all the studies reviewed is that most of them focused on a one-off sampling, usually resulting in a very limited number of isolates or samples. Such small sample sizes would make it challenging to draw strong conclusions and would require further investigations. Furthermore, many studies used either culture or sequencing and only a few used both methods. Using only the culture methods could underestimate the microbial load due to viable but non-culturable isolates, hence reducing the actual resistome reported. On the other hand, using only genomic approaches could overestimate the risk associated with AMR in wastewater. Nevertheless, the presence of any resistance genes and MGEs would signify the possible transmission to other related or even unrelated species. A summary of some studies on wastewater resistome in Africa is provided in Table 1.

Table 1. Summary of some studies on AMR in wastewater in Africa between 2012 and 2022.

Country	& Wastewater Type/Source	Duration of Study	Sample Size	Targeted Resistance	Phenotypic (P)/Genotypic (G) Resistance	Method	Reference
* South Africa	WWTP	Two campaigns—actual duration not mentioned	# Not indicated	Cefotaxime-resistance	P	Culture	[23]
Algeria	WWTP	3 days in 2 months	Not indicated	ESBLs and associated quinolone resistance	P, G	Culture; PCR	[24]
Botswana	WWTP	$ One-off sampling	one	Overall resistome	G	Shotgun metagenomics	[25]
Botswana	WWTP	Monthly for 1 year	72	General resistance—9 antibiotics tested	P	Culture	[26]
Burkina Faso	Urban channel	6 months	101	ESBLs	P	Culture	[27]
Burkina Faso	WWTP	Monthly for 5 months	15	General resistance—19 antibiotics	P	Culture	[28]
Cameroon	Open-air canals	One-off	6 (composite) samples	Overall resistome	G	Shotgun metagenomics	[29]
Ethiopia	Hospital wastewater	3 months	27	General resistance—13 antibiotics	P	Culture	[30]

Table 1. *Cont.*

Country	[&] Wastewater Type/Source	Duration of Study	Sample Size	Targeted Resistance	Phenotypic (P)/Genotypic (G) Resistance	Method	Reference
Ethiopia	Hospital wastewater	4 months	40 (composite samples)	General resistance—13 antibiotics	P	Culture	[31]
Ghana	WWTP	Monthly—6 months	30	General resistance	P	Culture	[32]
Kenya	University WWTP	4 months	Not mentioned	Overall resistome	P, G	Culture; whole-genome sequencing	[33]
Kenya	Septic tank	2 months	Not mentioned	General resistance	P	Culture	[34]
Kenya	WWTP	6 months (covering the dry and rainy seasons)	24	General resistance	P	Culture	[35]
Nigeria	Hospital WWTP	Weekly for 4 months	Not mentioned	ESBLs	P, G	Culture; PCR	Adekanmbi
Senegal	Slaughterhouse wastewater and WWTP	Not mentioned	Not mentioned	General resistance—16 antibiotics	P	Culture	[36]
South Africa	WWTP	7 months (Every two weeks)	81	Overall resistome	P, G	Culture; whole-genome sequencing	[37]
Tanzania	WWTP	2013/2014 (Not specific)	52	General resistance—14 antibiotics	P	Microdilution	[38]
Tunisia	WWTP	Not mentioned	Not mentioned	*intI1*, ARGs $bla_{CTX\text{-}M}$, bla_{TEM}, *qnr*A, *qnr*S, *sul* I, *erm*B	G	PCR	[39]
Uganda	Multiple sources	Not mentioned	Not mentioned	General resistance—15 antibiotics	P	Culture	[40]
Zambia	Wastewater ponds	Not mentioned	5 samples	General resistance—8 antibiotics	P	Culture	[41]
Zimbabwe	Abattoir wastewater	3 months	600 samples	General resistance—16 antibiotics	P	Culture	[42]

* Part of a multinational (22 countries) study in Europe, Asia, Africa, Australia, and North America. # A total of 472 samples were collected from all the countries. $ Analysed once and used to irrigate soil. Focus was not on the monitoring of the wastewater resistome, but the impact of the wastewater in the soil resistome. & Includes influent or effluent or both.

Despite the recognised role of WWTPs in AMR, studies on AMR in wastewater are not evenly distributed within the continent, with most of the studies reported in South Africa (Figure 1).

However, it is evident that wastewater as a reservoir and source of AMR is gaining attention in Africa, as seen by the increasing trend of studies focusing on wastewater (Figure 2).

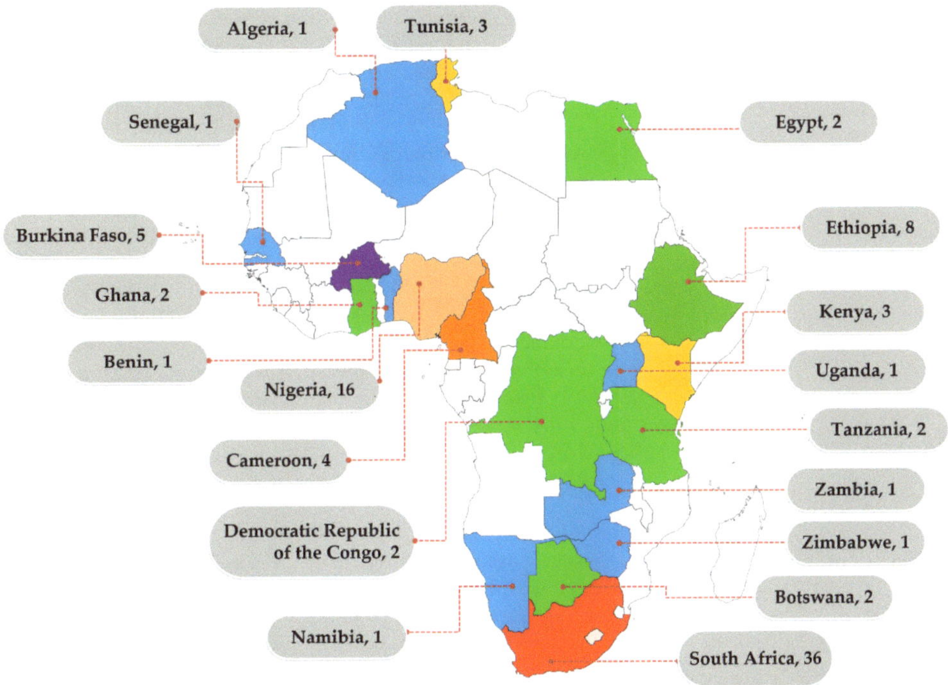

Figure 1. Distribution of African studies on AMR in wastewater between 2012 and 2022. Numbers represent the number of studies identified within the reviewed period. Only counties that reported at least one study in the review period are labelled.

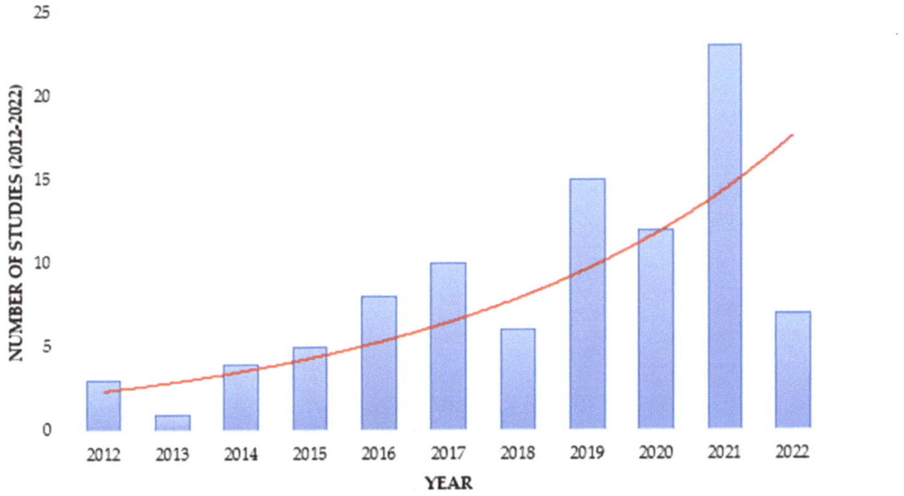

Figure 2. Trend in ARM studies focusing on wastewater. The red line shows the increasing trend within the reviewed period.

3. Case Study: South Africa

3.1. The South African Wastewater Resistome

A 2015 survey assessed antimicrobial use in inpatients in various hospitals globally and reported that over 50% of African patients received antibiotics [19]. However, a later study revealed a 55% inappropriate use of antimicrobials in some South African primary healthcare facilities [43]. Furthermore, South Africa is among the highest consumers of antimicrobials used in food animals. For example, the country consumed over 870 tons of antimicrobials in food-producing animals, and this quantity is estimated to increase to over 1100 tons by 2030, driven by increased demand for animal protein [19]. These use patterns could be responsible for the AMR rates observed within the country and could ultimately result in a significant discharge of chemically active pharmaceutical residues, ARB and ARGs into the environment through poorly treated or untreated WWTP effluents.

The distribution of WWTPs in South Africa is, Eastern Cape: 123, Free State: 96, Gauteng: 60, KwaZulu-Natal: 147, Limpopo: 64, Mpumalanga: 76, Northern Cape: 78, North-West: 48, and Western Cape: 158 [44]. According to the South African Green Drop evaluation, a WWTP should obtain an overall $\geq$ 90% Green Drop score to be considered in an excellent functional state [44]. However, according to the 2022 report, the country's WWTPs have experienced a massive decrease in functional capacity, with the number of WWTPs failing to meet these criteria, significantly increasing from those reported in the preceding report. Thus, monitoring WWTPs would provide an excellent way of determining the AMR burden within the country, and this has attracted interest from the South African scientific community in recent years.

3.2. Distribution of Studies by Province

Several studies have assessed AMR in South African wastewaters. However, a review of the literature between 2012 and 2022 revealed an uneven distribution of the studies within the country's nine regions, with KwaZulu-Natal and the Eastern Cape accounting for the bulk of the studies identified within the study period (Figure 3).

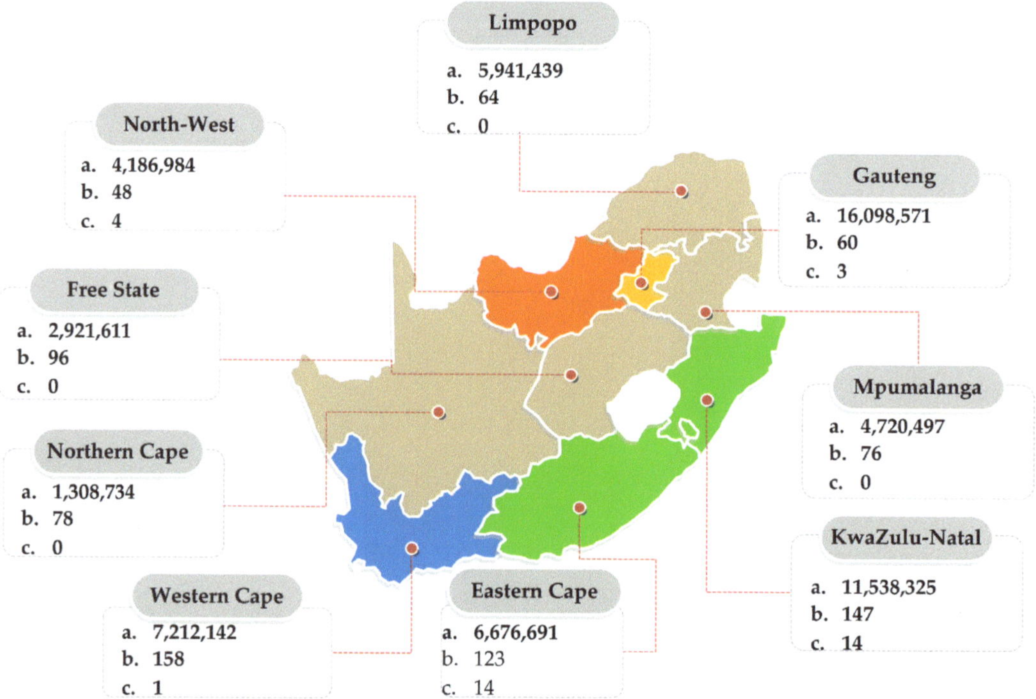

Figure 3. Distribution of South African studies on the wastewater resistome between 2012 and 2022. a = population (https://www.statssa.gov.za/publications/P0302/P03022022.pdf (accessed on 19 April 2023)); b = number of WWTPs in province [44]; c = number of studies.

Although 36 studies were identified on AMR in wastewater within the study period, not all of them focused on WWTPs (Figure 4). While most of the studies were on WWTPs, other sources of wastewater evaluated included hospital wastewater (HWW), abattoirs and domestic wastewater (DWW).

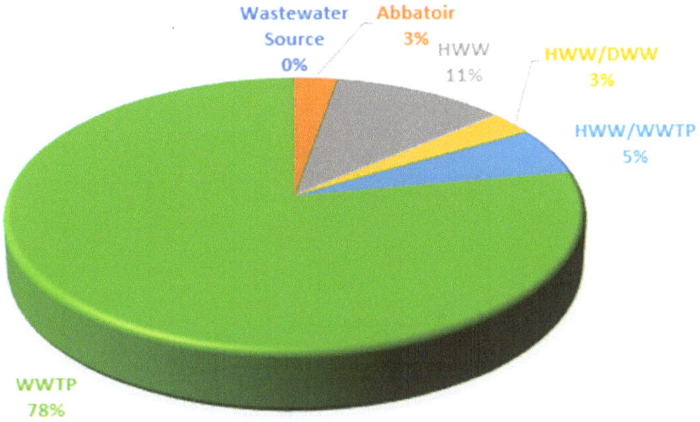

Figure 4. Various wastewater sources evaluated for AMR in South Africa between 2012 and 2022.

3.3. Micro-organisms Targeted

Microbial species in wastewater are diverse, and attempting to identify them all would not be practical, timewise, resource-wise or technically. Thus, using indicator organisms has been the gold standard for determining the microbial quality of microbially contaminated waters [45–49]. Apart from being a good faecal indicator, *Escherichia coli* has been identified as a good indicator of AMR in the environment, including wastewater [50]. Thus, in the current report, *E. coli* was the most identified organism in all the studies evaluated (Figure 5). However, the culture methods and media used for the identification of *E. coli* and other organisms differed considerably between studies (Table 2).

Table 2. Media and incubation conditions used for the identification of different micro-organisms in waterwater AMR studies in South Africa between 2012 and 2022.

Organism	Media	Incubation Temperature (°C)	Duration (Hours)	Reference
Brevibacillus spp.; *Paenibacillus* spp.	R2A media	Not mentioned (NM)	NM	[51]
Acinetobacter baumannii	Leeds Acinetobacter Medium	37	24	[52]
Acinetobacter baumannii; *Acinetobacter* spp.	CHROMagar Acinetobacter	37	18–24	[53,54]
Aeromonas, Exiguobacterium	Nutrient agar, Blood agar	NM	NM	[55]
Aeromonas spp.	Glutamate Starch Phenol-red (GSP) agar plates	37	24	[56]
Aeromonas spp.	Rimler-Shotts agar	37	20	[57]
Aeromonas spp.	Aeromonas spp. Isolation agar	37	24	[58]
Bacillus amyloliquefaciens	nutrient agar	37	18–24	[59]
Bacillus spp.	Nutrient agar, Blood agar	NM	NM	[55]
Bacillus spp.	R2A media	NM	NM	[51]
E. coli	Eosin methylene blue agar	37	24	[60]
E. coli	Membrane Fecal Coliform (mFC) agar supplemented with 4 mg/L or 8 mg/L cefotaxime antibiotic	37	24	[61]
E. coli	Chromocult Coliform Agar (Merck)	37	24	[62]
E. coli	*E. coli*-Coliforms Chromogenic medium	37	24	[63,64]
E. coli	CHROMagar ECC	37	24	[65]
E. coli	*E. coli*-coliform selective agar	37	24	[66]
E. coli	Chromogenic agar *	37	24	[67]
E. coli	Colilert-18^{TM}	37	24	[68]
Enterobacteriaceae	Violet Red Bile Glucose (VRBG) agar	37	18	[69]
Enterococcus spp.	R2A media	NM	NM	[51]

Table 2. *Cont.*

Organism	Media	Incubation Temperature (°C)	Duration (Hours)	Reference
Enterococcus spp.	KF-Streptococcus agar containing 1 mL of 2,3,5-Triphenyltetrazolium chloride	37	48	[70]
Enterococcus spp.	chromogenic 51,759 HiCrome™ Rapid Enterococci Agar media	37	24–48	[71]
Enterococcus spp.	Tryptic Soy Broth	37	18	[67]
Enterococcus spp.	Bile Aesculin Azide Agar	37	24	[67]
Enterococcus spp.	CHROMagar™ VRE, BBL™ Enterococcosel™ Broth	37 ± 2 °C	18 to 24	[72]
Enterococcus spp.	Enterolert™	41	24–48	[68]
Klebsiella spp.	Nutrient agar, Blood agar	NM	NM	[55]
Klebsiella spp.	HiCrome Klebsiella selective agar	35	24	[73]
Listeria spp.	Listeria Chromogenic agar	35	24–48	[57]
Pseudomonas aeruginosa	Mineral salt medium	30	18–24	[59]
Pseudomonas aeruginosa	CHROMagarTM Pseudomonas	37	24–48	[74]
Pseudomonas spp.	Nutrient agar, Blood agar	NM	NM	[55]
Pseudomonas spp.	R2A media	NM	NM	[51]
Pseudomonas spp.	Pseudomonas Isolation Agar	35	24–48	[75]
Pseudomonas spp.	Cetrimide agar	37	24	[58]
Pseudomonas spp.	Glutamate Starch Phenol-red (GSP) agar	37	24	[56]
Salmonella spp.	Salmonella-Shigella (SS) agar	37	24–48	[76]
Shewanella spp.	Nutrient agar, Blood agar	NM	NM	[55]
Staphylococcus aureus	Mannitol Salt Agar supplemented with cefoxitin.	Not mentioned (NM)	NM	[77]
Stenotrophomonas maltophilia	Stenotrophomonas selective agar base with Vancomycin Imipenem Amphotericin B (VIA) supplement	37	18 to 24	[54]
Vibrio spp.	thiosulfate-citrate–bile salt-sucrose (TCBS) agar	37	24	[63,78,79]

* Specific media was not mentioned.

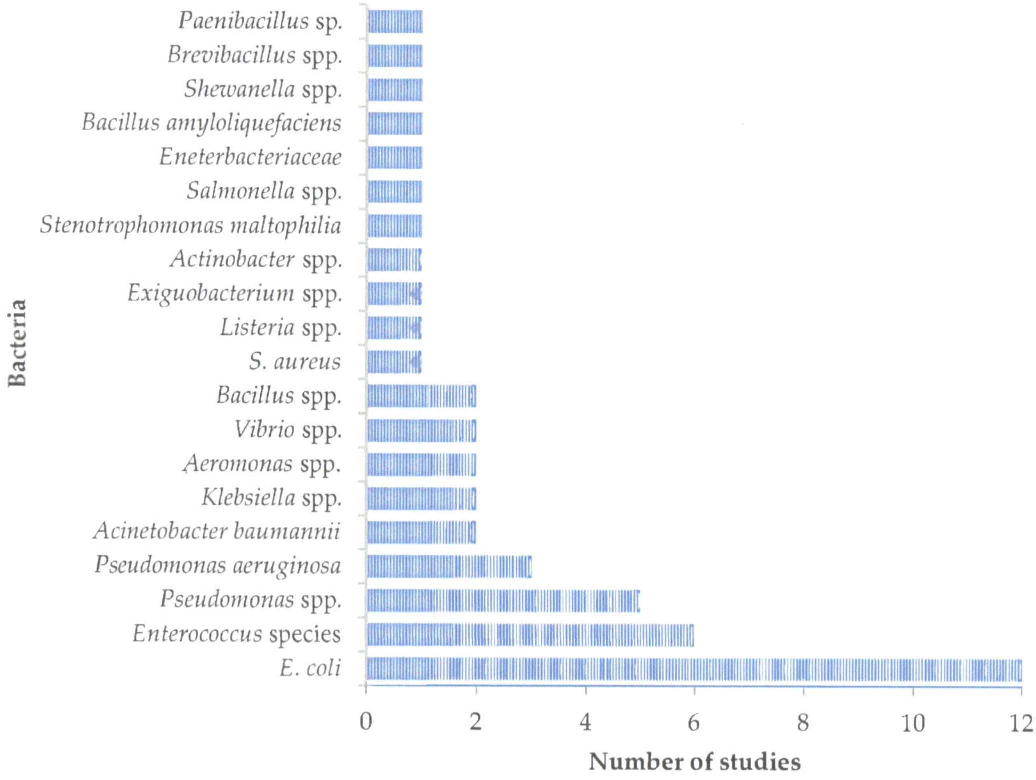

Figure 5. Main micro-organisms identified in South African wastewater (2012–2022).

3.4. AMR Determination Methods

The methods used to determine AMR in wastewater samples depend on the aim of the study. Determination of phenotypic resistance is performed using the disk diffusion, agar dilution or broth dilution method [80]. Although disk diffusion is commonly used, automated systems using mainly the broth dilution method have been developed. An example is the VITEK system [81,82].

On the other hand, genotypic resistance is achieved through polymerase chain reaction (PCR) using specific primers to target specific genes [83]. However, this method could be time-consuming and labour-intensive when dealing with many organisms and may require further sequencing of amplified genes to further differentiate them, like with the *tet* genes conferring resistance to tetracycline [60]. Furthermore, recent advances in molecular techniques have allowed the detection of resistance genes in whole populations directly from environmental samples without the need for culture [84].

Finally, whole-genome sequencing (WGS) has been used in cases where high-resolution characterisation of specific isolates is required, as this approach can lead to the identification of novel genes and mutations related to AMR [85].

In the studies reviewed in the current report, the most used method was disk diffusion as most studies focused on phenotypic resistance. Furthermore, the disk diffusion is cost-effective, and flexible, allowing visual growth observation, correct inoculum, mixed (contaminated) cultures and other irregularities [86]. Although the broth dilution method has the added advantage of providing the minimum bactericidal concentration (MBC), the minimum concentration of an antimicrobial that eliminates 99.9% of bacteria [87], this method is more valuable in clinical settings where treatment is required. This could influence its reduced use in the studies evaluated here, as they focused on environmental samples. Where genotypic resistance was investigated, this was mostly achieved through PCR (conventional and real-time). Only a few studies used metagenomics or WGS. There is no doubt that WGS provides an unprecedented level of detail regarding AMR, something that cannot be achieved with culture and other molecular techniques [88]. However, the cost of sequencing and the need for highly skilled bioinformaticians are major impediments to its routine use within the African continent. The VITEK automated system was only used for isolate identification and not for the determination of AMR. Although this system is highly automated and time-efficient, allowing the simultaneous analysis of hundreds of samples [87], the cost of instrumentation could be challenging for most researchers in Africa due to a lack of sufficient research funds. A summary of South African studies that focused specifically on WWTPs between 2012 and 2022 is provided in Table 3.

Table 3. Summary of AMR studies on WWTPs in South Africa (2012–2022).

Organism(s)	Antibiotics Tested (*n* = Number Tested)	Phenotypic Resistance	Genotypic Resistance	Method	Reference
E. coli	*n* = 23: Amoxicillin/clavulanic acid, amoxicillin, amikacin, ampicillin, cefepime, cephalothin, cefotaxime, cefoxitin, cefixime, nalidixic acid, ceftazidime, cephalexin, cefuroxime, chloramphenicol, ciprofloxacin, gentamicin, imipenem, meropenem, nitrofurantoin, piperacillin, tetracycline, tigecycline, trimethoprim/Sulfamethoxazole.	Amoxicillin/clavulanic acid, amoxicillin, amikacin, ampicillin, cefepime, cephalothin, cefotaxime, cefoxitin, cefixime, ceftazidime, cephalexin, cefuroxime, chloramphenicol, ciprofloxacin, gentamicin, imipenem, meropenem, nitrofurantoin, piperacillin, tetracycline, tigecycline, nalidixic acid, trimethoprim/Sulfamethoxazole.	*TEM*, *SHV*, CTX-M	DD/PCR-Sanger Sequencing	[60]
E. coli	*n* = 8: Meropenem, colistin, amoxicillin/clavulanic, ciprofloxacin, nitrofurantoin trimethoprim/sulfamethoxazol, gentamicin, tetracycline.	Colistin, amoxicillin-clavulanic, ciprofloxacin, trimethoprim-sulphamethoxazole, gentamicin, tetracycline, nitrofurantoin.	*TEM*, *SHV*, CTX-M, *VIM*, *OXA*-1, *KPC*-2, *NDM*-1	DD/PCR	[61]

Table 3. *Cont.*

Organism(s)	Antibiotics Tested (*n* = Number Tested)	Phenotypic Resistance	Genotypic Resistance	Method	Reference
S. aureus	*n* = 20: Amikacin, Gentamicin, Amoxicillin/clavulanic acid, Ampicillin, Oxacillin, Penicillin, Imipenem, Cefoxitin, Cefozolin, Ciprofloxacin, Norfloxacin, Vancomycin, Clindamycin, Lincomycin, Azithromycin, Erythromycin, Chloramphenicol, Rifampicin, Tetracycline Sulfamethoxazole/trimethoprim.	Amikacin, Gentamicin, Amoxicillin/clavulanic acid, Ampicillin, Oxacillin, Penicillin, Imipenem, Cefoxitin, Cefozolin, Norfloxacin, Vancomycin, Clindamycin, Lincomycin, Azithromycin, Erythromycin, Chloramphenicol, Rifampicin, Sulfamethoxazole/trimethoprim, Tetracycline.	*aac(6′)/aph(2″)*, *blaZ*, *erm*C, *msr*A and *tet*K,	DD/PCR	[77]
Klebsiella spp.	*n* = 16: Amoxicillin-clavulanic acid, piperacillin-tazobactam, cefotaxime, ceftazidime, cefalexin, cefoxitin, ertapenem, meropenem, doripenem, imipenem, aztreonam, ciprofloxacin, norfloxacin, moxifloxacin, gentamicin, tobramycin.	Amoxicillin-clavulanic acid, piperacillin-tazobactam, cefotaxime, ceftazidime, cefalexin, cefoxitin, ertapenem, doripenem, aztreonam, ciprofloxacin, norfloxacin, moxifloxacin, gentamicin, tobramycin.		DD	[73]
Aeromonas spp.	*n* = 20: Ciprofloxacin, Trimethoprim, Ofloxacin, Chloramphenicol, Penicillins, Clindamycin, Ampicillin-sulbactam, Ampicillin, Gentamicin, Nalidixic acid, Cefotaxime, Nitrofurantoin, Oxacillin, Sulphamethoxazole, Cephalothin, Erythromycin, Tetracycline, Minocycline, vancomycin, Rifamycin.	Ciprofloxacin, Trimethoprim, Chloramphenicol, Penicillins, Clindamycin, Ampicillin-sulbactam, Oxacillin, Ampicillin, Gentamicin, Nalidixic acid, Cefotaxime, Nitrofurantoin, Sulphamethoxazole, Cephalothin, Erythromycin, Tetracycline, Minocycline, vancomycin, Rifamycin.	blaP1class A β-lactamase (*pse1-PSE-1/CARB-2*), *bla*$_{TEM}$, *Tet*C, Class 1 integron, Class 2 integron	DD/PCR	[56]
Listeria spp.	*n* = 24: Penicillin, Cephalothin, Gentamicin, Kanamycin, Amikacin, Ertapenem, Meropenem, Cefotaxime, Ceftriaxone, Vancomycin, Clindamycin, Erythromycin, Nitrofurantoin, Ampicillin, Colistin, Nalidixic acid, Mixofloxacin, Fusidic Acid Ciprofloxacin, Trimethoprim, Tetracycline, Streptomycin, Fosfomycin Chloramphenicol.	Penicillin, Cephalothin, Kanamycin, Ertapenem, Cefotaxime, Ceftriaxone, Vancomycin, Clindamycin, Erythromycin, Nitrofurantoin, Ampicillin, Colistin, Nalidixic acid, Mixofloxacin, Trimethoprim, Tetracycline,		DD	[57]
Aeromonas spp.		Penicillin, Cephalothin, Kanamycin, Ertapenem, Meropenem, Cefotaxime, Ceftriaxone, Vancomycin, Clindamycin, Erythromycin, Nitrofurantoin, Ampicillin, Colistin, Nalidixic acid, Mixofloxacin, Trimethoprim, Tetracycline, Streptomycin, Chloramphenicol, Fosfomycin, Fusidic Acid.			
E. coli	*n* = 13: Ampicillin, amoxicillin, cephalothin, cefazolin, ceftazidime, tetracycline, doxycycline, chloramphenicol, amikacin, gentamicin, nalidixicacid, norfloxacin, fosfomycin.	Ampicillin, amoxicillin, cephalothin, ceftazidime, tetracycline, doxycycline, chloramphenicol, nalidixic acid, norfloxacin, fosfomycin.		DD	[62]
Klebsiella *Bacillus* *Pseudomonas* *Aeromonas* *Exiguobacterium* *Shewanella* spp.	*n* = 6: Vancomycin, kanamycin, trimethoprim, oxytetracycline, amoxicillin and chloramphenicol.	Vancomycin, kanamycin, trimethoprim, oxytetracycline, amoxicillin and chloramphenicol.		BD	[55]
Enterococcus spp.	*n* = 1: Vancomycin		*erm*(B) *was*, VREfm, *van*A (*van*A, *van*HA, *van*RA, *van*SA, *van*YA and *van*ZA gene clusters), *van*G (*van*RG), vanN (*van*RN) and *van*L (*van*SL), *van*C (*van*C1XY, *van*SC, *van*RC and *van*XYC), *isa*(A), *et*(M), *aac(6′)-Ii*	WGS	[72]

Table 3. *Cont.*

Organism(s)	Antibiotics Tested (*n* = Number Tested)	Phenotypic Resistance	Genotypic Resistance	Method	Reference
Enterobacteriaceae	*n* = 18: Doxycycline, tetracycline, ampicillin, gentamicin, meropenem amoxicillin/clavulanic acid, amikacin, nitrofurantoin, cefuroxime, cefotaxime, norfloxacin, ciprofloxacin, chloramphenicol, nalidixic acid, colistin sulphate, polymyxin, trimethoprim-sulfamethoxazole, imipenem.	Gentamycin, neomycin, penicillin G, nitrofurantoin, polymyxin B, cefuroxime.	ESBL (*bla*$_{CTX-M}$, *bla*$_{TEM}$, *bla*$_{SHV}$, *bla*$_{GES}$, *bla*$_{IMP}$, *bla*$_{KPC}$, *bla*$_{VIM}$, *bla*$_{OXA-1-like}$,*bla*$_{PER}$, *bla*$_{OXA-48-like}$, and *bla*$_{VEB}$), pAmpC (bla$_{ACC}$, bla$_{EBC}$, *bla*$_{FOX}$,*bla*$_{CIT}$, *bla*$_{DHA}$, and *bla*$_{MOX}$), non-β-lactam (*aad*A, *cat*I,*cat*II, *str*A, *sul*I, *sul*II, *tet*A, *tet*B, *tet*C, *tet*D, *tet*K, and *tet*M)	DD/PCR	[69]
E. coli	*n* = 18: Ampicillin, amikacin, imipenem, meropenem, streptomycin, ciprofloxacin, chloramphenicol, nalidixic, tetracycline, trimethoprim, norfloxacin, Sulfamethoxazole, gentamycin, neomycin, penicillin G, nitrofurantoin, polymyxin B, cefuroxime.		*bla*$_{TEM}$, *bla*$_{SHV}$, *bla*$_{Z}$, *bla*$_{CTX-M}$, *aad*A, *str*A, *tet*A, *tet*B, *tet*K and *tet*M,	DD/PCR	[63]
Vibrio spp.		Ampicillin, amikacin, imipenem, meropenem, streptomycin, chloramphenicol, ciprofloxacin, nalidixic, tetracycline, trimethoprim, norfloxacin, Sulfamethoxazole, gentamycin, neomycin, penicillin G, nitrofurantoin, polymyxin B, cefuroxime.			
Enterococcus spp.	*n* = 14: Chloramphenicol, tetracycline, ampicillin, nitrofurantoin, ciprofloxacin, levofloxacin, imipenem, linezolid, erythromycin, quinupristin-dalfopristin, tigecycline, trimethoprim-sulfamethoxazole, vancomycin, teicoplanin.		*lsa*(A), *msr*(C), *msr*(D), *erm*(B), and *mef*(A), *tet*(S), *tet*(M), and *tet*(L), *aac(60)-aph(200)*, *ant(6)-Ia*, *aph(30)-*III, *aac(60)-Iid*, *aac(60)-Iih*, *dfr*G	DD/WGS	[37]
E. coli	*n* = 17: Ampicillin, amikacin, imipenem, meropenem, streptomycin, cefotaxime, chloramphenicol, cephalexin, ciprofloxacin, nalidixic acid, tetracycline, norfloxacin, gentamicin, cefuroxime, polymyxin B, colistin sulfate, and nitrofurantoin.	Ampicillin, amikacin, streptomycin, chloramphenicol, ciprofloxacin, cephalexin, nalidixic acid, tetracycline, norfloxacin, gentamicin, cefuroxime, cefotaxime, polymyxin B, colistin sulfate, and nitrofurantoin.	*str*A, *aad*A, *cat* I, *cat* II, *cml*A1, *ampC*, *bla*$_{Z}$, *bla*$_{TEM}$, *tet*A, *tet*B, *tet*C, *tet*D, *tet*K, *tet*M	DD/PCR	[64]
Aeromonas spp.	*n* = 12: Ampicillin, ceftazidime, cefixime, polymyxin B, colistin, ciprofloxacin, levofloxacin, ofloxacin, minocycline, meropenem, imipenem, trimethoprim-sulphamethoxazole.	Ampicillin, ceftazidime, cefixime, polymyxin B, colistin, ciprofloxacin, levofloxacin, minocycline, meropenem, imipenem, trimethoprim-sulphamethoxazole.	*bla*$_{TEM}$, *bla*$_{AmpC}$, *AmpC*/$_{blaOXA}$, *mcr*-1,	DD/PCR	[58]
Pseudomonas spp.		Ampicillin, ceftazidime, cefixime, polymyxin B, colistin, ciprofloxacin, levofloxacin, ofloxacin, minocycline, meropenem, imipenem, trimethoprim-sulphamethoxazole.			
Enterococci			*erm*A,*erm*B and *erm*C, *tet*K, *tet*M and *tet*L, *van*A, *van*B and *van*C, *aph(3′)-IIIa*, *ant(4′)-Ia*,*aac(6′)-Ie-aph(2″)-Ia*	PCR	[71]
Vibrio spp.	*n* = 13: Imipenem, nalidixic acid, erythromycin, gentamicin, Sulfamethoxazole, cefuroxime, penicillin G, chloramphenicol, polymyxin B, trimethoprim-sulfamethoxazole, tetracycline, meropenem and trimethoprim.	Nalidixic acid, erythromycin, Sulfamethoxazole, cefuroxime, penicillin G, chloramphenicol, polymyxin B, trimethoprim-sulfamethoxazole, tetracycline and trimethoprim.		DD	[78]
Salmonella spp.	*n* = 20: Cephalothin, Imipenem, Cefoxitin, Cefuroxime, Piperacillin, Ampicillin, Cefixime, Ceftazidime, Aztreonam, Gentamycin, Amikacin, Streptomycin, Chloramphenicol, Tetracycline, Ciprofloxacin, Norfloxacin, Nalidixic acid, Nitrofurantoin, Sulfamethoxazole Trimethoprim/Sulfamethoxazole.	Imipenem, Piperacillin, Ampicillin, Cefixime, Ceftazidime, Streptomycin, Nalidixic acid, Sulfamethoxazole.		DD	[76]

Table 3. *Cont.*

Organism(s)	Antibiotics Tested (*n* = Number Tested)	Phenotypic Resistance	Genotypic Resistance	Method	Reference
Pseudomonas spp.	*n* = 19: Ampicillin, cefotaxime, cephalothin, cefepime, chloramphenicol, clindamycin, erythromycin, gentamicin, minocycline, nalidixic acid, nitrofurantoin, ofloxacin, oxacillin, penicillin G, rifampin, sulphamethoxazole, tetracycline, vancomycin, ampicillin-sulbactam.	Ampicillin, cefotaxime, cephalothin, cefepime, chloramphenicol, clindamycin, minocycline, nalidixic acid, nitrofurantoin, oxacillin, penicillin G, rifampin, sulphamethoxazole, tetracycline, vancomycin, ampicillin-sulbactam.		DD	[75]
Enterococcus spp.	*n* = 11: Ampicillin, amoxicillin, penicillin, neomycin, streptomycin, vancomycin, chloramphenicol, ciprofloxacin, tetracycline, trimethoprim, erythromycin.	Ampicillin, amoxicillin, penicillin, neomycin, streptomycin, vancomycin, chloramphenicol, ciprofloxacin, tetracycline, trimetho-prim, erythromycin.		DD	[70]
E. coli	*n* = 9: Ampicillin, penicillin, ciprofloxacin, tetracycline, trimethoprim, cefotaxime, ceftazidime, imipenem and meropenem.	Ampicillin, penicillin, ciprofloxacin, tetracycline, trimethoprim, cefotaxime, ceftazidime.	*Alr*, bla_{TEM}, bla_{SHV} and $bla_{CTX\text{-}M}$	DD/PCR	[65]
Bacillus, *Pseudomonas*, *Enterococcus*, *Brevibacillus*, *Paenibacillus*	*n* = 3 Penicillin G, vancomycin, erythromycin.	Vancomycin Erythromycin Penicillin G		DD	[51]
E. coli	*n* = 12: Amoxicillin, Cefuroxime, Gentamicin, Doxycycline, Ciprofloxacin, Ofloxacin, Trimithoprime, Menopenem, Colistin sulphate, Erythromycin, Clindamy-cin, Sulphamethoxazole.	Amoxicillin, Cefuroxime, Gentamicin, Doxycycline, Ciprofloxacin, Ofloxacin, Trimithoprime, Menopenem, Colistin sulphate, Erythromycin, Clindamy-cin, Sulphamethoxazole.		DD	[67]
Pseudomonas spp.	*n* = 20: Penicillins, clinamycins, ciprofloxacin, rafamycin, trimethoprim, sulphamethoxazole, gentamicin, chloramphenicol, tetracycline, erythromycin, minocycline, vacomycin, cefotaxime, nalidixic acid, nitrofurantoin, cephalothin, ofloxacin, ampicillin, ampicillin-sulbactam, oxacillin.	Penicillins, clinamycins, rafamycin, trimethoprim, sulphamethoxazole, chloramphenicol, tetracycline, minocycline, vacomycin, cefotaxime, nalidixic acid, nitrofurantoin, cephalothin, ampicillin, ampicillin-sulbactam, oxacillin.	bla_{TEM}, bla_{OXA}, bla_{AmpC}, *TetC*,	DD/PCR	[89]
Escherichia coli *Enterococcus* spp.	*n* = 22: Amikacin, ampicillin, azithromycin, amoxicillin-clavulanic acid, cefepime, cefotaxime, cefoxitin, ceftazidime, ceftriaxone, cephalexin, ciprofloxacin, chloramphenicol, gentamicin, imipenem, meropenem, nalidixic acid, piperacillin-tazobactam, tetracycline, tigecycline, trimethoprim-sulfamethoxazole.				[68]
	n = 16: Imipenem, Ampicillin, tetracycline, Nitrofurantoin, quinupristin-dalfopristin, tigecycline, Linezolid, ciprofloxacin, trimethoprim-sulfamethoxazole, Levofloxacin, Teicoplanin, vancomycin, Gentamycin, Streptomycin, Erythromycin, chloramphenicol.				

DD = Disk diffusion; BD = Broth dilution; PCR = Polymerase chain reaction; WGS = Whole-genome sequencing.

3.5. Water Research Funding

One of the driving factors in research is the availability of funds. For example, the Water Research Commission (WRC) funds most water-related projects in South Africa. This section identifies past WRC projects, and their main aims, to identify similar studies that have been reported on AMR in WWTPs (Table 4). Based on their database, of all these studies, only one focused on antimicrobial resistance in WWTPs (https://search.wrc.org.za/#!/ (accessed on 3 February 2023)). This archive revealed that only a single project was specifically funded relating to the wastewater resistome.

Table 4. Past WRC-funded projects.

SN	Report Number	Project Title	Year	Aim	WWTP	AST
1	1126/1/05	Enteric pathogens in water sources and stools of residents in the Venda region of the Limpopo Province	2005	Identify and characterise enteric pathogens in water sources and stool samples of residents in the Venda region of the Limpopo Province	No	Yes
2	1967/1/13	Investigations into the existence of unique environmental *Escherichia coli* populations	2013	Identify and characterise *E. coli* from chosen localities and different samples	No	No
3	2138/1/16	An investigation into the presence of free-living amoebae and amoeba-resistant bacteria in drinking water distribution systems of health care institutions in Johannesburg, South Africa	2016	To establish the occurrence of free-living amoebae and amoeba resistant bacteria within the drinking water distribution system in health care facilities in Johannesburg and also highlight the potential human health risk implication thereof	Yes	No
4	2432/1/18	Cholera Monitoring and Response Guidelines	2018	The development of cholera monitoring and response guidelines for inclusion in the water resource monitoring programme.	Yes	Yes
5	2585/1/19	Antibiotic-resistant bacteria and genes in drinking water. Implications for drinking water production and quality monitoring	2019	Identify and characterise microbial parameters in drinking water systems	No	Yes
6	2610/1/18	Microplastics in freshwater water environments	2018	Identify and characterise microplastics in freshwater, drinking water and groundwater	No	No
7	2706/1/21	Measurement of water pollution determining the sources and changes of microbial contamination and impact on food safety from farming to retail level for fresh vegetables	2021	To determine the link between water pollution and crop contamination and to determine sources of microbial product contamination, and assess the impact on food safety from farming to retail for selected fresh vegetable supply chains	No	Yes
8	2733/1/20	Substances of emerging concern in South African aquatic ecosystems	2020	Identify and evaluate different contaminants of emerging concern in different water sources	Yes	No
9	1655/1/10	Identification of Arsenic Resistance Genes in Micro-organisms from Maturing Fly Ash-Acid Mine Drainage Neutralised Solids	2011	To isolate micro-organisms resistant to arsenic from matured AMD-FA neutralized solids, to characterize their arsenic resistance systems and to assess whether these organisms pose a potential 'threat' to the sustained use of 'Neutralization Solids'	No	No

Table 4. *Cont.*

SN	Report Number	Project Title	Year	Aim	WWTP	AST
10	KV 360/16	A Scoping Study on the Levels of Antimicrobials and Presence of Antibiotic-Resistant Bacteria in Drinking Water	2016	To provide an overview of the levels of antimicrobials and the presence of antibiotic-resistant bacteria in selected drinking water treatment systems (drinking water production facilities)	No	Yes
11	TT 742/1/17	Emerging contaminants in wastewater treated for direct potable reuse: the human health risk priorities in South Africa	2018	Identify and evaluate different contaminants of emerging concern in different water sources	Yes	No
12		The epidemiology and cost of treating diarrhoea in South Africa		Identify and characterise enteric pathogens in water sources and stool samples of residents in the Venda region of the Limpopo Province	No	Yes

4. Identifying Knowledge Gaps

4.1. Spatial (Geographical) Gaps

Studies on the WWTP resistome in South Africa have been dominated by two provinces—KwaZulu-Natal and Eastern Cape. Very few studies have been conducted in provinces such as the North-West and Gauteng, while others such as Mpumalanga and Limpopo did not perform such studies within the reviewed period. This provides an incomplete picture of the country's WWTP resistome. This gap could be due to the non-functioning of most WWTPs in these locations, especially in rural settings.

4.2. Methodological Gaps and Associated Challenges

The sampling frequency is not standardised; lower samples may exclude seasonal variation. Infectious diseases requiring antimicrobial treatment, such as diarrhoea usually follow a seasonal pattern [90]. This means that antibiotic consumption would vary based on these seasons. This could therefore affect the type and frequency of resistance observed in wastewater. One-off samplings recorded by Gumede et al. [60] would paint an incomplete picture of the wastewater resistome.

On the other hand, Molale-Tom and Bezuidenhout [70] sampled in a single month (May), while Mbanga et al. [68] sampled for seven months, cutting across different seasons, although both studies focused on *Enterococcus* spp. Furthermore, WWTPs experience periods of peak and low flow [91]. The sampling time could therefore affect the abundance and frequency of AMR, which would be missed with limited sampling. However, none of the studies reviewed indicated the sampling times.

The number and the type of antibiotics tested vary per study, even when the same organisms were tested. For example, Gumede et al. [60], Adegoke et al. [61], Pillay and Olaniran [62], Adefisoye and Okoh [64], and Nzima et al. [65] tested 23, 8, 13, 17 and 9 antibiotics, respectively, although they were all working on *E. coli*. Furthermore, Adegoke et al. [61] tested for colistin which was not tested by the other studies, while Pillay and Olaniran [62] included norfloxacin and fosfomycin in their panel.

These two factors would pose a significant challenge when comparing different studies.

The studies reviewed indicated that the most used detection method was disk diffusion and, in some cases, combined with PCR. However, this creates a knowledge gap regarding the various genes implicated in the observed phenotypic resistance. Although it has been shown that discrepancies exist between phenotypic and genotypic resistance, some organisms may be phenotypically susceptible to the tested antibiotics yet possess genes that could be expressed under appropriate environmental stress, as observed in WWTP settings.

Moreover, culture-based approaches would introduce selection bias, as only a subset of isolates is usually selected for downstream analysis. This would also be the case with WGS, where a selected number of isolates would be subjected to sequencing. On the other hand, metagenomic approaches would identify genes in a total population, regardless of the micro-organisms. Despite the advantages of genomic methods for AMR monitoring, these methods were only used in very few studies during the review period.

This methodological gap is probably fuelled by two main factors: the cost of performing advanced genomic studies and the lack of technical skills, including bioinformatic skills for analysing genomic data.

4.3. Micro-organisms Gap

Gram-positive and Gram-negative bacteria differ in the structure of their outer membranes, a characteristic that affects their response to antibiotics. Thus, because of an extra outer layer, Gram-negative bacteria have been reported to be more antibiotic-resistant than their Gram-positive counterparts [92,93]. However, most of the evaluated studies focused on *E. coli* (Gram-negative), while a few assessed *Enterococcus* spp. (Gram-positive).

Despite the greater medical importance of Gram-negatives, Gram-positive bacteria could serve as important reservoirs of ARGs within WWTPs. This reliance on *E. coli* alone is also due to the simplicity of its isolation and characterisation, which make it a suitable organism for monitoring AMR. However, determining the WWTP resistome using *E. coli* alone could lead to gross underestimation of AMR in these milieus.

4.4. Reporting Gap

Research findings should be made available for consumption by the general public and relevant stakeholders as this would foster the implementation of such findings for the benefit of humanity and its environment [94,95]. However, while the studies reviewed here were journal articles published in scholarly outlets, such information does not usually get to the grassroots people, who are more impacted by the problems investigated. Furthermore, even with the scientific publications, the analysis gaps identified earlier significantly affect the overall information available on AMR in WWTPs due to the non-standard nature of the studies. For example, repositories containing the various resistances identified in the studies are unavailable within the country.

5. Proposed Future Perspective

It is evident that wastewater-based monitoring of AMR is gaining significant ground globally, including in South Africa. However, this could still be challenging in many African countries as most LMICs lack structured sewer systems. However, in places such as South Africa where such facilities are available:

(i). There is a need to standardise protocols for assessing the WWTP resistome. This should consider the sampling regime, the sampling frequency, the organisms targeted, which antibiotics need to be tested and which methods should be used.

(ii). There is a need to build capacity in sequencing technologies and bioinformatics, given the recent drift of the science to big data analysis.

(iii). Funding must be made available to researchers as sequencing technologies are not yet widespread in the country, and the cost of using these facilities is still considerably high.

(iv). Reporting of works on AMR in WWTPs needs to be improved, and there is a need to create a repository that would serve as a referral point for future studies.

Author Contributions: Conceptualization, N.P., A.L.K.A. and A.N.T.; methodology, A.L.K.A. and T.B.; validation, N.P. and A.N.T.; formal analysis, A.L.K.A.; investigation, A.L.K.A. and T.B.; data curation, N.P., A.N.T. and T.B.; writing—original draft preparation, A.L.K.A.; writing—review and editing, A.L.K.A.; project administration, N.P.; funding acquisition, N.P. All authors have read and agreed to the published version of the manuscript.

Funding: This research was funded by the South African Water Research Commission, grant number C2022/2023-00991. The APC was funded by the University of Venda.

Institutional Review Board Statement: Not applicable.

Informed Consent Statement: Not applicable.

Data Availability Statement: Not applicable.

Conflicts of Interest: The authors declare no conflict of interest. The funders had no role in the design of the study; in the collection, analyses, or interpretation of data; in the writing of the manuscript; or in the decision to publish the results.

References

1. UN United Nations Meeting on Antimicrobial Resistance. *Bull. World Health Organ.* **2016**, *94*, 638–639. [CrossRef]
2. World Health Organization United Nations High-Level Meeting on Antimicrobial Resistance. Available online: https://apps.who.int/mediacentre/events/2016/antimicrobial-resistance/en/index.html (accessed on 14 April 2023).
3. WHO. *Antimicrobial Resistance and the United Nations Sustainable Development Cooperation Framework. Guidance for United Nations Country Teams*; WHO Press: Geneva, Switzerlan, 2021; pp. 1–24.
4. Stanton, I.C.; Bethel, A.; Frances, A.; Leonard, C.; Gaze, W.H.; Garside, R. Existing Evidence on Antibiotic Resistance Exposure and Transmission to Humans from the Environment: A Systematic Map. *Environ. Evid.* **2022**, *11*, 8. [CrossRef]
5. Essack, S.Y.; Sartorius, B. Global Antibiotic Resistance: Of Contagion, Confounders, and the COM-B Model. *Lancet Planet. Health* **2018**, *2*, e376–e377. [CrossRef]
6. De Sosa, J.A.; Byarugaba, D.K.; Amabile-Cuevas, C.F.; Hsueh, P.R.; Kariuki, S.; Okeke, I.N. *Antimicrobial Resistance in Developing Countries*; Springer: New York, NY, USA, 2010; ISBN 9780387893709.
7. Tiseo, K.; Huber, L.; Gilbert, M.; Robinson, T.P.; Van Boeckel, T.P. Global Trends in Antimicrobial Use in Food Animals from 2017 to 2030. *Antibiotics* **2020**, *9*, 918. [CrossRef]
8. Kubone, P.Z.; Mlisana, K.P.; Govinden, U.; Abia, A.L.K.; Essack, S.Y. Antibiotic Susceptibility and Molecular Characterization of Uropathogenic *Escherichia coli* Associated with Community-Acquired Urinary Tract Infections in Urban and Rural Settings in South Africa. *Trop. Med. Infect. Dis.* **2020**, *5*, 176. [CrossRef]
9. *WHO Global Action Plan on Antimicrobial Resistance*; WHO Document Production Services; WHO: Geneva, Switzerland, 2015.
10. Chereau, F.; Opatowski, L.; Tourdjman, M.; Vong, S. Risk Assessment for Antibiotic Resistance in South East Asia. *BMJ* **2017**, *358*, j3393. [CrossRef]
11. O'Neill, J. The Review on Antimicrobial Resistance Chaired by Jim O'Neill. 2015. Available online: https://amr-review.org/sites/default/files/Report-52.15.pdf (accessed on 3 February 2023).
12. Proia, L.; Anzil, A.; Borrego, C.; Farrè, M.; Llorca, M.; Sanchis, J.; Bogaerts, P.; Balcázar, J.L.; Servais, P. Occurrence and Persistence of Carbapenemases Genes in Hospital and Wastewater Treatment Plants and Propagation in the Receiving River. *J. Hazard. Mater.* **2018**, *358*, 33–43. [CrossRef]
13. Moslah, B.; Hapeshi, E.; Jrad, A.; Fatta-Kassinos, D.; Hedhili, A. Pharmaceuticals and Illicit Drugs in Wastewater Samples in North-Eastern Tunisia. *Environ. Sci. Pollut. Res.* **2018**, *25*, 18226–18241. [CrossRef]
14. Sinthuchai, D.; Boontanon, S.K.; Boontanon, N.; Polprasert, C. Evaluation of Removal Efficiency of Human Antibiotics in Wastewater Treatment Plants in Bangkok, Thailand. *Water Sci. Technol.* **2016**, *73*, 182–191. [CrossRef]
15. Li, X.; Shi, H.; Li, K.; Zhang, L.; Gan, Y. Occurrence and Fate of Antibiotics in Advanced Wastewater Treatment Facilities and Receiving Rivers in Beijing, China. *Front. Environ. Sci. Eng.* **2014**, *8*, 888–894. [CrossRef]
16. Zhang, Y.; Marrs, C.F.; Simon, C.; Xi, C. Wastewater Treatment Contributes to Selective Increase of Antibiotic Resistance among *Acinetobacter* spp. *Sci. Total Environ.* **2009**, *407*, 3702–3706. [CrossRef]
17. Omuferen, L.O.; Maseko, B.; Olowoyo, J.O. Occurrence of Antibiotics in Wastewater from Hospital and Convectional Wastewater Treatment Plants and Their Impact on the Effluent Receiving Rivers: Current Knowledge between 2010 and 2019. *Environ. Monit. Assess.* **2022**, *194*, 306. [CrossRef]
18. Nkengasong, J.N.; Tessema, S.K. Africa Needs a New Public Health Order to Tackle Infectious Disease Threats. *Cell* **2020**, *183*, 296–300. [CrossRef]
19. Sriram, A.; Kalanxhi, E.; Kapoor, G.; Craig, J.; Ruchita Balasubramanian, S.B.; Criscuolo, N.; Hamilton, A.; Klein, E.; Tseng, K.; Van Boeckel, T.; et al. The State of the World's Antibiotics in 2021: A Global Analysis of Antimicrobial Resistance and Its Drivers; 2021. Available online: https://onehealthtrust.org/publications/reports/the-state-of-the-worlds-antibiotic-in-2021/ (accessed on 3 February 2023).

20. Delgado-Blas, J.F.; Valenzuela Agüi, C.; Marin Rodriguez, E.; Serna, C.; Montero, N.; Saba, C.K.S.; Gonzalez-Zorn, B. Dissemination Routes of Carbapenem and Pan-Aminoglycoside Resistance Mechanisms in Hospital and Urban Wastewater Canalizations of Ghana. *mSystems* **2022**, *7*, e01019–e01021. [CrossRef]
21. Akpan, S.N.; Odeniyi, O.A.; Adebowale, O.O.; Alarape, S.A.; Adeyemo, O.K. Antibiotic Resistance Profile of Gram-Negative Bacteria Isolated from Lafenwa Abattoir Effluent and Its Receiving Water (Ogun River) in Abeokuta, Ogun State, Nigeria. *Onderstepoort J. Vet. Res.* **2020**, *87*, 1–6. [CrossRef]
22. Tesfaye, H.; Alemayehu, H.; Desta, A.F.; Eguale, T. Antimicrobial Susceptibility Profile of Selected Enterobacteriaceae in Wastewater Samples from Health Facilities, Abattoir, Downstream Rivers and a WWTP in Addis Ababa, Ethiopia. *Antimicrob. Resist. Infect. Control* **2019**, *8*, 134. [CrossRef]
23. Marano, R.B.M.; Fernandes, T.; Manaia, C.M.; Nunes, O.; Morrison, D.; Berendonk, T.U.; Kreuzinger, N.; Telson, T.; Corno, G.; Fatta-Kassinos, D.; et al. A Global Multinational Survey of Cefotaxime-Resistant Coliforms in Urban Wastewater Treatment Plants. *Environ. Int.* **2020**, *144*, 106035. [CrossRef]
24. Alouache, S.; Estepa, V.; Messai, Y.; Ruiz, E.; Torres, C.; Bakour, R. Characterization of ESBLs and Associated Quinolone Resistance in *Escherichia coli* and *Klebsiella pneumoniae* Isolates from an Urban Wastewater Treatment Plant in Algeria. *Microb. Drug Resist.* **2014**, *20*, 30–38. [CrossRef]
25. Onalenna, O.; Rahube, T.O. Assessing Bacterial Diversity and Antibiotic Resistance Dynamics in Wastewater Effluent-Irrigated Soil and Vegetables in a Microcosm Setting. *Heliyon* **2022**, *8*, e09089. [CrossRef]
26. Tapela, K.; Rahube, T. Isolation and Antibiotic Resistance Profiles of Bacteria from Influent, Effluent and Downstream: A Study in Botswana. *Afr. J. Microbiol. Res.* **2019**, *13*, 279–289. [CrossRef]
27. Soré, S.; Sawadogo, Y.; Bonkoungou, J.I.; Kaboré, S.P.; Béogo, S.; Sawadogo, C.; Bationo, B.G.; Ky, H.; Madingar, P.D.-M.; Ouédraogo, A.S.; et al. Detection, Identification and Characterization of Extended-Spectrum Beta-Lactamases Producing Enterobacteriaceae in Wastewater and Salads Marketed in Ouagadougou, Burkina Faso. *Int. J. Biol. Chem. Sci.* **2020**, *14*, 2746–2757. [CrossRef]
28. Abasse, O.; Boukaré, K.; Sampo, E.; Bouda, R.; CISSE, H.; Stéphane, K.; Odetokun, I.; Sawadogo, A.; Henri Nestor, B.; Savadogo, A. Spread and Antibiotic Resistance Profile of Pathogens Isolated from Human and Hospital Wastewater in Ouagadougou. *Microbes Infect. Dis.* **2022**, *3*, 318–331. [CrossRef]
29. Bougnom, B.P.; McNally, A.; Etoa, F.X.; Piddock, L.J. Antibiotic Resistance Genes Are Abundant and Diverse in Raw Sewage Used for Urban Agriculture in Africa and Associated with Urban Population Density. *Environ. Pollut.* **2019**, *251*, 146–154. [CrossRef]
30. Mekengo, B.M.; Hussein, S.; Ali, M.M. Distribution and Antimicrobial Resistance Profile of Bacteria Recovered from Sewage System of Health Institutions Found in Hawassa, Sidama Regional State, Ethiopia: A Descriptive Study. *SAGE Open Med.* **2021**, *9*, 205031212110390. [CrossRef]
31. Asfaw, T.; Negash, L.; Kahsay, A.; Weldu, Y. Antibiotic Resistant Bacteria from Treated and Untreated Hospital Wastewater at Ayder Referral Hospital, Mekelle, North Ethiopia. *Adv. Microbiol.* **2017**, *7*, 871–886. [CrossRef]
32. Adomako, L.A.B.; Yirenya-Tawiah, D.; Nukpezah, D.; Abrahamya, A.; Labi, A.K.; Grigoryan, R.; Ahmed, H.; Owusu-Danquah, J.; Annang, T.Y.; Banu, R.A.; et al. Reduced Bacterial Counts from a Sewage Treatment Plant but Increased Counts and Antibiotic Resistance in the Recipient Stream in Accra, Ghana—A Cross-Sectional Study. *Trop. Med. Infect. Dis.* **2021**, *6*, 79. [CrossRef]
33. Wawire, S.A.; Reva, O.N.; O'Brien, T.J.; Figueroa, W.; Dinda, V.; Shivoga, W.A.; Welch, M. Virulence and Antimicrobial Resistance Genes Are Enriched in the Plasmidome of Clinical *Escherichia coli* Isolates Compared with Wastewater Isolates from Western Kenya. *Infect. Genet. Evol.* **2021**, *91*, 104784. [CrossRef]
34. Mutuku, C. Antibiotic Resistance Profiles among Enteric Bacteria Isolated from Wastewater in Septic Tanks 2017. *Am. Sci. Res. J. Eng. Technol. Sci.* **2017**, *27*, 99–107.
35. Song'oro, E.; Nyerere, A.; Magoma, G.; Gunturu, R. Occurrence of Highly Resistant Microorganisms in Ruai Wastewater Treatment Plant and Dandora Dumpsite in Nairobi County, Kenya. *Adv. Microbiol.* **2019**, *9*, 479–494. [CrossRef]
36. Alpha, A.D.; Delphine, B.; Fatou, T.L.; Mbaye, M.; Mohamed, M.S.; Moussa, D.; Yacine, S.; Monique, K.; Rianatou, A.; Yaya, T.; et al. Prevalence of Pathogenic and Antibiotics Resistant *Escherichia coli* from Effluents of a Slaughterhouse and a Municipal Wastewater Treatment Plant in Dakar. *African J. Microbiol. Res.* **2017**, *11*, 1035–1042. [CrossRef]
37. Mbanga, J.; Amoako, D.G.; Abia, A.L.K.; Allam, M.; Ismail, A.; Essack, S.Y. Genomic Analysis of *Enterococcus* spp. Isolated from a Wastewater Treatment Plant and Its Associated Waters in Umgungundlovu District, South Africa. *Front. Microbiol.* **2021**, *12*, 648454. [CrossRef]
38. Mhongole, O.J.; Mdegela, R.H.; Kusiluka, L.J.M.; Forslund, A.; Dalsgaard, A. Characterization of *Salmonella* spp. from Wastewater Used for Food Production in Morogoro, Tanzania. *World J. Microbiol. Biotechnol.* **2017**, *33*, 42. [CrossRef]
39. Rafraf, I.D.; Lekunberri, I.; Sànchez-Melsió, A.; Aouni, M.; Borrego, C.M.; Balcázar, J.L. Abundance of Antibiotic Resistance Genes in Five Municipal Wastewater Treatment Plants in the Monastir Governorate, Tunisia. *Environ. Pollut.* **2016**, *219*, 353–358. [CrossRef]
40. Afema, J.A.; Byarugaba, D.K.; Shah, D.H.; Atukwase, E.; Nambi, M.; Sischo, W.M. Potential Sources and Transmission of *Salmonella* and Antimicrobial Resistance in Kampala, Uganda. *PLoS ONE* **2016**, *11*, e0152130. [CrossRef]
41. Mubbunu, L.; Siyumbi, S.; Katongo, C.; Mwambungu, A. Waste Water as Reservoir of Antibiotic Resistant Micro-Organisms: A Case of Luanshya Waste Water Ponds. *Int. J. Res. Med. Health Sci.* **2014**, *4*, 9.

42. Gufe, C.; Ndlovu, M.N.; Sibanda, Z.; Makuvara, Z.; Marumure, J. Prevalence and Antimicrobial Profile of Potentially Pathogenic Bacteria Isolated from Abattoir Effluents in Bulawayo, Zimbabwe. *Sci. African* **2021**, *14*, e01059. [CrossRef]
43. Gasson, J.; Blockman, M.; Willems, B. Antibiotic Prescribing Practice and Adherence to Guidelines in Primary Care in the Cape Town Metro District, South Africa. *S. Afr. Med. J.* **2018**, *108*, 304–310. [CrossRef]
44. DWS—South African Department of Water and Sanitation. *Green Drop National Report 2022*; Department of Water Affairs: Pretoria, South Africa, 2022.
45. Devane, M.L.; Moriarty, E.; Weaver, L.; Cookson, A.; Gilpin, B. Fecal Indicator Bacteria from Environmental Sources; Strategies for Identification to Improve Water Quality Monitoring. *Water Res.* **2020**, *185*, 116204. [CrossRef]
46. Liang, L.; Goh, S.G.; Vergara, G.G.R.V.; Fang, H.M.; Rezaeinejad, S.; Chang, S.Y.; Bayen, S.; Lee, W.A.; Sobsey, M.D.; Rose, J.B.; et al. Alternative Fecal Indicators and Their Empirical Relationships with Enteric Viruses, *Salmonella enterica*, and *Pseudomonas aeruginosa* in Surface Waters of a Tropical Urban Catchment. *Appl. Environ. Microbiol.* **2015**, *81*, 850–860. [CrossRef]
47. Field, K.G.; Samadpour, M. Fecal Source Tracking, the Indicator Paradigm, and Managing Water Quality. *Water Res.* **2007**, *41*, 3517–3538. [CrossRef]
48. Saxena, G.; Bharagava, R.N.; Kaithwas, G.; Raj, A. Microbial Indicators, Pathogens and Methods for Their Monitoring in Water Environment. *J. Water Health* **2015**, *13*, 319–339. [CrossRef]
49. Harwood, V.; Shanks, O.; Koraijkic, A.; Verbyla, M.; Ahmed, W.; Iriate, M. General and Host- Associated Bacterial Indicators of Faecal Pollution. 2017. Available online: https://www.waterpathogens.org/book/bacterial-indicators (accessed on 3 February 2023).
50. Anjum, M.F.; Schmitt, H.; Börjesson, S.; Berendonk, T.U.; Donner, E.; Stehling, E.G.; Boerlin, P.; Topp, E.; Jardine, C.; Li, X.; et al. The Potential of Using *E. coli* as an Indicator for the Surveillance of Antimicrobial Resistance (AMR) in the Environment. *Curr. Opin. Microbiol.* **2021**, *64*, 152–158. [CrossRef]
51. Coetzee, I.; Bezuidenhout, C.C.; Bezuidenhout, J.J. Triclosan Resistant Bacteria in Sewage Effluent and Cross-Resistance to Antibiotics. *Water Sci. Technol.* **2017**, *76*, 1500–1509. [CrossRef]
52. Eze, E.C.; El Zowalaty, M.E.; Pillay, M. Antibiotic Resistance and Biofilm Formation of *Acinetobacter baumannii* Isolated from High-Risk Effluent Water in Tertiary Hospitals in South Africa. *J. Glob. Antimicrob. Resist.* **2021**, *27*, 82–90. [CrossRef]
53. Mapipa, Q.; Digban, T.O.; Nnolim, N.E.; Nontongana, N.; Okoh, A.I.; Nwodo, U.U. Molecular Characterization and Antibiotic Susceptibility Profile of *Acinetobacter baumannii* Recovered from Hospital Wastewater Effluents. *Curr. Microbiol.* **2022**, *79*, 123. [CrossRef]
54. Govender, R.; Amoah, I.D.; Kumari, S.; Bux, F.; Stenström, T.A. Detection of Multidrug Resistant Environmental Isolates of *Acinetobacter* and *Stenotrophomonas maltophilia*: A Possible Threat for Community Acquired Infections? *J. Environ. Sci. Heal. Part A Toxic/Hazardous Subst. Environ. Eng.* **2020**, *56*, 213–225. [CrossRef]
55. Mann, B.C.; Bezuidenhout, J.J.; Bezuidenhout, C.C. Biocide Resistant and Antibiotic Cross-Resistant Potential Pathogens from Sewage and River Water from a Wastewater Treatment Facility in the North-West, Potchefstroom, South Africa. *Water Sci. Technol.* **2019**, *80*, 551–562. [CrossRef]
56. Igbinosa, I.H.; Okoh, A.I. Antibiotic Susceptibility Profile of *Aeromonas* Species Isolated from Wastewater Treatment Plant. *Sci. World J.* **2012**, *2012*, 764563. [CrossRef]
57. Olaniran, A.O.; Nzimande, S.B.T.; Mkize, N.G. Antimicrobial Resistance and Virulence Signatures of *Listeria* and *Aeromonas* Species Recovered from Treated Wastewater Effluent and Receiving Surface Water in Durban, South Africa. *BMC Microbiol.* **2015**, *15*, 234. [CrossRef]
58. Govender, R.; Amoah, I.D.; Adegoke, A.A.; Singh, G.; Kumari, S.; Swalaha, F.M.; Bux, F.; Stenström, T.A. Identification, Antibiotic Resistance, and Virulence Profiling of *Aeromonas* and *Pseudomonas* Species from Wastewater and Surface Water. *Environ. Monit. Assess.* **2021**, *193*, 294. [CrossRef]
59. Ndlovu, T.; Rautenbach, M.; Vosloo, J.A.; Khan, S.; Khan, W. Characterisation and Antimicrobial Activity of Biosurfactant Extracts Produced by *Bacillus amyloliquefaciens* and *Pseudomonas aeruginosa* Isolated from a Wastewater Treatment Plant. *AMB Express* **2017**, *7*, 108. [CrossRef]
60. Gumede, S.N.; Abia, A.L.K.; Amoako, D.G.; Essack, S.Y. Analysis of Wastewater Reveals the Spread of Diverse Extended-Spectrum β-Lactamase-Producing *E. coli* Strains in Umgungundlovu District, South Africa. *Antibiotics* **2021**, *10*, 860. [CrossRef]
61. Adegoke, A.A.; Madu, C.E.; Aiyegoro, O.A.; Stenström, T.A.; Okoh, A.I. Antibiogram and Beta-Lactamase Genes among Cefotaxime Resistant *E. coli* from Wastewater Treatment Plant. *Antimicrob. Resist. Infect. Control* **2020**, *9*, 46. [CrossRef]
62. Pillay, L.; Olaniran, A.O. Assessment of Physicochemical Parameters and Prevalence of Virulent and Multiple-Antibiotic-Resistant *Escherichia coli* in Treated Effluent of Two Wastewater Treatment Plants and Receiving Aquatic Milieu in Durban, South Africa. *Environ. Monit. Assess.* **2016**, *188*, 260. [CrossRef]
63. Adefisoye, M.A.; Okoh, A.I.; Africa, S.; Adefisoye, M.A.; Okoh, A.I. Ecological and Public Health Implications of the Discharge of Multidrug-Resistant Bacteria and Physicochemical Contaminants from Treated Wastewater Effluents in the Eastern Cape, South Africa. *Water* **2017**, *9*, 562. [CrossRef]
64. Adefisoye, M.A.; Okoh, A.I. Identification and Antimicrobial Resistance Prevalence of Pathogenic *Escherichia coli* Strains from Treated Wastewater Effluents in Eastern Cape, South Africa. *Microbiologyopen* **2016**, *5*, 143–151. [CrossRef]

65. Nzima, B.; Adegoke, A.A.; Ofon, U.A.; Al-Dahmoshi, H.O.M.; Saki, M.; Ndubuisi-Nnaji, U.U.; Inyang, C.U. Resistotyping and Extended-Spectrum Beta-Lactamase Genes among *Escherichia coli* from Wastewater Treatment Plants and Recipient Surface Water for Reuse in South Africa. *New Microbes New Infect.* **2020**, *38*, 100803. [CrossRef]
66. Osuolale, O.; Okoh, A. Human Enteric Bacteria and Viruses in Five Wastewater Treatment Plants in the Eastern Cape, South Africa. *J. Infect. Public Health* **2017**, *10*, 541–547. [CrossRef]
67. Igwaran, A.; Iweriebor, B.C.; Okoh, A.I. Molecular Characterization and Antimicrobial Resistance Pattern of *Escherichia coli* Recovered from Wastewater Treatment Plants in Eastern Cape South Africa. *Int. J. Environ. Res. Public Health* **2018**, *15*, 1237. [CrossRef]
68. Mbanga, J.; Abia, A.L.K.; Amoako, D.G.; Essack, S.Y. Longitudinal Surveillance of Antibiotic Resistance in *Escherichia coli* and *Enterococcus* spp. From a Wastewater Treatment Plant and Its Associated Waters in KwaZulu-Natal, South Africa. *Microb. Drug Resist.* **2021**, *27*, 904–918. [CrossRef]
69. Fadare, F.T.; Okoh, A.I. Distribution and Molecular Characterization of ESBL, PAmpC β-Lactamases, and Non-β-Lactam Encoding Genes in Enterobacteriaceae Isolated from Hospital Wastewater in Eastern Cape Province, South Africa. *PLoS ONE* **2021**, *16*, e0254753. [CrossRef]
70. Molale-Tom, L.G.; Bezuidenhout, C.C. Prevalence, Antibiotic Resistance and Virulence of *Enterococcus* spp. From Wastewater Treatment Plant Effluent and Receiving Waters in South Africa. *J. Water Health* **2020**, *18*, 753–765. [CrossRef] [PubMed]
71. Hamiwe, T.; Kock, M.M.; Magwira, C.A.; Antiabong, J.F.; Ehlers, M.M. Occurrence of Enterococci Harbouring Clinically Important Antibiotic Resistance Genes in the Aquatic Environment in Gauteng, South Africa. *Environ. Pollut.* **2019**, *245*, 1041–1049. [CrossRef] [PubMed]
72. Ekwanzala, M.D.; Dewar, J.B.; Kamika, I.; Momba, M.N.B. Comparative Genomics of Vancomycin-Resistant *Enterococcus* spp. Revealed Common Resistome Determinants from Hospital Wastewater to Aquatic Environments. *Sci. Total Environ.* **2020**, *719*, 137275. [CrossRef] [PubMed]
73. King, T.L.B.; Schmidt, S.; Essack, S.Y. Antibiotic Resistant *Klebsiella* spp. from a Hospital, Hospital Effluents and Wastewater Treatment Plants in the UMgungundlovu District, KwaZulu-Natal, South Africa. *Sci. Total Environ.* **2020**, *712*, 135550. [CrossRef]
74. Hosu, M.C.; Vasaikar, S.; Okuthe, G.E.; Apalata, T. Molecular Detection of Antibiotic-Resistant Genes in *Pseudomonas aeruginosa* from Nonclinical Environment: Public Health Implications in Mthatha, Eastern Cape Province, South Africa. *Int. J. Microbiol.* **2021**, *2021*, 8861074. [CrossRef]
75. Odjadjare, E.E.; Igbinosa, E.O.; Mordi, R.; Igere, B.; Igeleke, C.L.; Okoh, A.I. Prevalence of Multiple Antibiotics Resistant (MAR) *Pseudomonas* Species in the Final Effluents of Three Municipal Wastewater Treatment Facilities in South Africa. *Int. J. Environ. Res. Public Health* **2012**, *9*, 2092–2107. [CrossRef]
76. Odjadjare, E.C.; Olaniran, A.O. Prevalence of Antimicrobial Resistant and Virulent *Salmonella* spp. in Treated Effluent and Receiving Aquatic Milieu of Wastewater Treatment Plants in Durban, South Africa. *Int. J. Environ. Res. Public Health* **2015**, *12*, 9692–9713. [CrossRef]
77. Ramessar, K.; Olaniran, A.O. Antibiogram and Molecular Characterization of Methicillin-Resistant *Staphylococcus aureus* Recovered from Treated Wastewater Effluent and Receiving Surface Water in Durban, South Africa. *World J. Microbiol. Biotechnol.* **2019**, *35*, 142. [CrossRef]
78. Okoh, A.I.; Sibanda, T.; Nongogo, V.; Adefisoye, M.; Olayemi, O.O.; Nontongana, N. Prevalence and Characterisation of Non-Cholerae *Vibrio* Spp. in Final Effluents of Wastewater Treatment Facilities in Two Districts of the Eastern Cape Province of South Africa: Implications for Public Health. *Environ. Sci. Pollut. Res.* **2015**, *22*, 2008–2017. [CrossRef]
79. Olayinka Osuolale, A.O. Isolation and Antibiotic Profile Of Pakistan. *J. Nutr.* **2018**, *10*, 982–986.
80. Jiang, L. Comparison of Disk Diffusion, Agar Dilution, and Broth Microdilution for Antimicrobial Susceptibility Testing of Five Chitosans. *Fujian Agric. For. Univ. China* **2011**, 24–27.
81. Cartwright, E.J.P.; Paterson, G.K.; Raven, K.E.; Harrison, E.M.; Gouliouris, T.; Kearns, A.; Pichon, B.; Edwards, G.; Skov, R.L.; Larsen, A.R.; et al. Use of Vitek 2 Antimicrobial Susceptibility Profile to Identify MecC in Methicillin-Resistant *Staphylococcus aureus*. *J. Clin. Microbiol.* **2013**, *51*, 2732–2734. [CrossRef]
82. Kuchibiro, T.; Komatsu, M.; Yamasaki, K.; Nakamura, T.; Niki, M. Evaluation of the VITEK2 AST–XN17 Card for the Detection of Carbapenemase—Producing *Enterobacterales* in Isolates Primarily Producing Metallo β—Lactamase. *Eur. J. Clin. Microbiol. Infect. Dis.* **2022**, *41*, 723–732. [CrossRef]
83. Vasala, A.; Hytönen, V.P.; Laitinen, O.H. Modern Tools for Rapid Diagnostics of Antimicrobial Resistance. *Front. Cell. Infect. Microbiol.* **2020**, *10*, 308. [CrossRef]
84. Ekwanzala, M.D.; Dewar, J.B.; Momba, M.N.B. Environmental Resistome Risks of Wastewaters and Aquatic Environments Deciphered by Shotgun Metagenomic Assembly. *Ecotoxicol. Environ. Saf.* **2020**, *197*, 110612. [CrossRef]
85. Mbanga, J.; Amoako, D.G.; Abia, A.L.K.; Fatoba, D.; Essack, S. Genomic Analysis of Antibiotic-Resistant Enterobacter Spp. from Wastewater Sources in South Africa: The First Report of the Mobilisable Colistin Resistance Mcr-10 Gene in Africa. *Ecol. Genet. Genomics* **2021**, *21*, 100104. [CrossRef]
86. Coorevits, L.; Boelens, J.; Claeys, G. Direct Susceptibility Testing by Disk Diffusion on Clinical Samples: A Rapid and Accurate Tool for Antibiotic Stewardship. *Eur. J. Clin. Microbiol. Infect. Dis.* **2015**, *34*, 1207–1212. [CrossRef]
87. Gajic, I.; Kabic, J.; Kekic, D.; Jovicevic, M.; Milenkovic, M.; Mitic Culafic, D.; Trudic, A.; Ranin, L.; Opavski, N. Antimicrobial Susceptibility Testing: A Comprehensive Review of Currently Used Methods. *Antibiotics* **2022**, *11*, 427. [CrossRef]

88. Hendriksen, R.S.; Bortolaia, V.; Tate, H.; Tyson, G.H.; Aarestrup, F.M.; McDermott, P.F. Using Genomics to Track Global Antimicrobial Resistance. *Front. Public Health* **2019**, *7*, 242. [CrossRef]
89. Igbinosa, I.H.; Nwodo, U.U.; Sosa, A.; Tom, M.; Okoh, A.I. Commensal *Pseudomonas* Species Isolated from Wastewater and Freshwater Milieus in the Eastern Cape Province, South Africa, as Reservoir of Antibiotic Resistant Determinants. *Int. J. Environ. Res. Public Health* **2012**, *9*, 2537–2549. [CrossRef] [PubMed]
90. Gonzales, L.; Joffre, E.; Rivera, R.; Sjöling, Å.; Svennerholm, A.M.; Iñiguez, V. Prevalence, Seasonality and Severity of Disease Caused by Pathogenic *Escherichia coli* in Children with Diarrhoea in Bolivia. *J. Med. Microbiol.* **2013**, *62*, 1697–1706. [CrossRef] [PubMed]
91. Munksgaard, D.G.; Young, J.C. Flow and Load Variations at Wastewater Treatment Plants. *J. Water Pollut. Control Fed.* **1980**, *52*, 2131–2144.
92. Alhumaid, S.; Al Mutair, A.; Al Alawi, Z.; Alzahrani, A.J.; Tobaiqy, M.; Alresasi, A.M.; Bu-Shehab, I.; Al-Hadary, I.; Alhmeed, N.; Alismail, M.; et al. Antimicrobial Susceptibility of Gram-Positive and Gram-Negative Bacteria: A 5-Year Retrospective Analysis at a Multi-Hospital Healthcare System in Saudi Arabia. *Ann. Clin. Microbiol. Antimicrob.* **2021**, *20*, 43. [CrossRef]
93. Jubeh, B.; Breijyeh, Z.; Karaman, R. Resistance of Gram-Positive Bacteria to Current Antibacterial Agents and Overcoming Approaches. *Molecules* **2020**, *25*, 2888. [CrossRef] [PubMed]
94. Edwards, D.J. Dissemination of Research Results: On the Path to Practice Change. *Can. J. Hosp. Pharm.* **2015**, *68*, 465–468. [CrossRef]
95. Ross-Hellauer, T.; Tennant, J.P.; Banelytė, V.; Gorogh, E.; Luzi, D.; Kraker, P.; Pisacane, L.; Ruggieri, R.; Sifacaki, E.; Vignoli, M. Ten Simple Rules for Innovative Dissemination of Research. *PLoS Comput. Biol.* **2020**, *16*, e1007704. [CrossRef]

antibiotics

MDPI

Review

Evolution and Emergence of Antibiotic Resistance in Given Ecosystems: Possible Strategies for Addressing the Challenge of Antibiotic Resistance

Ramganesh Selvarajan [1,*], Chinedu Obize [2], Timothy Sibanda [3], Akebe Luther King Abia [4,5,*] and Haijun Long [1]

1 Laboratory of Extraterrestrial Ocean Systems (LEOS), Institute of Deep-Sea Science and Engineering, Chinese Academy of Sciences, Sanya 572000, China
2 Centre d'étude de la Forêt, Institut de Biologie Intégrative et des Systèmes, Université Laval, Québec City, QC G1V 0A6, Canada
3 School of Molecular and Cell Biology, Faculty of Science, University of the Witwatersrand, Johannesburg 2050, South Africa
4 Department of Microbiology, Venda University, Thohoyando 1950, South Africa
5 Environmental Research Foundation, Westville 3630, South Africa
* Correspondence: ramganesh.presidency@gmail.com (R.S.); lutherkinga@yahoo.fr (A.L.K.A.)

Abstract: Antibiotics were once considered the magic bullet for all human infections. However, their success was short-lived, and today, microorganisms have become resistant to almost all known antimicrobials. The most recent decade of the 20th and the beginning of the 21st century have witnessed the emergence and spread of antibiotic resistance (ABR) in different pathogenic microorganisms worldwide. Therefore, this narrative review examined the history of antibiotics and the ecological roles of antibiotics, and their resistance. The evolution of bacterial antibiotic resistance in different environments, including aquatic and terrestrial ecosystems, and modern tools used for the identification were addressed. Finally, the review addressed the ecotoxicological impact of antibiotic-resistant bacteria and public health concerns and concluded with possible strategies for addressing the ABR challenge. The information provided in this review will enhance our understanding of ABR and its implications for human, animal, and environmental health. Understanding the environmental dimension will also strengthen the need to prevent pollution as the factors influencing ABR in this setting are more than just antibiotics but involve others like heavy metals and biocides, usually not considered when studying ABR.

Keywords: antimicrobial-resistant bacteria; antimicrobial resistance genes; public health; environmental health; horizontal gene transfer; One Health; mitigating strategies; resistome; genomics; evolution

check for updates

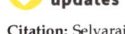

Citation: Selvarajan, R.; Obize, C.; Sibanda, T.; Abia, A.L.K.; Long, H. Evolution and Emergence of Antibiotic Resistance in Given Ecosystems: Possible Strategies for Addressing the Challenge of Antibiotic Resistance. *Antibiotics* **2023**, *12*, 28. https://doi.org/10.3390/antibiotics12010028

Academic Editor: Jie Fu

Received: 27 November 2022
Revised: 20 December 2022
Accepted: 23 December 2022
Published: 24 December 2022

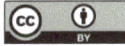

1. Introduction

The term "antibiotics" refers to the substances naturally produced by microorganisms such as actinomycetes, bacteria or fungi, which can inhibit the growth of other microorganisms and destroy their cells [1]. The introduction of antibiotics into clinical practice was the most incredible clinical breakthrough forward of the 20th century [2]. The introduction of the first antibiotics hugely impacted the treatment of various life-threatening bacterial infections and society by reducing morbidity and mortality [3]. Nonetheless, the most recent decade of the 20th century and the beginning of the 21st century have witnessed the emergence and spread of ABR in different pathogenic bacteria worldwide [4]. Continuous misuse of these valuable compounds has rapidly increased antimicrobial resistance in various pathogens that are effectively untreatable [2]. Thus, some organisms have become resistant to more than one antibiotic simultaneously and have been referred to as multidrug-resistant (MDR); some organisms are even resistant to all known antibiotics and are termed pan-drug resistant [5]. Furthermore, although initially developed to describe *Mycobacterium tuberculosis* strains resistant to first-line of treatment—"resistance to the first-line agents, isoniazid and rifampicin, to a fluoroquinolone and to at least one of the three-second-line parenteral drugs", the term extremely drug resistance evolved to define any organism resistant to any standard antimicrobial treatment regimen [5]. Although modern scientific technologies have boosted humanity's hope regarding developing new antibiotics, the current scenario shows few novel antibiotics under development. Simultaneously, antibiotic-resistant bacteria that endure antibiotic treatment are getting increasingly regular, making accessible antibiotics ineffectual. Hence, humanity is confronted by significant adverse public and environmental health impacts. This review examines the history of antibiotics and the ecological roles of antibiotics, and their resistance. In addition, this article adds information on the evolution of bacterial antibiotic resistance in different environments, including aquatic and terrestrial ecosystems, and modern tools used for its identification. Further, the review argues the ecotoxicological impact of antibiotic-resistant bacteria and public health concerns. Finally, it concludes with the possible strategies for addressing the challenge of antibiotic resistance.

2. History of Antibiotics

Since the dawn of time, bacterial infections have had a predominant spot in human diseases [3] and caused death in humans. During ancient times (earlier 1640), Greeks and Indians used molds and other plants to treat wounds and infections, while farmers in Russia used warm soils to cure infected wounds. The doctors from Sumerian and Babylonian used beer soup mixed with turtle shells and snakeskins and a mixture of frog bile and sour milk to treat diseases. Likewise, the Sri Lankan army used oil cake (sweetmeat) as a desiccant and antibacterial agent. Despite the lack of a clear idea about the reason for these illnesses, there were consistent attempts to battle them.

Microorganisms exist in an unfathomably wide variety. The most prominent microbiologists, including Louis Pasteur (1822–1895) and Robert Koch (1843–1910), strongly believed that microbes must develop lethal weapons ("antibiosis") to combat their rivals to thrive in a competitive environment, and that those that go through the competition have developed resistance to their opponents' weapons. They reasoned that because the soil contains the greatest variety of microorganisms, this is where these mechanisms would be most effective. A scientist named Selman Waksman (1888–1973) coined the term "antibiotic" (meaning "against life") in 1942. He explained that it is something microorganisms make at low concentrations to kill or inhibit the growth of other organisms. The term was used throughout the subsequent 20 years per the abovementioned specification. Although the term is still in use, it has expanded to include the many semi- and fully-synthetic "antibiotics" developed by the pharmaceutical industry.

Rudolph Emmerich and Oscar Löw, two German researchers, created the first antibiotic, pyocyanase, in the late 1890s. It was produced by growing the bacterium *Pseudomonas aeruginosa* in a lab and had questionable efficacy and safety when used to treat cholera and typhus. Later, Salvarsan, an arsenic-based medication discovered by Paul Ehrlich in 1909, was effective against the syphilis-causing bacterium *Treponema pallidum*. In other words, this finding paved the way for future research and development of antimicrobial drugs [6]. Penicillin, derived from the fungus *Penicillium*, was the first antibiotic supplied to doctors in the 1940s. As its development was preceded by years of study and observation during World War II, it is commonly referred to as "a child of the war" [1]. By the late 1940s and early 1950s, antibiotic chemotherapy was well tolerated in clinical medicine after the discovery of streptomycin and tetracycline from *Actinomycetes*. In addition to being efficient against the bacillus causing tuberculosis, these medicines were also effective against other pathogenic bacteria [3]. In this context, the filamentous actinomycetes (64%) were the primary source of most naturally occurring antibiotics, followed by the bacterial and fungal species (Table 1). On the other hand, synthetic derivatives are believed to be efficient against pathogenic microbes.

Table 1. Natural and Synthetic antimicrobials from 1910–2010 [2,7].

Year of Discovery	Microorganisms			Synthetic Antimicrobials
	Actinomycetes	Bacteria	Fungi	
1910–1940				Salvarsan Sulfonamides sufapyridine
1940	Streptomycin Aminoglycosides Tetrecyclines Amphenicols	Polypeptides Bacitracin	Penicillins	Sulfones Salicylates
1950	Macrolides Glycopeptides Tuberactinomycins	Polymyxins		Nitrofurans Pyridinamides
1960	Ansamycins Lincosamides Streptogramins Cycloserine		Fusidic acid Cephalosporins Enniatins	Quinolones Azoles Thioamides Ethambutol Phenazines Diaminopyrimidines
1970	Phosphonates Fosfomycin			
1980	Carbapenems	Mupirocin Monobactams		
2000	Lipopetides		Pleuromutilins	Oxazolidinones linezolid
2010	Liparmycins			Diarylquinolines

First-generation cephalosporins, including parenteral medications like cephalothin (1964) and cefazolin (1970) and oral medications like cephalexin (1967), are the most effective against Gram-positive bacteria, methicillin-susceptible staphylococci, and non-enterococcus streptococci [3]. Unlike first-generation cephalosporins, which are effective against Gram-positive and Gram-negative bacteria, second-generation cephalosporins are more successful in the clinic against Gram-negative bacteria such as *Hemophilus influenzae*, *Enterobacter aerogenes*, and some *Neisseria* spp. [8–10]. Further, extended-spectrum cephalosporins such as cefpirome (1983), cefepime (1987), and cefaclidine (1989) have enhanced action against *Enterobacter* spp., *Citrobacter freundii*, *Serratia marcescens*, and severe *P. aeruginosa* infections [11–13]. Antibiotics gradually established themselves as life-saving medications. In the middle of the 20th century, a large increase in the number of novel antibiotic compounds developed for medical use was observed. Between the years 1935 and 1968, a total of 12 new classes were introduced. However, there was a significant decline in the number of new classes after this; between 1969 and 2003, merely two new classes were developed [14].

3. Rise of Antimicrobial Resistance

The term "antimicrobial resistance" (AMR) is used to describe the ability of bacteria and other microorganisms to resist the adverse effects of an antimicrobial to which they were formerly susceptible [15]. Antimicrobial resistance (AMR) was first noted in staphylococci, streptococci, and gonococci; penicillin-resistant *S. aureus* emerged in 1942 following the introduction of penicillin as a commercial antibiotic in 1941 [16]. However, in the early 1930s, Sulphonamide-resistant *Streptococcus pyogenes* appeared in human clinical settings. Later in the 1950s, the problem of multidrug-resistant enteric bacteria became evident [17]. Furthermore, methicillin, which is linked to penicillin and is a semi-synthetic antibiotic, was marketed in 1960 to treat *S. aureus* infections resistant to penicillin. Conversely, in the very same year, methicillin resistance emerged in *S. aureus* [18]. Since their introduction in the 1980s, fluoroquinolones have revolutionized the treatment of bacterial infections. Initially intended for use against Gram-negative bacteria, the emergence of fluoroquinolone resistance has shown that these medications have also been applied to combat Gram-positive infections, most notably among methicillin-resistant strains [19]. Furthermore, although Vancomycin has been on the market for 44 years, in 2002, clinical isolates of Vancomycin-resistant *S. aureus* (VRSA) emerged [20].

A rise in deaths worldwide is attributed to bacteria resistant to multiple antibiotics. For example, there are over 63,000 annual deaths in the United States of America (USA) due to hospital-acquired bacterial infections [21]. Further, in 2019, the Centre for Disease Control (CDC) reported that over 2.8 million antibiotic-resistant infections occurred annually in the United States, leading to over 35,000 deaths [22]. The Indian Council of Medical Research (ICMR) released its annual report on antimicrobial resistance in 2020, which stated that the overall proportion of MRSA throughout the country had reached 42.1% in 2019, representing an increase of nearly 10% compared to the previous year [23]. According to the latest Global Antimicrobial Resistance and Use Surveillance System (GLASS) project report, data from South and Southeast Asian countries (such as India, Bangladesh, and Pakistan) reflect a considerable rise in antibiotic resistance levels. For instance, carbapenem-resistant *Acinetobacter* was found to be exceptionally high in Pakistan (66.9%), followed by India (59.4%). Similarly, the highest prevalence of carbapenem-resistant *E. coli* and carbapenem-resistant *K. pneumonia* was recorded in India (16.4% and 34.2%, respectively), followed by Bangladesh (9.2% and 11.2%) and Pakistan (6.2% and 11.3%) respectively. The other MDR pathogens, such as fluoroquinolone-resistant *Salmonella* sp. (80.3%) and MRSA (65%), were recorded as high in Pakistan [24]. According to the Antimicrobial Resistance Surveillance System (CARSS) and the China Antimicrobial Surveillance Network (CHINET), the antimicrobial resistance profiles of gram-negative bacilli are higher in China. There has been an increase in the incidence of carbapenem-resistant *Klebsiella pneumoniae* since 2005, and the prevalence of extended-spectrum-lactamases and antimicrobial resistance in *Acinetobacter baumannii* are both concerning. Furthermore, the incidence of methicillin-resistant *Staphylococcus aureus* and vancomycin-resistant *Pseudomonas aeruginosa* both declined between 2005 and 2017 [25]. According to a report published by the European Antimicrobial Resistance Surveillance Network (EARS-Net), between 2015 and 2019, there were shifts in the frequency of antimicrobial resistance throughout the European Union. These changes were based on the species of bacteria, with *E. coli* being the most common (44.2%), followed by *S. aureus* (20.6%), *K. pneumoniae* (11.3%), *Enterococcus faecalis* (6.8%), *P. aeruginosa* (5.6%), *Streptococcus pneumoniae* (5.3%), *E. faecium* (4.5%), and *Acinetobacter* spp. (1.7%) [22].

Due to limited resources and the difficulty of monitoring medicine supply systems within and outside their borders, many African countries struggle to protect their populations from unsafe and substandard/counterfeit medicines. Several African countries have not yet banned oral artemisinin monotherapies for uncomplicated malaria, for example. This is a major risk for developing resistance to artemisinin-based combination therapies [26]. In all African regions, *S. aureus*, *Klebsiella* sp., *E. coli*, and *S. pneumoniae* exhibited lower resistance to carbapenems and fluoroquinolones than other antibiotic combinations. In West Africa, *Klebsiella* spp. resistance to ciprofloxacin was greater than in other regions [27]. In conclusion, antimicrobial resistance has emerged as a severe threat to human health in the last decades, responsible for an estimated 700,000 annual deaths worldwide; is is anticipated to result in millions of deaths by 2050 if not adequately addressed [28].

4. What Caused These Organisms in the Environment to Develop Resistance to Multiple Drugs?

Bacteria are distinct in that they can acquire genes from the parent microorganism during division (vertical gene transfer) and from the larger community (horizontal gene transfer), first demonstrated for aminoglycoside resistance [29]. This horizontal gene transfer has been observed at every major taxonomic rank, even between bacteria and archaea. A strain that was once susceptible may acquire and transfer resistance to a new species or genus. Most antibacterial resistance genes are carried on plasmids (Table 2) and other mobile genetic

that confer resistance to fosfomycin and chloramphenicol have been identified in class IV integrons [101]. However, current research is limited to class I integron and Gram-negative bacteria. Class I integron on Gram-positive microorganisms, along with classes II, III and IV, has barely been touched, making such concerns unnoticed about antibiotic resistance determinants. Further, the complex origin of antibiotic resistance still hinges on several factors. These include antibiotic overuse and abuse, inaccurate diagnosis, inappropriate antibiotic medicating, loss of responsiveness in patients, patients self-medicating, poor healthcare settings, lack of personal hygiene, and pervasive agricultural use [102,103].

5. Mechanisms of Antibiotic Resistance

The development of antibiotic resistance is a natural ecological phenomenon and the product of billions of years of evolution. However, much attention has been focused on antibiotic resistance in pathogenic organisms encountered in hospitalized patients and bacteria responsible for adverse health effects [104]. In addition, microbes in pristine environments, such as caves and permafrost, have been studied and found to develop resistance in the absence of human interference. Antibiotics are used for a wide variety of bacterial infections in humans and animals. This promotes the generation of resistance or "immunity" genes in the producer organisms and the selection of resistance in environmental species. The presence of resistance in the natural environment may be a natural occurrence' this reservoir of resistance genes can be mobilized and transferred into human pathogens, worse the situation [105–107]. The presence of identical genes in both environmental and human bacteria demonstrates the movement of resistance genes from different environmental reservoirs, including aquatic and terrestrial environments, into human pathogens and vice versa. Furthermore, environmental microorganisms already have genes encoding resistance to antibiotics before they are widely used commercially [108,109].

The development of antibiotic resistance has brought to light a plethora of diverse and intricate mechanisms responsible for the genesis and propagation of antibiotic resistance among bacteria of the same species or even among bacteria of different species [110]. Important resistance mechanisms shown in Figure 1 include (i) antibiotic exclusion by the cell membrane, (ii) antibiotic modification and/or deactivation within the cell, (iii) reduced sensitivity of the cellular target, (iv) antibiotic exclusion from the cell, and (v) intracellular sequestration [111]. These multiple processes mediate antibiotic resistance enabling bacteria to become resistant to all currently available antibiotics. For instance, three biochemical pathways can lead to fluoroquinolone resistance; these pathways can exist in the same bacteria at the same time with increased expression and, often, increased resistance levels such as (i) overexpression of efflux pumps that effectively remove the drug from the cell, (ii) mutations in genes that encode the target site of fluoroquinolones (DNA gyrase and topoisomerase IV), and (iii) protection of the fluoroquinolone site of action by a protein named Qnr [112].

The most common resistance mechanism in Gram-negative bacteria is the production of beta-lactamases; in Gram-positive organisms, resistance is typically achieved by alteration of the target site, i.e., penicillin-binding proteins (PBPs) [112]. One of the unique mechanisms of antibiotic resistance is the efflux pumps system, which pumps antibiotics and other toxins out of the cell. This mechanism is crucial in bacteria becoming resistant to the antibiotic. On the other hand, Gram-negative bacteria acquire tetracycline resistance via efflux pump systems, specifically the *tet* efflux pumps, which export tetracyclines from cells through proton exchange [113]. Other MDR efflux pumps that extrude tetracycline are AcrAB-TolC and MexAB-OprM, found in *Enterobacteriaceae* and *P. aeruginosa* [114]. Finally, resistance to trimethoprim is caused by alterations in metabolic pathways, such as the increased production of dihydrofolate reductase, an enzyme that lacks the binding site for trimethoprim [115], and dihydropteroate synthase. This enzyme mediates resistance to sulfonamides [116]. Table 3 explains the different mechanisms is mediating antibiotic resistance.

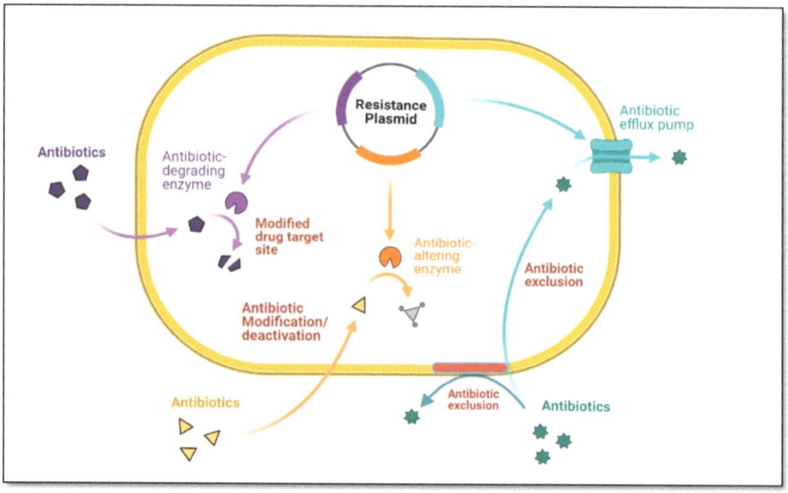

Figure 1. Antibiotic resistance mechanisms (Figure created using Bio-render).

Table 3. Different mechanisms of antibiotic resistance with examples.

Antimicrobial Agents	Mechanism of Action	Examples	References
Penicillins and cephalosporins	Enzymatic inactivation by β-lactamase; enzymatic modification by acylase and esterase; outer membrane protein deletion; alteration of penicillin-binding proteins	β-lactamase containing gram-negative rods	[117–119]
Monobactams	Enzymatic inactivation by β-lactamase	*Haemophilus influenza; Pseudomonas aeruginosa*	[120,121]
Carbapenems	Enzymatic inactivation by β-lactamase; outer-membrane protein deletion	*Neisseria gonorrhoea; A. baumannii; Citrobacter portucalensis; K. pneumoniae; Escherichia coli*	[122,123]
Carbacephems	Cell wall synthesis inhibition	*ESBL-producing Enterobacteria*	[124]
Imipenem	Decreased Cell membrane permeability	*Pseudomonas* sp.; *K.*	[125,126]
*Van*comycin	Inhibition of glycopeptides access	*S. aureus; Enterococcus* sp.	[127,128]
Trimethoprim	Increased production of dihydrofolate reductase; production of trimethoprim-insensitive dihydrofolate reductase	*Streptococcus agalactiae; E. coli; Burkholderia pseudomallei*	[129–131]
*Sul*fonamides	Increased production of p-aminobenzoic acid; increased production of pteridine; increased production of sulfonamide-insensitive dihydropteroate synthetase	*Haemophilus influenza; S. pneumoniae; S. pyogenes; Neisseria meningitidis*	[132]
Aminoglycosides	Enzymatic modification by acetylation, phosphorylation, and nucleotidylation; ribosomal alteration; diminished drug uptake	*Clostridium perfringens; Bacteroides fragilis; S. aureus; Bacillus cereus*	[133–135]
Chloramphenicol	Enzymatic inactivation by acetylation; decreased drug permeability	*Streptomyces venezuelae; Pseudomonas putida; Pneumococcus* sp.; *E. coli*	[136–139]
Macrolides	Enzymatic modification by esterase; alteration of 23S ribosomal RNA	*S. pneumoniae, S. aureus*	[137,140]
Lincosamides	Enzymatic modification by nucleotidylation or phosphorylation; alteration of 23S ribosomal RNA	*S. pneumoniae; S. agalactiae; Acinetobacter baumannii*	[140–142]
Tetracyclines	Active efflux preceded by chemical modification; ribosomal alterations	*E. coli, Shigella* sp., *S. pneumoniae, S.s aureus, Clostridium perfringens, Helicobacter pylori*	[143,144]
Quinolones	Alteration of subunit A of DNA gyrase; decreased drug permeability	*Stenotrophomonas maltophilia; Pseudomonas* species; *Enterobacteriaceae*	[145–147]

6. Antibiotic Resistance in Different Environments

Excessive antibiotic use results in antibiotics being released into different environments, including aquatic and terrestrial environments. The reduced effectiveness of antibiotics against human and animal pathogens is a significant concern raised by the widespread release of antibiotics into these environments. Globally, the public and scientific community are becoming increasingly concerned about antibiotics in the given environment [148].

6.1. Aquatic Environments

Freshwater ecosystems are among the natural settings that have the potential to become contaminated with antibiotics released into the environment by a wide range of sources, including agricultural runoffs, sewage discharges, and leaching from nearby farms [148]. Mobile genetic elements (MGEs) encoding antibiotic resistance spread quickly through horizontal gene transfer (HGT) in aquatic environments [149] and have played an essential role in the development and spread of resistant bacteria into the environment, which can cause infections in both humans and animals. Water bodies like rivers, streams, wastewater effluents, and lakes are connected ecological habitats that have received increased scrutiny recently due to evidence that they play a significant role in spreading antibiotic-resistant genes [21].

6.1.1. Wastewater

Wastewater Treatment Plants

Wastewater treatment plants (WWTPs) are a repository for numerous organic compounds, nutrients, and metals [150]. Traditional wastewater treatment plants are very effective at removing organic compounds and nutrients from wastewater but are not designed to eliminate antibiotics [151]. It was previously thought that biological or chemical degradation, or sorption to sludge, removed some antibiotics that inevitably made their way to WWTPs from both human and animal usages [152]. Some approximations can be made using hydrophobicity and partitioning coefficients for the propensity of antibiotics to sorb to organic matter in WWTPs [153]. For instance, sulfonamides and trimethoprim are shown to have a lower sorption potential than fluoroquinolones and tetracyclines, but both sorb strongly to solids. As evidence, a study found that tetracycline concentrations across ten Chinese WWTPs were much lower than sulfonamide concentrations [154]. While biodegradation plays another significant role in antibiotic removal during wastewater treatment, it is typically seen to be less important than sorption in the removal of the most common antibiotics studied [153,155]. Despite this, sulfonamides and several beta-lactams [153,156] exhibit low sorption characteristics and have an important removal mechanism through the biodegradation process. Although there are many stages of treatment in place at WWTPs, antibiotics in wastewater are not entirely removed and/or degraded, leading to persistent accumulation. For instance, wastewater treatment facilities have been singled out as a potential origin of HGT, contributing to the development of antibiotic resistance, which in turn increases the concentration and overexpression of antibiotic resistance genes (ARGs) in the wastewater system [157].

The effluents from WWTPs contain high concentrations of antibiotic-resistant bacteria (ARB) and ARGs [157], typically found in aquatic environments. For instance, WWTP processes can harbor resistant and MDR bacteria such as *Enterobacteriaceae*, *P. aeruginosa*, *E. coli*, and *Acinetobacter* sp. [158]. However, various clinically significant ARBs, including MRSA, VRE, and a few Gram-negative bacteria, have been identified. These bacteria produced ESBLs and were resistant to fluoroquinolones and carbapenems [159,160]. Martins da Costa et al. [161] studied antimicrobial resistance in *Enterococcus* spp. and reported that biological treatment at WWTPs was ineffective in preventing the spread of MDR enterococci from urban sewage and sludge in Portugal. In addition to resistant bacteria found with culture-dependent methods, genes conferring resistance to all antibiotic classes have been found in WWTPs effluents globally using culture-independent methods. For example, 30 ARGs encoding resistance to tetracycline, sulphonamides, quinolones, and macrolides were found in the activated sludge of two WWTPs in China. Additionally, ten ARGs were significantly increased compared to the abundance of the *16S rRNA* genes [162]. Similarly, a survey of 16 urban WWTPs across ten European countries found a wide range of ARGs in the effluent, including *sul*1, *tet*M, $bla_{OXA\text{-}58}$, bla_{TEM}, $bla_{OXA\text{-}48}$, $bla_{CTX\text{-}M\text{-}32}$, *mcr*-1, $bla_{CTX\text{-}M\text{-}15}$, and $bla_{KPC\text{-}3}$ and reported that the majority of ARGs were found in water bodies downstream from WWTP discharge points [163].

Hospital and Pharmaceutical Wastewater

Since the widespread use of antibiotics in hospitals leads to the excretion of their active forms into the environment, clinical sewage has long been recognized as a significant source of antimicrobial resistance determinants in aquatic environments [164]. Similarly, substantial amounts of antibiotics, and other compounds in pharmaceutical wastewater exert selection pressure even at concentrations well below therapeutic levels [165]. Many recent investigations have focused on pharmaceutical wastewater (PWW) and hospital wastewater (HWW) to examine the resistomes and the associated health risk [166–169]. For instance, Obayiuwana and Ibekwe reported that PWW exhibited a variety of ARGs, including *cat*A1 (58.3%); *sul*I (31.7%); *tet*E (30%); *aac(3)-IV* (28.3%); *erm*C (20%); bla_{TEM}, $bla_{CTX\text{-}M}$, $bla_{NDM\text{-}1}$ at (18.3% each), encoding resistance to chloramphenicol, sulfonamides, tetracycline, aminoglycoside, macrolide-lincosamide-streptogramin, and β-lactams and penicillins, respectively [170]. Another recent meta-analysis of HWW revealed a similar pattern, with high levels of resistance genes to carbapenems, sulfonamides, tetracyclines, and mobile genetic elements. From 2014 to 2018, there was a significant decline in the number of resistance genes to ESBLs, carbapenems, sulfonamides, and glycopeptides, while there was an increase in the number of genes that were resistant to tetracycline [171]. Many previous studies have highlighted the need to increase wastewater treatment capacity in developing countries, focusing on hospital wastewater. Since untreated wastewater is sometimes used to irrigate crops, this could result in the spread of resistant bacteria to the food supply and the local population. Although this poses no immediate risk to produce, the more prevalent these bacteria are, the more likely AMR might spread, especially among immune-compromised individuals or those undergoing surgery. The global COVID-19 pandemic has recently resulted in a spike in demand for antibiotics. This is because a sizable subset of COVID-19 patients also required antimicrobial therapy for secondary bacterial or fungal infection [172]. This increased the concentrations and diversity of these pharmaceuticals in HWW. Therefore, inadequate disposal of non-metabolized antibiotics into hospital sewage systems is also a source of antibiotic-resistant microbes in the aquatic environment.

6.1.2. Rivers and Groundwater

Rivers are potential compartments where environmental, human, and animal-related bacteria can coexist, at least in the short term, because they receive ARB from various sources, such as WWTPs, urban runoff, and industrial or agricultural activities [173]. In addition, ARGs can be released or spread by ARB and are relatively stable and accessible to other bacteria, resulting in the evolution of a new generation of bacteria resistant to antibiotics [174].

Genes for aminoglycoside resistance, such as *aac*, *aph*, and *ant*, are widely dispersed throughout many different genera, including *Aeromonas*, *Escherichia*, *Vibrio*, *Salmonella*, and *Listeria* spp., which have been isolated from river water [175]. Similarly, ARGs encoding resistance to other aminoglycoside group antibiotics, such as phosphotransferase genes encoding resistance to neomycin (*npt*II) and streptothricin (*str*AB), have also been detected in river water in Canada [176] and India [177]. Microorganisms in river water with high concentrations of antibiotics due to urban and agricultural activities were found to carry sulphonamide resistance genes like *sul*I, II, III, and A [178]. However, there is evidence that some rivers have ARGs, including stretches showing no pollution. The four *sul* genes (*sul*I, II, III, and A) found in bacteria isolated from a pristine river suggest that *sul*I, as a component of class I integrons, can be disseminated and transferred horizontally within and between bacterial species in river water [179].

Antibiotics can make their way into the groundwater and even a water supply that people drink *via* surface water [180]. Not surprisingly, antibiotic exposure in groundwater was less than in surface water [181]. However, there is substantial evidence in the scientific literature linking microbial contamination of groundwater to adverse public health outcomes [182–185]. According to a recent review by Murphy et al. [186], there is strong epidemiological evidence of disease transmission due to groundwater contamination on a global scale, with an annual estimate of 35.2–59.4 million cases of acute gastrointestinal infection potentially attributable to groundwater consumption. The global disease burden is already high, and the potential implications of groundwater-borne ARB are even more alarming.

6.1.3. Marine System

The oceanic ecosystem has received the least attention among the aquatic environments. There is a possibility that antibiotic release is not subject to significant selection in oceans because of the high diffusion rates. However, the presence of AMR in marine environments can potentially be caused by one of three different mechanisms. The first way is transporting ARB from terrestrial sources to coastal environments via runoff. In this scenario, ARGs should be present in bacterial taxa that are generally not found in the ocean. The second mechanism is antimicrobial resistance selection due to anthropogenic antibiotic runoff, which encourages naturally occurring bacteria to become resistant to the antibiotics. The third factor is the development of antibiotic resistance as a direct result of the production of antibiotics in marine environments [187]. Using metagenomic sequencing, a recent baseline study found ARGs in 12 coastal environmental samples from the urban coastline of Kuwait. The authors detected 402 ARGs in these samples, with the most common being *pat*A, *ade*F, *Erm*E, *Erm*F, *Tae*A, *tet*X, *mph*D, *bcr*C, *srm*B, *mtr*D, *bae*S, *Erm*30, *van*TE, *VIM-7*, *Acr*F, *ANT4*-1a, *tet*33, *ade*B, *efm*A, and *rps*L. The beta-lactams (cephalosporins and penam) elicited the highest levels of resistance, and 46% of the genes originated from Proteobacteria. Also, ESKAPEE pathogens (*Enterococcus faecium*, *S. aureus*, *K. pneumonia*, *Acinetobacter baumannii*, *Pseudomonas aeruginosa*, *Enterobacter* sp., and *Escherichia coli*) were found in low concentrations [188]. Nonetheless, future research into MGEs and integrons will be necessary to monitor the spread of ARGs in the marine ecosystem and assess their impact on human health.

6.1.4. Factors Affecting Antibiotic Resistance in the Aquatic Environment

Antibiotic migration, transformation, and fate are analogous to and consistent with ARG transfer and accumulation in the environment (Figure 2) [189]. Antibiotics have been implicated in various studies as a critical factor in the spread of ARGs between species [190,191]. In Beijing, the *sul* gene correlated well with the concentrations of selected sulfamethazine [192]. Still, in the study by Xu et al. [190], no such correlation was found for the same set of ten sulfonamide antibiotics. Based on these results, it is possible to conclude that antibiotics are used to target the effects they have on ARGs.

Heavy metals in the environment are also crucial in the horizontal transfer of ARGs, alongside antibiotics as the most direct source of selection pressure. Specifically, metal ions increase the permeability of cell membranes, which in turn promote the horizontal transfer of ARGs through oxidative stress, the SOS response, and the production of reactive oxygen species (ROS) [193]. There is growing evidence that the co-selection of heavy metals significantly impacts the dispersal and propagation of ARG in the natural environment. Co-selection between ARB and other pathogens could be facilitated by heavy metals used in livestock and fisheries [194]. Recently, certain metal nanoparticles (nano-alumina and Nano-TiO2) have been commonly detected as new pollutants in various environments; studies have shown that nanoparticles and heavy metals can promote the conjugate transfer of ARGs in the environment [195,196]. Other than these factors, other factors such as non-antibiotic antimicrobial chemicals, microbial community diversity, and environmental physical and chemical properties also play significant roles in AR transmission in the aquatic environment [193].

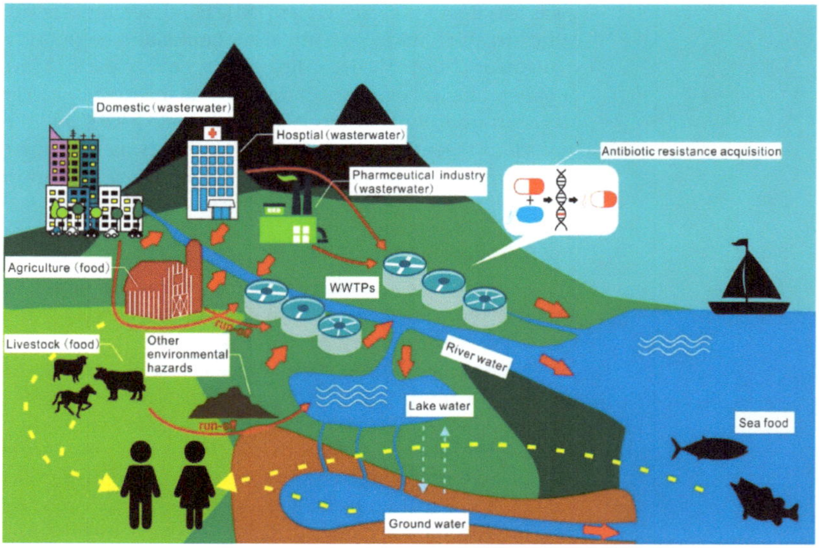

Figure 2. Migration, transformation, and the fate of antibiotics and their resistance in the given environment.

6.2. Terrestrial Environments

The origin of ARGs in the terrestrial environment can be traced back to spontaneous mutations and HGT, just as in the aquatic ecosystem [197]. However, the impact of antibiotics in the soil on persistence and vertical or horizontal gene transport is influenced by co-selection [197,198] and other factors such as antibiotic structure, hydrophobicity, mobility, and biodegradability [199]. It has been shown, for instance, that resident, non-pathogenic soil microbial species can better acquire ARGs in the presence of non-antibiotic stressors like heavy metals, microplastics, and pesticides [197,200,201]. This is due to a phenomenon known as cross- and co-resistance. The terms "cross-resistance" and "co-resistance" refer to two forms of resistance that can develop when the same process reduces susceptibility to antibiotics and non-antibiotics, respectively [199,202].

6.2.1. Sludge Manure

The sludge produced as a by-product of WWTPs can be used as a plant fertilizer or a substrate for improving soil remediation [203]. Using sewage sludge as manure is unquestionably an effective waste management strategy. Sewage sludge is rich in nutrients and organic matter, making it a good candidate for this use. However, sewage sludge harbors microorganisms resistant to multiple antibiotics, metals, plastics, and organic contaminants that pose severe threats to human and environmental health [199,204]. Recent years have witnessed a particular interest in the putative ecotoxicological effects of pharmaceuticals in the environment [198,205]. A recent assessment of treated sewage sludge used for agricultural purposes revealed the presence and accumulation of antibiotics with potential acute and short-term environmental risks [206]. In addition, compounds harmful to the environment, such as heavy metals, are frequently revealed in treated and untreated wastewater sludge [204]. In principle, antibiotics consumed by humans and animals are not entirely metabolized and are released into WWTPs as either parent or partially metabolized compounds. Together with heavy metals, residual antibiotics are not completely removed by WWTPs [207], even in advanced wastewater treatment systems that employ anaerobic digestion, coagulation, lime stabilization, membrane bioreactors, and inactivation and disinfection processes [204,208]. Therefore, if the sludge materials are deployed as manure, these compounds eventually get to the soil in concentrations relative to the treatment method and the source of waste materials. A combination of anaerobic, aerobic, and inactivation treatment strategies appears to be more effective for containing the spread of ARGs from wastewater treatment system sludge [204].

6.2.2. Agricultural System

A sustainable strategy for conserving freshwater is the reuse of treated wastewater for agricultural irrigation [209]. However, wastewater irrigation is another important source of ARGs in agricultural systems. Multiple studies have shown that irrigating with wastewater increases the abundance of multidrug-resistant microorganisms and ARGs in agricultural fields [185,207,210,211]. Several ARGs conferring resistance to rifampicin, chloramphenicol, tetracycline, trimethoprim, β-lactams, aminoglycosides, fluoroquinolones, and sulfonamides, as well as tetracycline- and sulfonamide-resistant bacteria have been detected in wastewater effluent [212].

The risk of ARG spread from agricultural systems into the food chain is also of great concern. For instance, antibiotics from wastewater irrigation can accumulate in edible vegetables and, if ingested, can trigger adaptive resistance in the gut microbiome [213]. In addition, Onalenna and Rahube [214] revealed that wastewater irrigation influenced a structural shift in microbial communities and increased the spread and persistence of beta-lactamases in irrigated soil and edible vegetables. Furthermore, the distribution and persistence of ARGs from wastewater irrigation are not limited to topsoils and edible plants; the accumulation of antibiotic residues in a treated wastewater-irrigated field was found to promote the spread and persistence of ARGs among groundwater microbial communities [185]. ARG detection and spread at this depth highlight the importance of monitoring agricultural systems to control the burden of antibiotic resistance in the environment effectively.

Accordingly, one important factor determining ARG spread from wastewater irrigation is the influence of seasonal variation. Pu et al. [207] reported that the abundance of ARGs in treated wastewater was higher in summer than in winter. Based on the study of Sun et al. [215], seasonal variation impacts the nutrient content of WWTP influent, and this has a corresponding effect on the assembly mechanisms and structure of important microbial species that contribute to the removal of nutrients, pesticides, antibiotics, and other undesirable compounds during wastewater treatment. Thus, a significant change in the assembly of important microbial phylotypes due to seasonal variation reduces the efficiency of WWTPs. Overall, removing ARGs and ARB in both sludge manure and irrigation wastewater requires advancement in WWTP technologies and the development of policies that could reduce antibiotics' misuse. This is critical because the selective pressure of residual antibiotics on microbial communities is what triggers the spread of ARGs in WWTP systems and agricultural fields.

6.2.3. Manure from Livestock and Pesticides

Antibiotics are widely employed in animal breeding industries for disease prevention and treatment. However, such use could lead to the development of ABR in this sector. For example, Abdalla et al. used the farm-to-fork approach to investigate the presence of antibiotic-resistant *E. coli* in intensive pig farming in South Africa [216]. The authors analyzed 1044 pure isolates and observed an 88.5% resistance to at least one of the 20 antibiotics tested. Of greater concern in this study was that the organisms were resistant to most of the antibiotics listed in the WHO list of critically important antibiotics. Similarly, Molechan et al. used the same approach in intensive poultry farming in South Africa and found that close to 80% of all *Enterococcus* species isolated in their study were resistant to at least one of the antibiotics tested [217]. Most antibiotics used by animals (and humans) are excreted in partially metabolized or unmetabolized forms [218]. Thus, as a direct consequence, livestock manure is an important reservoir of multidrug-resistant microorganisms and ARGs. Fatoba et al. revealed that soil before chicken manure application had fewer multidrug-resistant *Enterococcus* species (10%) than soil after manure application (67.7%) [219]. However, though livestock manure is rich in nutrients and improves soil quality [220], it is also a source of undesirable materials, including antibiotics, ARG, multidrug-resistant microorganisms, and heavy metals [221]. The quantity of these materials that can be released into agricultural systems depends on the source of the livestock manure [222], the frequency of application, and soil depth [223]. For example, a recent study revealed that poultry and pig manure holds the largest reservoir of ARGs, antibiotics, and heavy metals compared to sheep and cattle manure [224]. Also, the accumulation of high-risk ARGs in topsoil depended on the frequency of manure application and the microbial communities, while the vertical migration of ARG was driven by variations in soil properties [223]. Furthermore, as with sludge manure, the spread and persistence of ARGs through livestock manure are also influenced by the co-selection of non-antibiotics like heavy metals and biocides. For example, in the co-selection of heavy metal and antibiotics resistance, Cu and Zn were the heavy metals with the strongest influence on ARG proliferation [207].

Pesticides or biocides are used to control soil-borne plant pathogens, including nematodes, oomycetes, fungi, bacteria, and other plant pathogenic groups. However, sub-lethal levels of biocides in agricultural systems impact the metabolic functionality of the soil microbiota and contribute to the evolution of microbial antibiotic resistance [225,226]. Just as with other non-antibiotic compounds like heavy metals and microplastics, pesticide stress aids the acquisition of ARGs in agricultural systems through several mechanisms, including gene mutation induction, activation of efflux pumps, and outer membrane pores inhibition [226]. For example, the co-exposure of streptomycin and pesticide in some *E. coli* strains, including O157:H7 and O103:H2, induced the emergence of significantly stronger streptomycin-resistant mutants [227]. Further, Shahid and Khan [228] demonstrated a correlation between pesticide resistance and antibiotic resistance among bacterial species recovered from the rhizosphere of edible crops. In most cases, sub-lethal pesticide levels increased the proportion of MGEs that aided the distribution of ARGs, influenced the HGT of ARGs and supported conjugation by increasing cell membrane permeability [197]. Overall, the influence of pesticides on the evolution of ARGs can be controlled by drafting policy documents for the safe use of pesticides in agricultural fields.

6.2.4. Factors Affecting Antibiotic Persistence in the Terrestrial Environment

Cross- and co-resistance phenomena are important factors that determine the spread and persistence of ARGs in the terrestrial environment. Several studies have demonstrated the association between environmental ARGs and non-antibiotic compounds like heavy metals, microplastics, and pesticides [198,229–231]. For example, microplastics in activated sludge systems have been shown to inhibit the removal of ARGs [232] and increase microbial cooperation. Similarly, the pattern of antibiotic spread in activated sludge systems of WWTPs has been demonstrated [233]. According to the findings, stress from high concentrations of heavy metals promoted the spread of ARGs, firstly, through conjugation and subsequently through vertical gene transfer, with gram-negative bacteria detected as the highest recipients of resistant plasmids due to the selection pressure of heavy metals. Accordingly, Niu et al. [234] revealed that the passivation of heavy metals led to effective control of the abundance of bacitracin resistance genes in soil compost. Also, reducing the occurrence of cross- and co-resistance using adsorbents like biochar and clay minerals have been demonstrated as a good strategy for managing the acquisition of ARGs in the environment [235].

Other factors that influence the spread of ARGs from sludge and wastewater irrigation include the design of the WWTPs, the source of the WWTP influent, seasonal variation that impacts important microbial phylotypes, and other abiotic factors like pH and electrical conductivity [236,237]. Redesigning WWTPs to include steps that effectively remove antibiotics and other compounds of concern, like heavy metals and microplastics, could effectively reduce the spread of ARG in both wastewater sludge and effluents used for agricultural purposes, while effective policies for the administration of antibiotics in livestock farming could minimize the transfer of ARGs into agricultural systems.

6.3. Tools Used for Antibiotic Resistance Studies

One of the key issues with studying resistomes and ARGs is that only a significant fraction of microbial species can be grown under laboratory conditions [238]. However, culture remains the gold standard tool for every microbiologist. Therefore, studies investigating phenotypic resistance would require culturing the microorganisms and then determining their resistance to selected antimicrobials using disk-diffusion or agar dilution methods [239]. Despite the success achieved with this approach, working with a large number of samples is challenging. Therefore, automated systems like the VITEK2 Compact system have been developed. Apart from determining the susceptibility of microorganisms, this system has the added advantage of determining the organism's identity [240]. However, the need to culture the organisms before determining their resistance profiles limits these culture-based techniques as the resistome of a large microbial population cannot easily be determined. Therefore,, next-generation DNA sequencing (NGS) and other 'omics' tools are especially helpful in resistome research because some microbial species harboring ARGs are viable but non-cultivable. The *16S rRNA* gene profile PCR assay is a common method for investigating the resistome. In computational analysis, ARG profiles are linked to the microbial population using the *16S rRNA* gene as taxonomic identity markers. The use of taxonomic markers in resistome research has some drawbacks, the most significant of which is the insufficient depth of its sequences; most markers provide an accurate estimate only to the family or genus level, but not the species level [241]. Nevertheless, an integrated approach that utilizes *16S rRNA*, metagenomics, and other tools can shed light on the interactions and dynamics of the resistome in bacteria communities, whereas *16S rRNA* genes alone are limited in their ability to achieve this goal.

Next-generation sequencing techniques like high throughput shotgun metagenomics are valuable when assessing the resistome of entire populations. This involves sequencing total genomes extracted from a population and analysing the resulting files using different bioinformatic pipelines such as PRAP (Pan Resistome Analysis Pipeline) [242]. While metagenomics is a powerful tool for investigating ARG abundance at the population level, it is more difficult because it requires significantly more computational resources than are needed to analyse the *16S rRNA* gene. Another significant restriction is that the mere presence of a gene does not ensure that it is functional or expressed by the microbial cells. Integrating metagenomics with other methods, such as functional metagenomics, could help fill this information gap [243]. Functional metagenomics does not necessitate a prior understanding of environmental ARGs. The main techniques include growth in diffusion chambers or expressing metagenomic genes in surrogate hosts for biochemical studies. These methods are not limited to any particular culture because they can also be used on non-cultivable organisms [244]. The most significant drawback is using ARGs in surrogate expression systems, which removes them from their natural environment. Functional metagenomics causes far more disruption to the natural environment than other techniques, such as *16S rRNA* gene sequencing and metagenomics [245]. Future resistome research will most likely be driven by combined functional metagenomics and culturomics techniques, particularly when used with third-generation sequencing or Nanopore sequencing techniques [243].

Protein studies can offer a profound understanding of enzyme activity and the function of proteins in microbial cells that make up the resistome. Few reports on antibiotic resistance in microbial populations found in the environment have been analysed using metaproteomics or metabolomics [246]. Unlike metagenomics and metatranscriptomics, which are made easier by developments in NGS, metaproteomics and metabolomics depend on technologies that make only incremental leaps forward. These technologies include two-dimensional or differential in-gel electrophoresis, liquid chromatography with mass spectrometry, or MALDI-TOF [247,248]. To make these methods applicable to future resistome studies, there is a need for advancements in high throughput sampling techniques.

Using metaproteomics and metabolomics in resistome research can answer questions about the mechanisms involved in developing resistomes, although the scope of this research is limited. Figure 3 depicts modern techniques used in resistome studies.

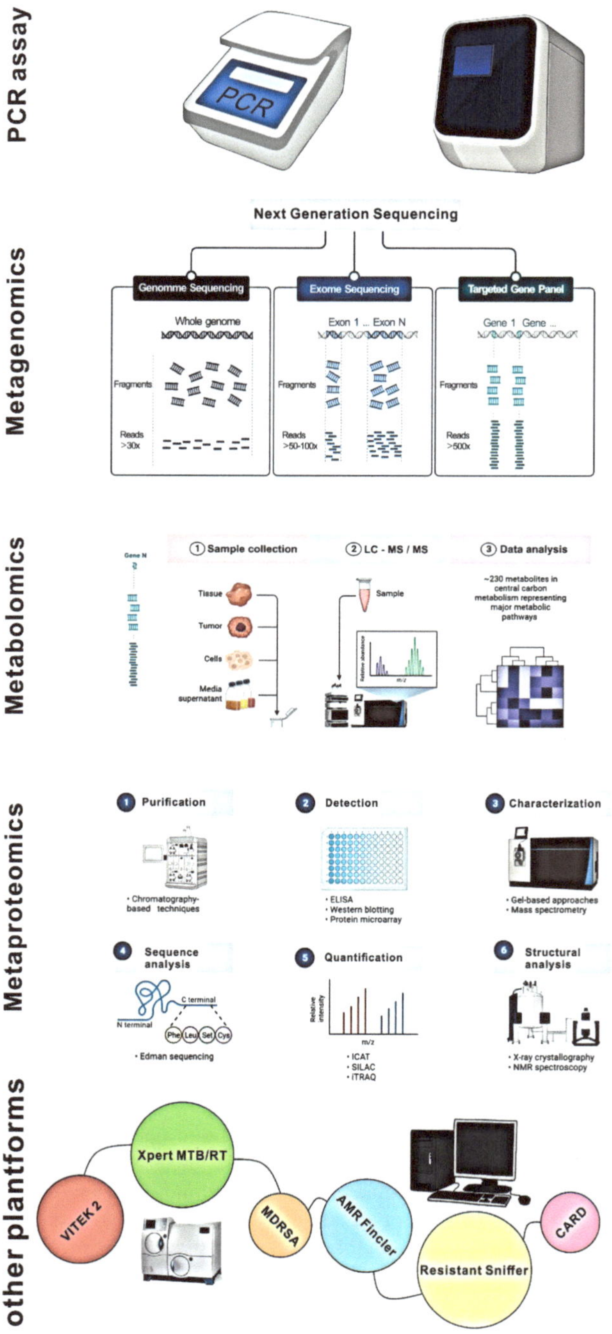

Figure 3. Modern tools used for resistome identification analysis.

6.4. Ecotoxicological Impact of Antibiotics and Antibiotic-Resistant Bacteria

The persistence of antibiotics in the environment can alter the ecosystem's community structure and ecological function, including biomass and biodiversity, as well as the survival, reproduction, metabolism and population of organisms [249]. Multiple investigations have demonstrated that antibiotics may have physiological effects on non-target organisms like plants and other living organisms. For instance, many antibiotic classes have been found to share common receptors in plants; these include those that inhibit chloroplast replication (fluoroquinolones), transcription and translation (tetracyclines, macrolides, lincosamides, P-aminoglycosides, and pleuromutilins), metabolic pathways (folate biosynthesis, *sul*fonamides, and triclosan), and sterol biosynthesis (triclosan and other classes of statin-type blood lipid regulators) [250]. Similarly, numerous studies have evaluated the effects of antibiotics on non-target sensitive organisms like zebrafish, Daphnia, algae, mussels, and other aquatic organisms and have reported general toxicity indicators like LC_{50}, EC_{50}, and mean inhibitory concentration (IC_{50}) [251]. However, existing standard ecotoxicology tests used in the regulatory assessment of pharmaceuticals have been questioned due to possible inadequacies in capturing ecologically significant effects [252]. Due to a lack of information, a thorough analysis of environmental risks cannot be conducted at this time. There is still a dearth of primary data on antibiotics and ARGs' environmental fate and impacts. Such information must be readily available to conduct accurate risk assessments and implement effective risk management programs.

7. Antibiotic-Resistant Bacteria and Human Health Concerns

Antibiotic resistance or drug resistance is a worldwide public health crisis requiring immediate action. In 2019, antimicrobial resistance was linked to 4.95 million deaths, 1.27 million of which were attributed to drug-resistant illnesses alone. Without concerted action, this number might exceed ten million by 2050, costing more than USD 100 trillion [253]. In recent decades, many pathogenic bacteria have evolved into multi-drug resistant (MDR) bacteria. For instance, the US Centre for Disease Control and Prevention (CDC) released a list of the top public threats in 2015, which included drug-resistant diseases and classified them as Urgent, Serious, or concerning threats (Table 4). Four urgent threats include carbapenem-resistant *Enterobacteriaceae* and *Acinetobacter*, drug-resistant *N. gonorrhoeae* and *Clostridium difficile*, causing numerous deaths annually in the US and other countries. Serious infections include those indicated in Table 4, such as methicillin-resistant *S. aureus* (MRSA) and *van*comycin-resistant *Enterococcus* (VRE) infections and extremely drug-resistant tuberculosis (XDR-TB). Other members of this category include *S. pneumoniae*, which accounts for most bacterial pneumonia and meningitis worldwide, and *Acinetobacter*, *Campylobacter*, fluconazole-resistant *Candida*, *Enterobacteriaceae* (*Pseudomonas aeruginosa*, *Salmonella* (both typhi and non-typhi) generating a beta-lactamase that has extensive activity against most penicillins and cephalosporins. It is estimated that this group is responsible for around 22,500 deaths annually in the United States. In addition, the presence of streptococci resistant to erythromycin and clindamycin is viewed as "of concern" [16]. While these concerns focus more on human consumption of antibiotics, it should be noted that these problematic organisms could also originate from animal sources—directly through contact with infected animals or indirectly through the consumption of contaminated animal products. For example, hospitalized pets have been recognized as significant reservoirs and sources of carbapenem-resistant bacteria, including *Acinetobacter* spp. [254], implying a possible direct transmission from these animals to humans. These carbapenem-resistant bacteria have also been identified in food animals [255,256], meaning that indirect transmission to humans could occur through the consumption of these animals as a protein source.

Table 4. Public threat status of different antimicrobial-resistant organisms.

Threat Status	Organism	Estimated Clinical Cases Per Year	Estimated Healthcare Cost (US Dollars)	Descriptions
Urgent	Carbapenem-resistant *Acinetobacter*	8500 (700)	281 million	Carbapenem-resistant *Acinetobacter* causes pneumonia and wound, bloodstream, and urinary tract infections. Nearly all these infections happen in patients who recently received care in a healthcare facility
	Clostridioides difficile (*C. difficile*)	223,900 (12,800)	1 billion	*C. difficile* causes life-threatening diarrhoea and colitis (inflammation of the colon), mostly in people who have had both recent medical care and antibiotics.
	Carbapenem-resistant *Enterobacterales* (CRE)	13,100 (1100)	130 million	CRE are a major concern for patients in healthcare facilities. Some *Enterobacterales* are resistant to nearly all antibiotics, leaving more toxic or less effective treatment options.
	Drug-resistant *N. gonorrhoeae* (*N. gonorrhoeae*)	550,000	133.4 million	*N. gonorrhoeae* causes the sexually transmitted disease *Gonorrhoea* that can result in life-threatening ectopic pregnancy and infertility and can increase the risk of getting and giving HIV.
Serious	Drug-resistant *Campylobacter*	448,400 (70)	270 million	*Campylobacter* usually causes diarrhoea (often bloody), fever, and abdominal cramps and can spread from animals to people through contaminated food, especially raw or undercooked chicken
	ESBL-producing *Enterobacterales*	197,400 (9100)	1.2 billion	ESBL-producing *Enterobacterales* are a concern in healthcare settings and the community. They can spread rapidly and cause or complicate infections in healthy people. ESBLs are enzymes that break down commonly used antibiotics, such as penicillins and cephalosporins, making them ineffective.
	Vancomycin-resistant *Enterococcus* (VRE)	54,500 (5400)	539 million	*Enterococci* can cause severe infections for patients in healthcare settings, including bloodstream, surgical site, and urinary tract infections.
	Multidrug-resistant *Pseudomonas aeruginosa* (*P. aeruginosa*)	32,600 (2700)	767 million	*P. aeruginosa* infections usually occur in people with weakened immune systems and can be particularly dangerous for patients with chronic lung diseases.
	Drug-resistant non-typhoidal *Salmonella*	212,500 (70)	400 million	Non-typhoidal *Salmonella* can spread from animals to people through food and usually causes diarrhoea, fever, and abdominal cramps. Some infections spread to the blood and can have life-threatening complications.
	Drug-resistant *Salmonella* serotype Typhi	4100 (<5)	11 to 21 million	*Salmonella* Typhi causes severe typhoid fever, which can be life-threatening. Most people in the U.S. become infected while traveling to countries where the disease is common.
	Drug-resistant *Shigella*	77,000 (<5)	93 million	*Shigella* spreads in feces through direct contact or contaminated surfaces, food, or water. Most people with *Shigella* infections develop diarrhoea, fever, and stomach cramps.
	Methicillin-resistant *S. aureus* (MRSA)	323,700 (10,600)	1.7 billion	*S. aureus* are common bacteria that spread in healthcare facilities and the community. In addition, MRSA can cause difficult-to-treat staph infections because of resistance to some antibiotics.

Table 4. *Cont.*

Threat Status	Organism	Estimated Clinical Cases Per Year	Estimated Healthcare Cost (US Dollars)	Descriptions
	Drug-resistant *S. pneumoniae*	900,000 (3600)	4 billion	*S. pneumoniae* causes pneumococcal disease, ranging from ear and sinus infections to pneumonia and bloodstream infections
	Drug-resistant Tuberculosis	847 (62)	1.6 million	TB is caused by *M. tuberculosis*. It is among the most common infectious diseases and a frequent cause of death worldwide.
Concerning	Erythromycin-resistant Group A *Streptococcus (GAS)*	5400 (450)	2.6 million	GAS can cause many infections ranging from minor illnesses to severe and deadly diseases, including strep throat, pneumonia, flesh-eating infections, and sepsis.
	Clindamycin-resistant Group B *Streptococcus (GBS)*	13,000 (720)	NA	GBS can cause severe illness in people of all ages.
Watch list	Azole-resistant *Aspergillus fumigatus*	NA	NA	*Aspergillus fumigatus*, a ubiquitously distributed opportunistic pathogen, is the leading agent of aspergillosis, ranking first among fungal killers.
	Drug-resistant *Mycoplasma genitalium*			*Mycoplasma genitalium* is one of the important causes of non-gonococcal urethritis.
	Drug-resistant *Bordetella perstussis*			Pertussis (whooping cough), a highly contagious respiratory illness caused by *Bordetella pertussis*

8. Strategies for Addressing the Challenge of Antibiotic Resistance

The challenge posed by antibiotic-resistant bacteria can be categorized into five primary intervention strategies within the human and veterinary sectors. In the first place, infection prevention and control principles continue to be the cornerstone in the fight against the spread of ABR [22]. Second, vaccinations are a critical tool for preventing infections and decreasing the demand for antibiotics. Although new vaccine initiatives are being developed for *S. aureus*, *E. coli*, and others, vaccines are only available for one of the six leading pathogens (*S. pneumoniae*) [257]. Third, reducing exposure to antibiotics for purposes other than treating human disease is an essential potential risk-reduction strategy. An increase in ABR in humans has been linked to the widespread use of antibiotics in agriculture, though the exact cause-and-effect relationship is still up for debate [258]. Intensive farming imposes stress on food animals, forcing farmers to use antibiotics to treat their animals [259]. However, treating individual sick animals is challenging; hence, providing antibiotics to all animals on a farm prophylactically through their feed and water helps reduce the disease burden and improves animal health. This is not without consequences, as ABR is favoured under such conditions. Combating this phenomenon would require the observation of stringent biosecurity measures [260] and the use of alternatives to antimicrobials to treat sick animals [261]. Fourth, antibiotics should not be used to treat viral infections unless necessary. For antimicrobial use can be reduced or stopped when necessary, it is critical to establish mechanisms that facilitate rapid and accurate diagnosis of disease by clinicians [262]. Finally, it is essential to continue investing in the pipeline for developing new antibiotics and providing access to second-line antibiotics in areas that do not have widespread access [263]. It is an urgent priority to identify strategies that can reduce the burden of bacterial ABR across a wide range of settings or specifically tailored to the available resources and the leading pathogen–drug combinations in a particular setting.

The environmental dimension of ABR remains the least addressed component in the fight against this global ill. This is partly because the environment presents a more complex scenario involving numerous stressors than humans and animals. Nevertheless, wastewater treatment plants have been recognized as hotspots for the dissemination of ABR in the environment. Therefore, improving the quality of the effluents from these plants would reduce the discharge of polluted waters containing antimicrobial-resistant pathogens and ARGs into receiving water bodies. This is, however, challenging for areas in low- and middle-income countries where such facilities are unavailable. Nevertheless, greater sensitization and the provision of mobile toilets could prevent open defecation and pollution of the environment.

Although these strategies have been presented separately, it must be noted that for effective, sustainable solutions to be achieved in the fight against ABR, firm collaborations and communication must be established between actors in the One Health triad—humans, animals, and the environment.

9. Conclusions

Antibiotic resistance remains a significant challenge threatening human, animal and environmental health. Although ABR has increased over the years due to the indiscriminate use of antibiotics in human and veterinary settings, ABR is also shown to be a natural process, with resistance genes discovered in pristine environments with little or no human interference. Furthermore, although less studied, the environmental dimension of ABMR constitutes a significant reservoir as a source of ABR through horizontal and vertical transfer, with plasmids and other mobile genetic elements playing a crucial role in this process. Within the environment, other less-considered factors like heavy metals and pesticides also play an important role in selection pressure, inducing resistance in previously susceptible environmental organisms. Furthermore, wastewater treatment plants remain major contributors of ARB and ARGs in the environment. Given the broad distribution of ABR, solutions aiming to curb this ill should be multifacet, involving antimicrobial stewardship in humans and animals, prevention of environmental pollution and promoting the discovery of new antibiotics, among others.

Author Contributions: Conceptualization, All authors; methodology, R.S. and C.O.; validation, T.S. and H.L.; formal analysis, R.S., C.O., A.L.K.A. and T.S.; investigation, All authors; data curation, R.S., T.S. and H.L.; writing—original draft preparation, R.S.; writing—review and editing, R.S., C.O., A.L.K.A., T.S. and H.L. All authors have read and agreed to the published version of the manuscript.

Funding: This research received no external funding. The APC was funded by A.L.K.A. (University of Venda) and T.S. (University of the Witwatersrand).

Institutional Review Board Statement: Not applicable.

Informed Consent Statement: Not applicable.

Data Availability Statement: All articles reviewed have been included in the reference list.

Conflicts of Interest: The authors declare no conflict of interest.

References

1. Kourkouta, L.; Tsaloglidou, A.; Koukourikos, K.; Iliadis, C.; Plati, P.; Dimitriadou, A. History of Antibiotics. *Sumer. J. Med. Healthc.* **2018**, *1*, 51–54. [CrossRef]
2. Hutchings, M.I.; Truman, A.W.; Wilkinson, B. Antibiotics: Past, Present and Future. *Curr. Opin. Microbiol.* **2019**, *51*, 72–80. [CrossRef] [PubMed]
3. Zaffiri, L.; Gardner, J.; Toledo-Pereyra, L.H. History of Antibiotics. from Salvarsan to Cephalosporins. *J. Investig. Surg.* **2012**, *25*, 67–77. [CrossRef]
4. Alnemri, A.R.; Almaghrabi, R.H.; Alonazi, N.; Alfrayh, A.R. Current Paediatric Research. *Curr. Pediatr. Res.* **2016**, *20*, 169–173.
5. Magiorakos, A.P.; Srinivasan, A.; Carey, R.B.; Carmeli, Y.; Falagas, M.E.; Giske, C.G.; Harbarth, S.; Hindler, J.F.; Kahlmeter, G.; Olsson-Liljequist, B.; et al. Multidrug-Resistant, Extensively Drug-Resistant and Pandrug-Resistant Bacteria: An International Expert Proposal for Interim Standard Definitions for Acquired Resistance. *Clin. Microbiol. Infect.* **2012**, *18*, 268–281. [CrossRef] [PubMed]
6. Bosch, F.; Rosich, L. The Contributions of Paul Ehrlich to Pharmacology: A Tribute on the Occasion of the Centenary of His Nobel Prize. *Pharmacology* **2008**, *82*, 171–179. [CrossRef] [PubMed]
7. Walsh, C.T.K.; Wright, G. Introduction: Antibiotic Resistance. *Chem. Rev.* **2005**, *105*, 391–394. [CrossRef]

8. Derry, J.E. Evaluation of Cefaclor. *Am. J. Hosp. Pharm.* **1981**, *38*, 54–58. [CrossRef]
9. Drehobl, M.; Bianchi, P.; Keyserling, C.H.; Tack, K.J.; Griffin, T.J. Comparison of Cefdinir and Cefaclor in Treatment of Community-Acquired Pneumonia. *Antimicrob. Agents Chemother.* **1997**, *41*, 1579–1583. [CrossRef]
10. Schaad, U.B.; Suter, S.; Gianella-Borradori, A.; Pfenninger, J.; Auckenthaler, R.; Bernath, O.; Cheseaux, J.-J.; Wedgwood, J. A Comparison of Ceftriaxone and Cefuroxime for the Treatment of Bacterial Meningitis in Children. *N. Engl. J. Med.* **1990**, *322*, 141–147. [CrossRef]
11. Deal, E.N.; Micek, S.T.; Reichley, R.M.; Ritchie, D.J. Effects of an Alternative Cefepime Dosing Strategy in Pulmonary and Bloodstream Infections Caused by Enterobacter Spp, Citrobacter Freundii, and Pseudomonas Aeruginosa: A Single-Center, Open-Label, Prospective, Observational Study. *Clin. Ther.* **2009**, *31*, 299–310. [CrossRef] [PubMed]
12. McNabb, J.; Quintiliani, R.; Nightingale, C.H.; Nicolau, D.P. Comparison of the Bactericidal Activity of Trovafloxacin and Ciprofloxacin, Alone and in Combination with Cefepime, against Pseudomonas Aeruginosa. *Chemotherapy* **2000**, *46*, 383–389. [CrossRef] [PubMed]
13. Endimiani, A.; Perez, F.; Bonomo, R.A. Cefepime: A Reappraisal in an Era of Increasing Antimicrobial Resistance. *Expert Rev. Anti. Infect. Ther.* **2008**, *6*, 805–824. [CrossRef] [PubMed]
14. Conly, J.M.; Johnston, B.L. Where Are All the New Antibiotics? The New Antibiotic Paradox. *Can. J. Infect. Dis. Med. Microbiol.* **2005**, *16*, 159–160. [CrossRef] [PubMed]
15. Zaman, S.B.; Hussain, M.A.; Nye, R.; Mehta, V.; Mamun, K.T.; Hossain, N. A Review on Antibiotic Resistance: Alarm Bells Are Ringing. *Cureus* **2017**, *9*, e1403. [CrossRef] [PubMed]
16. Dodds, D.R. Antibiotic Resistance: A Current Epilogue. *Biochem. Pharmacol.* **2017**, *134*, 139–146. [CrossRef]
17. Levy, S.B.; Marshall, B. Antibacterial Resistance Worldwide: Causes, Challenges and Responses. *Nat. Med.* **2004**, *10*, S122–S129. [CrossRef] [PubMed]
18. Durand, G.A.; Raoult, D.; Dubourg, G. Antibiotic Discovery: History, Methods and Perspectives. *Int. J. Antimicrob. Agents* **2019**, *53*, 371–382. [CrossRef]
19. Lowy, F.D. Antimicrobial Resistance: The Example of Staphylococcus Aureus. *J. Clin. Investig.* **2003**, *111*, 1265–1273. [CrossRef]
20. Appelbaum, P.C. The Emergence of Vancomycin-intermediate and Vancomycin-resistant Staphylococcus Aureus. *Clin. Microbiol. Infect.* **2006**, *12*, 16–23. [CrossRef]
21. Aminov, R.I.; Mackie, R.I. Evolution and Ecology of Antibiotic Resistance Genes. *FEMS Microbiol. Lett.* **2007**, *271*, 147–161. [CrossRef] [PubMed]
22. European Centre for Disease Prevention and Control. *Antimicrobial Resistance in the EU/EEA (EARS-Net)—Annual Epidemiological Report 2019*; ECDC: Stockholm, Sweden, 2020; Available online: https://www.ecdc.europa.eu/en/publications-data/surveillance-antimicrobial-resistance-europe-2019#:~{}:text=EARS%2DNet%20data%20for%202019,aureus%20(20.6%25)%2C%20K (accessed on 1 November 2022).
23. Indian Council of Medical Research. *AMR and Surveillance Network Annual Report. January 2019 to December 2019*; ICMR: New Delhi, India, 2020; Available online: https://main.icmr.nic.in/sites/default/files/guidelines/AMRSN_annual_report_2020.pdf (accessed on 14 October 2022).
24. WHO. *WHO Global Antimicrobial Resistance and Use Surveillance System (GLASS) Report: 2021*; World Health Organization: Geneva, Switzerland, 2021.
25. Hu, F.; Zhu, D.; Wang, F.; Wang, M. Current Status and Trends of Antibacterial Resistance in China. *Clin. Infect. Dis.* **2018**, *67*, 128–134. [CrossRef] [PubMed]
26. Ndihokubwayo, J.B.; Yahaya, A.A.; Desta, A.T.; Ki-Zerbo, G.; Odei, E.A.; Keita, B.; Pana, A.P.; Nkhoma, W. Antimicrobial Resistance in the African Region: Issues, Challenges and Actions Proposed. *African Health Monit.* **2013**, *16*, 27–30.
27. Tadesse, B.T.; Ashley, E.A.; Ongarello, S.; Havumaki, J.; Wijegoonewardena, M.; Gonzalez, I.J.; Dittrich, S. Antimicrobial Resistance in Africa: A Systematic Review. *BMC Infect. Dis.* **2017**, *17*, 616. [CrossRef] [PubMed]
28. Uddin, T.M.; Chakraborty, A.J.; Khusro, A.; Zidan, B.M.R.M.; Mitra, S.; Emran, T.B.; Dhama, K.; Ripon, M.K.H.; Gajdács, M.; Sahibzada, M.U.K. Antibiotic Resistance in Microbes: History, Mechanisms, Therapeutic Strategies and Future Prospects. *J. Infect. Public Health* **2021**, *14*, 1750–1766. [CrossRef]
29. Benveniste, R.; Davies, J. Aminoglycoside Antibiotic-Inactivating Enzymes in Actinomycetes Similar to Those Present in Clinical Isolates of Antibiotic-Resistant Bacteria. *Proc. Natl. Acad. Sci. USA* **1973**, *70*, 2276–2280. [CrossRef]
30. Bennett, P.M. Plasmid Encoded Antibiotic Resistance: Acquisition and Transfer of Antibiotic Resistance Genes in Bacteria. *Br. J. Pharmacol.* **2008**, *153*, S347–S357. [CrossRef]
31. Firth, N.; Skurray, R.A. Mobile Elements in the Evolution and Spread of Multiple-Drug Resistance in Staphylococci. *Drug Resist. Updat.* **1998**, *1*, 49–58. [CrossRef]
32. Cloeckaert, A.; Schwarz, S. Molecular Characterization, Spread and Evolution of Multidrug Resistance in Salmonella Enterica Typhimurium DT104. *Vet. Res.* **2001**, *32*, 301–310. [CrossRef]
33. Palmer, K.L.; Kos, V.N.; Gilmore, M.S. Horizontal Gene Transfer and the Genomics of Enterococcal Antibiotic Resistance. *Curr. Opin. Microbiol.* **2010**, *13*, 632–639. [CrossRef]
34. Schultsz, C.; Geerlings, S. Plasmid-Mediated Resistance in Enterobacteriaceae. *Drugs* **2012**, *72*, 1–16. [CrossRef] [PubMed]
35. Chang, C.; Huang, P.; Lu, P. The Resistance Mechanisms and Clinical Impact of Resistance to the Third Generation Cephalosporins in Species of Enterobacter Cloacae Complex in Taiwan. *Antibiotics* **2022**, *11*, 1153. [CrossRef]

36. Robicsek, A.; Jacoby, G.A.; Hooper, D.C. The Worldwide Emergence of Plasmid-Mediated Quinolone Resistance. *Lancet Infect. Dis.* **2006**, *6*, 629–640. [CrossRef] [PubMed]
37. Strahilevitz, J.; Jacoby, G.A.; Hooper, D.C.; Robicsek, A. Plasmid-Mediated Quinolone Resistance: A Multifaceted Threat. *Clin. Microbiol. Rev.* **2009**, *22*, 664–689. [CrossRef] [PubMed]
38. Pagano, M.; Martins, A.F.; Barth, A.L. Mobile Genetic Elements Related to Carbapenem Resistance in Acinetobacter Baumannii. *Braz. J. Microbiol.* **2016**, *47*, 785–792. [CrossRef]
39. Berglund, F.; Marathe, N.P.; Osterlund, T.; Bengtsson-Palme, J.; Kotsakis, S.; Flach, C.F.; Larsson, D.G.J.; Kristiansson, E. Identification of 76 Novel B1 Metallo-Beta-Lactamases through Large-Scale Screening of Genomic and Metagenomic Data. *Microbiome* **2017**, *5*, 134. [CrossRef]
40. Armin, S.; Fallah, F.; Navidinia, M.; Vosoghian, S. Prevalence of BlaOXA-1 and BlaDHA-1 AmpC β-Lactamase-Producing and Methicillin-Resistant Staphylococcus Aureus in Iran. *Arch. Pediatr. Infect. Dis.* **2017**, *5*, e36778.
41. Shaheen, B.W.; Nayak, R.; Boothe, D.M. Emergence of a New Delhi Metallo-β-Lactamase (NDM-1)-Encoding Gene in Clinical Escherichia Coli Isolates Recovered from Companion Animals in the United States. *Antimicrob. Agents Chemother.* **2013**, *57*, 2902–2903. [CrossRef]
42. Partridge, S.R.; Kwong, S.M.; Firth, N.; Jensen, S.O. Mobile Genetic Elements Associated with Antimicrobial Resistance. *Clin. Microbiol. Rev.* **2018**, *31*, e00088-17. [CrossRef]
43. Moosavian, M.; Rahimzadeh, M. Molecular Detection of Metallo-β-Lactamase Genes, BlaIMP-1, BlaVIM-2 and BlaSPM-1 in Imipenem Resistant Pseudomonas Aeruginosa Isolated from Clinical Specimens in Teaching Hospitals of Ahvaz, Iran. *Iran. J. Microbiol.* **2015**, *7*, 2.
44. Mollenkopf, D.F.; Stull, J.W.; Mathys, D.A.; Bowman, A.S.; Feicht, S.M.; Grooters, S.V.; Daniels, J.B.; Wittum, T.E. Carbapenemase-Producing Enterobacteriaceae Recovered from the Environment of a Swine Farrow-to-Finish Operation in the United States. *Antimicrob. Agents Chemother.* **2017**, *61*, e01298-16. [CrossRef]
45. Mathys, D.A.; Mathys, B.A.; Mollenkopf, D.F.; Daniels, J.B.; Wittum, T.E. Enterobacteriaceae Harboring AmpC (Bla CMY) and ESBL (Bla CTX-M) in Migratory and Nonmigratory Wild Songbird Populations on Ohio Dairies. *Vector-Borne Zoonotic Dis.* **2017**, *17*, 254–259. [CrossRef] [PubMed]
46. Johnson, A.P.; Woodford, N. Global Spread of Antibiotic Resistance: The Example of New Delhi Metallo-β-Lactamase (NDM)-Mediated Carbapenem Resistance. *J. Med. Microbiol.* **2013**, *62*, 499–513. [CrossRef] [PubMed]
47. Fleury, C.; Resman, F.; Rau, J.; Riesbeck, K. Prevalence, Distribution and Transfer of Small β-Lactamase-Containing Plasmids in Swedish Haemophilus Influenzae. *J. Antimicrob. Chemother.* **2014**, *69*, 1238–1242. [CrossRef]
48. Tayh, G.; Al Laham, N.; Fhoula, I.; Abedelateef, N.; El-Laham, M.; Elkader Elottol, A.; Ben Slama, K. Frequency and Antibiotics Resistance of Extended-Spectrum Beta-Lactamase (ESBLs) Producing Escherichia Coli and Klebsiella Pneumoniae Isolated from Patients in Gaza Strip, Palestine. *J. Med. Microbiol. Infect. Dis.* **2021**, *9*, 133–141. [CrossRef]
49. Von Wintersdorff, C.J.H.; Penders, J.; Van Niekerk, J.M.; Mills, N.D.; Majumder, S.; Van Alphen, L.B.; Savelkoul, P.H.M.; Wolffs, P.F.G. Dissemination of Antimicrobial Resistance in Microbial Ecosystems through Horizontal Gene Transfer. *Front. Microbiol.* **2016**, *7*, 173. [CrossRef] [PubMed]
50. Bassetti, M.; Merelli, M.; Temperoni, C.; Astilean, A. New Antibiotics for Bad Bugs: Where Are We? *Ann. Clin. Microbiol. Antimicrob.* **2013**, *12*, 22. [CrossRef] [PubMed]
51. Shirley, J.D.; Nauta, K.M.; Carlson, E.E. Live-Cell Profiling of Penicillin-Binding Protein Inhibitors in Escherichia Coli MG1655. *ACS Infect. Dis.* **2022**, *8*, 1241–1252. [CrossRef]
52. Pai, H.; Kim, M.R.; Seo, M.-R.; Choi, T.Y.; Oh, S.H. A Nosocomial Outbreak of Escherichia Coli Producing CTX-M-15 and OXA-30 β-Lactamase. *Infect. Control Hosp. Epidemiol.* **2006**, *27*, 312–314. [CrossRef]
53. Jamrozy, D.; Coll, F.; Mather, A.E.; Harris, S.R.; Harrison, E.M.; MacGowan, A.; Karas, A.; Elston, T.; Estée Török, M.; Parkhill, J. Evolution of Mobile Genetic Element Composition in an Epidemic Methicillin-Resistant Staphylococcus Aureus: Temporal Changes Correlated with Frequent Loss and Gain Events. *BMC Genomics* **2017**, *18*, 684. [CrossRef]
54. Evans, B.A.; Amyes, S.G.B. OXA β-Lactamases. *Clin. Microbiol. Rev.* **2014**, *27*, 241–263. [CrossRef] [PubMed]
55. Roshani, M.; Goodarzi, A.; Hashemi, A.; Afrasiabi, F.; Goudarzi, H.; Arabestani, M. Detection of QnrA, QnrB, and QnrS Genes in Klebsiella Pneumoniae and Escherichia Coli Isolates from Leukemia Patients. *Rev. Med. Microbiol.* **2022**, *33*, 14–19. [CrossRef]
56. Ghobadi, N.; HakimiAleni, R. Evaluation of Plasmid-Mediated Quinolone Resistance Genes And Biofilm Formation in Clinical Isolates of Escherichia Coli. *Exp. Anim. Biol.* **2022**, *10*, 77–86.
57. Redgrave, L.S.; Sutton, S.B.; Webber, M.A.; Piddock, L.J. V Fluoroquinolone Resistance: Mechanisms, Impact on Bacteria, and Role in Evolutionary Success. *Trends Microbiol.* **2014**, *22*, 438–445. [CrossRef]
58. Haque, T.A.; Urmi, U.L.; Islam, A.B.M.M.K.; Ara, B.; Nahar, S.; Mosaddek, A.S.M.; Lugova, H.; Kumar, S.; Jahan, D.; Rahman, N.A.A. Detection of Qnr Genes and GyrA Mutation to Quinolone Phenotypic Resistance of UTI Pathogens in Bangladesh and the Implications. *J. Appl. Pharm. Sci.* **2022**, *12*, 185–198. [CrossRef]
59. Yakout, M.A.; Ali, G.H. A Novel ParC Mutation Potentiating Fluoroquinolone Resistance in Klebsiella Pneumoniae and Escherichia Coli Clinical Isolates. *J. Infect. Dev. Ctries.* **2022**, *16*, 314–319. [CrossRef]
60. Truong-Bolduc, Q.C.; Wang, Y.; Reedy, J.L.; Vyas, J.M.; Hooper, D.C. Staphylococcus Aureus Efflux Pumps and Tolerance to Ciprofloxacin and Chlorhexidine Following Induction by Mupirocin. *Antimicrob. Agents Chemother.* **2022**, *66*, e01845-21. [CrossRef]

61. De Rossi, E.; Arrigo, P.; Bellinzoni, M.; Silva, P.E.A.; Martín, C.; Aínsa, J.A.; Guglierame, P.; Riccardi, G. The Multidrug Transporters Belonging to Major Facilitator Superfamily (MFS) in Mycobacterium Tuberculosis. *Mol. Med.* **2002**, *8*, 714–724. [CrossRef]
62. Montero, C.; Mateu, G.; Rodriguez, R.; Takiff, H. Intrinsic Resistance of Mycobacterium Smegmatis to Fluoroquinolones May Be Influenced by New Pentapeptide Protein MfpA. *Antimicrob. Agents Chemother.* **2001**, *45*, 3387–3392. [CrossRef]
63. Cattoir, V.; Poirel, L.; Aubert, C.; Soussy, C.-J.; Nordmann, P. Unexpected Occurrence of Plasmid-Mediated Quinolone Resistance Determinants in Environmental *Aeromonas* Spp. *Emerg. Infect. Dis.* **2008**, *14*, 231. [CrossRef]
64. Hu, X.; Yu, X.; Shang, Y.; Xu, H.; Guo, L.; Liang, Y.; Kang, Y.; Song, L.; Sun, J.; Yue, F. Emergence and Characterization of a Novel IncP-6 Plasmid Harboring Bla *Aeromonas* KPC-2. In *"One Health" Approach for Revealing Reservoirs and Transmission of Antimicrobial Resistance*; Frontiers Media SA: Lausanne, Switzerland, 2022.
65. Yamane, K.; Wachino, J.; Suzuki, S.; Kimura, K.; Shibata, N.; Kato, H.; Shibayama, K.; Konda, T.; Arakawa, Y. New Plasmid-Mediated Fluoroquinolone Efflux Pump, QepA, Found in an Escherichia Coli Clinical Isolate. *Antimicrob. Agents Chemother.* **2007**, *51*, 3354–3360. [CrossRef] [PubMed]
66. Hansen, L.H.; Jensen, L.B.; Sørensen, H.I.; Sørensen, S.J. Substrate Specificity of the OqxAB Multidrug Resistance Pump in Escherichia Coli and Selected Enteric Bacteria. *J. Antimicrob. Chemother.* **2007**, *60*, 145–147. [CrossRef] [PubMed]
67. Yokota, S.; Sato, K.; Kuwahara, O.; Habadera, S.; Tsukamoto, N.; Ohuchi, H.; Akizawa, H.; Himi, T.; Fujii, N. Fluoroquinolone-Resistant Streptococcus Pneumoniae Strains Occur Frequently in Elderly Patients in Japan. *Antimicrob. Agents Chemother.* **2002**, *46*, 3311–3315. [CrossRef] [PubMed]
68. Ferrándiz, M.J.; Fenoll, A.; Liñares, J.; De La Campa, A.G. Horizontal Transfer of ParC and GyrA in Fluoroquinolone-Resistant Clinical Isolates of Streptococcus Pneumoniae. *Antimicrob. Agents Chemother.* **2000**, *44*, 840–847. [CrossRef]
69. Zając, O.M.; Tyski, S.; Laudy, A.E. The Contribution of Efflux Systems to Levofloxacin Resistance in Stenotrophomonas Maltophilia Clinical Strains Isolated in Warsaw, Poland. *Biology* **2022**, *11*, 1044. [CrossRef]
70. Wu, C.-J.; Lu, H.-F.; Lin, Y.-T.; Zhang, M.-S.; Li, L.-H.; Yang, T.-C. Substantial Contribution of SmeDEF, SmeVWX, SmQnr, and Heat Shock Response to Fluoroquinolone Resistance in Clinical Isolates of Stenotrophomonas Maltophilia. *Front. Microbiol.* **2019**, *10*, 822. [CrossRef]
71. Sánchez, M.B.; Martínez, J.L. The Efflux Pump SmeDEF Contributes to Trimethoprim-Sulfamethoxazole Resistance in Stenotrophomonas Maltophilia. *Antimicrob. Agents Chemother.* **2015**, *59*, 4347–4348. [CrossRef]
72. Häussler, S.; Becker, T. The Pseudomonas Quinolone Signal (PQS) Balances Life and Death in Pseudomonas Aeruginosa Populations. *PLoS Pathog.* **2008**, *4*, e1000166. [CrossRef]
73. Hansen, S.; Lewis, K.; Vulic, M. Role of Global Regulators and Nucleotide Metabolism in Antibiotic Tolerance in Escherichia Coli. *Antimicrob. Agents Chemother.* **2008**, *52*, 2718–2726. [CrossRef]
74. Binda, E.; Marinelli, F.; Marcone, G.L. Old and New Glycopeptide Antibiotics: Action and Resistance. *Antibiotics* **2014**, *3*, 572–594. [CrossRef]
75. Yushchuk, O.; Binda, E.; Marinelli, F. Glycopeptide Antibiotic Resistance Genes: Distribution and Function in the Producer Actinomycetes. *Front. Microbiol.* **2020**, *11*, 1173. [CrossRef]
76. Kahne, D.; Leimkuhler, C.; Lu, W.; Walsh, C. Glycopeptide and Lipoglycopeptide Antibiotics. *Chem. Rev.* **2005**, *105*, 425–448. [CrossRef] [PubMed]
77. Abdelhady, W.; Bayer, A.S.; Seidl, K.; Moormeier, D.E.; Bayles, K.W.; Cheung, A.; Yeaman, M.R.; Xiong, Y.Q. Impact of Vancomycin on SarA-Mediated Biofilm Formation: Role in Persistent Endovascular Infections Due to Methicillin-Resistant Staphylococcus Aureus. *J. Infect. Dis.* **2014**, *209*, 1231–1240. [CrossRef] [PubMed]
78. Novais, C.; Coque, T.M.; Boerlin, P.; Herrero, I.; Moreno, M.A.; Dominguez, L.; Peixe, L. Vancomycin-Resistant Enterococcus Faecium Clone in Swine, Europe. *Emerg. Infect. Dis.* **2005**, *11*, 1985. [CrossRef] [PubMed]
79. Xiong, W.; Sun, Y.; Zhang, T.; Ding, X.; Li, Y.; Wang, M.; Zeng, Z. Antibiotics, Antibiotic Resistance Genes, and Bacterial Community Composition in Fresh Water Aquaculture Environment in China. *Microb. Ecol.* **2015**, *70*, 425–432. [CrossRef]
80. Schwarz, S.; Johnson, A.P. Transferable Resistance to Colistin: A New but Old Threat. *J. Antimicrob. Chemother.* **2016**, *71*, 2066–2070. [CrossRef]
81. Pang, Y.; Bosch, T.; Roberts, M.C. Single Polymerase Chain Reaction for the Detection of Tetracycline-Resistant Determinants Tet K and Tet L. *Mol. Cell. Probes* **1994**, *8*, 417–422. [CrossRef]
82. Showsh, S.A.; Andrews, R.E., Jr. Tetracycline Enhances Tn916-Mediated Conjugal Transfer. *Plasmid* **1992**, *28*, 213–224. [CrossRef]
83. Truong-Bolduc, Q.C.; Wang, Y.; Hooper, D.C. Role of *Staphylococcus aureus* Tet38 in Transport of Tetracycline and Its Regulation in a Salt Stress Environment. *J. Bacteriol.* **2022**, *204*, e00142-22. [CrossRef]
84. Mechler, L.; Herbig, A.; Paprotka, K.; Fraunholz, M.; Nieselt, K.; Bertram, R. A Novel Point Mutation Promotes Growth Phase-Dependent Daptomycin Tolerance in Staphylococcus Aureus. *Antimicrob. Agents Chemother.* **2015**, *59*, 5366–5376. [CrossRef]
85. Yee, R.; Cui, P.; Shi, W.; Feng, J.; Zhang, Y. Genetic Screen Reveals the Role of Purine Metabolism in Staphylococcus Aureus Persistence to Rifampicin. *Antibiotics* **2015**, *4*, 627–642. [CrossRef] [PubMed]
86. Bonnet, R. Growing Group of Extended-Spectrum β-Lactamases: The CTX-M Enzymes. *Antimicrob. Agents Chemother.* **2004**, *48*, 1–14. [CrossRef] [PubMed]
87. de Been, M.; Lanza, V.F.; de Toro, M.; Scharringa, J.; Dohmen, W.; Du, Y.; Hu, J.; Lei, Y.; Li, N.; Tooming-Klunderud, A. Dissemination of Cephalosporin Resistance Genes between Escherichia Coli Strains from Farm Animals and Humans by Specific Plasmid Lineages. *PLoS Genet.* **2014**, *10*, e1004776. [CrossRef] [PubMed]

88. Kristich, C.J.; Rice, L.B.; Arias, C.A. Enterococcal Infection—Treatment and Antibiotic Resistance. In *Enterococci from Commensals to Leading Causes of Drug Resistant Infection*; Gilmore, M.S., Clewell, D.B., Ike, Y., Shankar, N., Eds.; Massachusetts Eye and Ear Infirmary: Boston, MA, USA, 2014.
89. Bailey, A.M.; Webber, M.A.; Piddock, L.J. V Medium Plays a Role in Determining Expression of AcrB, MarA, and SoxS in Escherichia Coli. *Antimicrob. Agents Chemother.* **2006**, *50*, 1071–1074. [CrossRef] [PubMed]
90. Douard, G.; Praud, K.; Cloeckaert, A.; Doublet, B. The Salmonella Genomic Island 1 Is Specifically Mobilized in Trans by the IncA/C Multidrug Resistance Plasmid Family. *PLoS One* **2010**, *5*, e15302. [CrossRef] [PubMed]
91. Sheikh, A.F.; Shahin, M.; Shokoohizadeh, L.; Ghanbari, F.; Solgi, H.; Shahcheraghi, F. Emerge of NDM-1-Producing Multidrug-Resistant Pseudomonas Aeruginosa and Co-Harboring of Carbapenemase Genes in South of Iran. *Iran. J. Public Health* **2020**, *49*, 959.
92. He, J.; Li, C.; Cui, P.; Wang, H. Detection of Tn7-Like Transposons and Antibiotic Resistance in Enterobacterales from Animals Used for Food Production with Identification of Three Novel Transposons Tn6813, Tn6814, and Tn6765. *Front. Microbiol.* **2020**, *11*, 2049. [CrossRef]
93. Akrami, F.; Rajabnia, M.; Pournajaf, A. Resistance Integrons; A Mini Review. *Casp. J. Intern. Med.* **2019**, *10*, 370–376. [CrossRef]
94. Jones, R.N.; Kugler, K.C.; Pfaller, M.A.; Winokur, P.L. Characteristics of Pathogens Causing Urinary Tract Infections in Hospitals in North America: Results from the SENTRY Antimicrobial Surveillance Program, 1997. *Diagn. Microbiol. Infect. Dis.* **1999**, *35*, 55–63. [CrossRef]
95. Arakawa, Y.; Murakami, M.; Suzuki, K.; Ito, H.; Wacharotayankun, R.; Ohsuka, S.; Kato, N.; Ohta, M. A Novel Integron-like Element Carrying the Metallo-Beta-Lactamase Gene BlaIMP. *Antimicrob. Agents Chemother.* **1995**, *39*, 1612–1615. [CrossRef]
96. Lin, M.-F.; Liou, M.-L.; Tu, C.-C.; Yeh, H.-W.; Lan, C.-Y. Molecular Epidemiology of Integron-Associated Antimicrobial Gene Cassettes in the Clinical Isolates of Acinetobacter Baumannii from Northern Taiwan. *Ann. Lab. Med.* **2013**, *33*, 242–247. [CrossRef] [PubMed]
97. Guérin, E.; Jové, T.; Tabesse, A.; Mazel, D.; Ploy, M.-C. High-Level Gene Cassette Transcription Prevents Integrase Expression in Class 1 Integrons. *J. Bacteriol.* **2011**, *193*, 5675–5682. [CrossRef] [PubMed]
98. Deng, Y.; Bao, X.; Ji, L.; Chen, L.; Liu, J.; Miao, J.; Chen, D.; Bian, H.; Li, Y.; Yu, G. Resistance Integrons: Class 1, 2 and 3 Integrons. *Ann. Clin. Microbiol. Antimicrob.* **2015**, *14*, 45. [CrossRef] [PubMed]
99. Poirel, L.; Carattoli, A.; Bernabeu, S.; Bruderer, T.; Frei, R.; Nordmann, P. A Novel IncQ Plasmid Type Harbouring a Class 3 Integron from Escherichia Coli. *J. Antimicrob. Chemother.* **2010**, *65*, 1594–1598. [CrossRef] [PubMed]
100. Jamali, S. Integrons and Insertion Sequences Associated with Beta-Lactamases. In *Beta-Lactam Resistance in Gram-Negative Bacteria*; Springer: Berlin/Heidelberg, Germany, 2022; pp. 179–189.
101. Deylam Salehi, M.; Ferdosi-Shahandashti, E.; Yahyapour, Y.; Khafri, S.; Pournajaf, A.; Rajabnia, R. Integron-Mediated Antibiotic Resistance in Acinetobacter Baumannii Isolated from Intensive Care Unit Patients, Babol, North of Iran. *Biomed Res. Int.* **2017**, *2017*, 7157923. [CrossRef]
102. Chokshi, A.; Sifri, Z.; Cennimo, D.; Horng, H. Global Contributors to Antibiotic Resistance. *J. Glob. Infect. Dis.* **2019**, *11*, 36.
103. Sreeja, M.K.; Gowrishankar, N.L.; Adisha, S.; Divya, K.C. Antibiotic Resistance-Reasons and the Most Common Resistant Pathogens–a Review. *Res. J. Pharm. Technol.* **2017**, *10*, 1886. [CrossRef]
104. Blair, J.M.A.; Webber, M.A.; Baylay, A.J.; Ogbolu, D.O.; Piddock, L.J. V Molecular Mechanisms of Antibiotic Resistance. *Nat. Rev.* **2015**, *13*, 42–51. [CrossRef]
105. Decousser, J.W.; Poirel, L.; Nordmann, P. Characterization of a Chromosomally Encoded Extended-Spectrum Class A β-Lactamase from Kluyvera Cryocrescens. *Antimicrob. Agents Chemother.* **2001**, *45*, 3595–3598. [CrossRef]
106. Li, R.; Chan, E.W.-C.; Chen, S. Characterisation of a Chromosomally-Encoded Extended-Spectrum β-Lactamase Gene BlaPER-3 in Aeromonas Caviae of Chicken Origin. *Int. J. Antimicrob. Agents* **2016**, *47*, 103–105. [CrossRef]
107. Wellington, E.M.H.; Boxall, A.B.A.; Cross, P.; Feil, E.J.; Gaze, W.H.; Hawkey, P.M.; Johnson-Rollings, A.S.; Jones, D.L.; Lee, N.M.; Otten, W.; et al. The Role of the Natural Environment in the Emergence of Antibiotic Resistance in Gram-Negative Bacteria. *Lancet Infect. Dis.* **2013**, *13*, 155–165. [CrossRef] [PubMed]
108. Forsberg, K.J.; Reyes, A.; Wang, B.; Selleck, E.M.; Sommer, M.O.A.; Dantas, G. The Shared Antibiotic Resistome of Soil Bacteria and Human Pathogens. *Science* **2012**, *337*, 1107–1111. [CrossRef] [PubMed]
109. Perry, J.A.; Wright, G.D. The Antibiotic Resistance "Mobilome": Searching for the Link between Environment and Clinic. *Front. Microbiol.* **2013**, *4*, 138. [CrossRef] [PubMed]
110. Le, T.H.; Truong, T.; Tran, L.-T.; Nguyen, D.-H.; Pham, T.P.T.; Ng, C. Antibiotic Resistance in the Aquatic Environments: The Need for an Interdisciplinary Approach. *Int. J. Environ. Sci. Technol.* **2022**, 244. [CrossRef]
111. Marti, E.; Balcázar, J.L. Antibiotic Resistance in the Aquatic Environment. In *Comprehensive Analytical Chemistry*; Elsevier: Amsterdam, The Netherlands, 2013; Volume 62, pp. 671–684. ISBN 0166-526X.
112. Munita, J.M.; Arias, C.A. Mechanisms of Antibiotic Resistance. *Microbiol. Spectr.* **2016**, *4*, 2. [CrossRef]
113. Pagès, J.M.; Masi, M.; Barbe, J. Inhibitors of Efflux Pumps in Gram-Negative Bacteria. *Trends Mol. Med.* **2005**, *11*, 382–389. [CrossRef]
114. Srikumar, R.; Kon, T.; Gotoh, N.; Poole, K. Expression of Pseudomonas Aeruginosa Multidrug Efflux Pumps MexA-MexB-OprM and MexC-MexD-OprJ in a Multidrug-Sensitive Escherichia Coli Strain. *Antimicrob. Agents Chemother.* **1998**, *42*, 65–71. [CrossRef]
115. Huovinen, P. Trimethoprim Resistance. *Antimicrob. Agents Chemother.* **1987**, *31*, 1451–1456. [CrossRef]

116. Yun, M.-K.; Wu, Y.; Li, Z.; Zhao, Y.; Waddell, M.B.; Ferreira, A.M.; Lee, R.E.; Bashford, D.; White, S.W. Catalysis and Sulfa Drug Resistance in Dihydropteroate Synthase. *Science* **2012**, *335*, 1110–1114. [CrossRef]
117. Livermore, D.M. Mechanisms of Resistance to Cephalosporin Antibiotics. *Drugs* **1987**, *34*, 64–88. [CrossRef]
118. Livermore, D.M. Mechanisms of Resistance To-Lactam Antibiotics. *Scand. J. Infect. Dis.* **1991**, *78*, 7–16.
119. MacGowan, A.; Macnaughton, E. Antibiotic Resistance. *Medicine* **2017**, *45*, 622–628. [CrossRef]
120. Neu, H.C. The Crisis in Antibiotic Resistance. *Science* **1992**, *257*, 1064–1073. [CrossRef] [PubMed]
121. Brooun, A.; Liu, S.; Lewis, K. A Dose-Response Study of Antibiotic Resistance in Pseudomonas Aeruginosa Biofilms. *Antimicrob. Agents Chemother.* **2000**, *44*, 640–646. [CrossRef]
122. Oliveira, M.; Leonardo, I.C.; Nunes, M.; Silva, A.F.; Barreto Crespo, M.T. Environmental and Pathogenic Carbapenem Resistant Bacteria Isolated from a Wastewater Treatment Plant Harbour Distinct Antibiotic Resistance Mechanisms. *Antibiotics* **2021**, *10*, 1118. [CrossRef]
123. Suay-García, B.; Pérez-Gracia, M.T. Drug-Resistant Neisseria Gonorrhoeae: Latest Developments. *Eur. J. Clin. Microbiol. Infect. Dis.* **2017**, *36*, 1065–1071. [CrossRef]
124. Singh, A.; Shahid, M.; Khan, P.A.; Khan, H.M.; Sami, H. An Overview on Antibiotic Resistance in Gram-Negative Bacteria. In *Beta-Lactam Resistance in Gram-Negative Bacteria*; Springer Nature: Cham, Switzerland, 2022; pp. 3–15.
125. Schiavano, G.F.; Carloni, E.; Andreoni, F.; Magi, S.; Chironna, M.; Brandi, G.; Amagliani, G. Prevalence and Antibiotic Resistance of Pseudomonas Aeruginosa in Water Samples in Central Italy and Molecular Characterization of Opr D in Imipenem Resistant Isolates. *PLoS ONE* **2017**, *12*, e0189172. [CrossRef]
126. Ma, L.; Lu, P.-L.; Siu, L.K.; Hsieh, M.-H. Molecular Typing and Resistance Mechanisms of Imipenem-Non-Susceptible Klebsiella Pneumoniae in Taiwan: Results from the Taiwan Surveillance of Antibiotic Resistance (TSAR) Study, 2002–2009. *J. Med. Microbiol.* **2013**, *62*, 101–107. [CrossRef]
127. Hiramatsu, K. Vancomycin-Resistant Staphylococcus Aureus: A New Model of Antibiotic Resistance. *Lancet Infect. Dis.* **2001**, *1*, 147–155. [CrossRef]
128. Arias, C.A.; Murray, B.E. The Rise of the Enterococcus: Beyond Vancomycin Resistance. *Nat. Rev. Microbiol.* **2012**, *10*, 266–278. [CrossRef]
129. Schweizer, H.P. Mechanisms of Antibiotic Resistance in Burkholderia Pseudomallei: Implications for Treatment of Melioidosis. *Future Microbiol.* **2012**, *7*, 1389–1399. [CrossRef] [PubMed]
130. Brochet, M.; Couvé, E.; Zouine, M.; Poyart, C.; Glaser, P. A Naturally Occurring Gene Amplification Leading to Sulfonamide and Trimethoprim Resistance in Streptococcus Agalactiae. *J. Bacteriol.* **2008**, *190*, 672–680. [CrossRef] [PubMed]
131. Lauxen, A.I.; Kobauri, P.; Wegener, M.; Hansen, M.J.; Galenkamp, N.S.; Maglia, G.; Szymanski, W.; Feringa, B.L.; Kuipers, O.P. Mechanism of Resistance Development in E. Coli against TCAT, a Trimethoprim-Based Photoswitchable Antibiotic. *Pharmaceuticals* **2021**, *14*, 392. [CrossRef] [PubMed]
132. Sköld, O. Resistance to Trimethoprim and Sulfonamides. *Vet. Res.* **2001**, *32*, 261–273. [CrossRef]
133. Parulekar, R.S.; Sonawane, K.D. Insights into the Antibiotic Resistance and Inhibition Mechanism of Aminoglycoside Phosphotransferase from Bacillus Cereus: In Silico and in Vitro Perspective. *J. Cell. Biochem.* **2018**, *119*, 9444–9461. [CrossRef]
134. Pantosti, A.; Sanchini, A.; Monaco, M. Mechanisms of Antibiotic Resistance in Staphylococcus Aureus. *Futur. Microbiol.* **2007**, *2*, 323–334. [CrossRef]
135. Bryan, L.E.; Kowand, S.K.; Van Den Elzen, H.M. Mechanism of Aminoglycoside Antibiotic Resistance in Anaerobic Bacteria: Clostridium Perfringens and Bacteroides Fragilis. *Antimicrob. Agents Chemother.* **1979**, *15*, 7–13. [CrossRef]
136. Moreira, M.A.S.; Oliveira, J.A.; Teixeira, L.M.; Moraes, C.A. Detection of a Chloramphenicol Efflux System in Escherichia Coli Isolated from Poultry Carcass. *Vet. Microbiol.* **2005**, *109*, 75–81. [CrossRef]
137. Wolter, N.; Smith, A.M.; Farrell, D.J.; Schaffner, W.; Moore, M.; Whitney, C.G.; Jorgensen, J.H.; Klugman, K.P. Novel Mechanism of Resistance to Oxazolidinones, Macrolides, and Chloramphenicol in Ribosomal Protein L4 of the Pneumococcus. *Antimicrob. Agents Chemother.* **2005**, *49*, 3554–3557. [CrossRef]
138. Mosher, R.H.; Camp, D.J.; Yang, K.; Brown, M.P.; Shaw, W.V.; Vining, L.C. Inactivation of Chloramphenicol by O-Phosphorylation: A Novel Resistance Mechanism in Streptomyces Venezuelae Isp5230, a Chloramphenicol Producer. *J. Biol. Chem.* **1995**, *270*, 27000–27006. [CrossRef]
139. Fernández, M.; Conde, S.; de la Torre, J.; Molina-Santiago, C.; Ramos, J.-L.; Duque, E. Mechanisms of Resistance to Chloramphenicol in Pseudomonas Putida KT2440. *Antimicrob. Agents Chemother.* **2012**, *56*, 1001–1009. [CrossRef] [PubMed]
140. Shortridge, V.D.; Doern, G.V.; Brueggemann, A.B.; Beyer, J.M.; Flamm, R.K. Prevalence of Macrolide Resistance Mechanisms in Streptococcus Pneumoniae Isolates from a Multicenter Antibiotic Resistance Surveillance Study Conducted in the United States in 1994–1995. *Clin. Infect. Dis.* **1999**, *29*, 1186–1188. [CrossRef]
141. Bolukaoto, J.Y.; Monyama, C.M.; Chukwu, M.O.; Lekala, S.M.; Nchabeleng, M.; Maloba, M.R.B.; Mavenyengwa, R.T.; Lebelo, S.L.; Monokoane, S.T.; Tshepuwane, C.; et al. Antibiotic Resistance of Streptococcus Agalactiae Isolated from Pregnant Women in Garankuwa, South Africa. *BMC Res. Notes* **2015**, *8*, 6–12. [CrossRef]
142. Kyriakidis, I.; Vasileiou, E.; Pana, Z.D.; Tragiannidis, A. Acinetobacter Baumannii Antibiotic Resistance Mechanisms. *Pathogens* **2021**, *10*, 373. [CrossRef]
143. De Francesco, V.; Zullo, A.; Hassan, C.; Giorgio, F.; Rosania, R.; Ierardi, E. Mechanisms of Helicobacter Pylori Antibiotic Resistance: An Updated Appraisal. *World J. Gastrointest. Pathophysiol.* **2011**, *2*, 35. [CrossRef] [PubMed]

144. Roberts, M.C. Mechanisms of Bacterial Antibiotic Resistance and Lessons Learned from Environmental Tetracycline-Resistant Bacteria. In *Antimicrobial Resistance in the Environment*; John Wiley & Sons, Inc.: New York, NY, USA, 2011; pp. 93–121.
145. Nordmann, P.; Poirel, L. Emergence of Plasmid-Mediated Resistance to Quinolones in Enterobacteriaceae. *J. Antimicrob. Chemother.* **2005**, *56*, 463–469. [CrossRef] [PubMed]
146. Sánchez, M.B. Antibiotic Resistance in the Opportunistic Pathogen Stenotrophomonas Maltophilia. *Front. Microbiol.* **2015**, *6*, 658. [CrossRef]
147. Prince, A. Antibiotic Resistance of Pseudomonas Species. *J. Pediatr.* **1986**, *108*, 830–834. [CrossRef]
148. Nnadozie, C.F.; Odume, O.N. Freshwater Environments as Reservoirs of Antibiotic Resistant Bacteria and Their Role in the Dissemination of Antibiotic Resistance Genes. *Environ. Pollut.* **2019**, *254*, 113067. [CrossRef]
149. Marti, E.; Variatza, E.; Balcazar, J.L. The Role of Aquatic Ecosystems as Reservoirs of Antibiotic Resistance. *Trends Microbiol.* **2014**, *22*, 36–41. [CrossRef]
150. Naquin, A.; Shrestha, A.; Sherpa, M.; Nathaniel, R.; Boopathy, R. Presence of Antibiotic Resistance Genes in a Sewage Treatment Plant in Thibodaux, Louisiana, USA. *Bioresour. Technol.* **2015**, *188*, 79–83. [CrossRef] [PubMed]
151. Rowan, N.J. Defining Established and Emerging Microbial Risks in the Aquatic Environment: Current Knowledge, Implications, and Outlooks. *Int. J. Microbiol.* **2011**, *2011*, 462832. [CrossRef] [PubMed]
152. Michael, I.; Rizzo, L.; Mcardell, C.S.; Manaia, C.M.; Merlin, C.; Schwartz, T.; Dagot, C.; Fatta-kassinos, D. Urban Wastewater Treatment Plants as Hotspots for the Release of Antibiotics in the Environment: A Review. *Water Res.* **2012**, *47*, 957–995. [CrossRef] [PubMed]
153. Yang, S.-F.; Lin, C.-F.; Lin, A.Y.-C.; Hong, P.-K.A. Sorption and Biodegradation of Sulfonamide Antibiotics by Activated Sludge: Experimental Assessment Using Batch Data Obtained under Aerobic Conditions. *Water Res.* **2011**, *45*, 3389–3397. [CrossRef]
154. Ben, W.; Wang, J.; Cao, R.; Yang, M.; Zhang, Y.; Qiang, Z. Distribution of Antibiotic Resistance in the Effluents of Ten Municipal Wastewater Treatment Plants in China and the Effect of Treatment Processes. *Chemosphere* **2017**, *172*, 392–398. [CrossRef]
155. Dorival-García, N.; Zafra-Gómez, A.; Navalón, A.; González, J.; Vílchez, J.L. Removal of Quinolone Antibiotics from Wastewaters by Sorption and Biological Degradation in Laboratory-Scale Membrane Bioreactors. *Sci. Total Environ.* **2013**, *442*, 317–328. [CrossRef]
156. Li, B.; Zhang, T. Biodegradation and Adsorption of Antibiotics in the Activated Sludge Process. *Environ. Sci. Technol.* **2010**, *44*, 3468–3473. [CrossRef]
157. Rowe, W.P.M.; Baker-Austin, C.; Verner-Jeffreys, D.W.; Ryan, J.J.; Micallef, C.; Maskell, D.J.; Pearce, G.P. Overexpression of Antibiotic Resistance Genes in Hospital Effluents over Time. *J. Antimicrob. Chemother.* **2017**, *72*, 1617–1623. [CrossRef]
158. Kümmerer, K. Antibiotics in the Aquatic Environment–a Review–Part I. *Chemosphere* **2009**, *75*, 417–434. [CrossRef]
159. Sabaté, M.; Prats, G.; Moreno, E.; Ballesté, E.; Blanch, A.R.; Andreu, A. Virulence and Antimicrobial Resistance Profiles among Escherichia Coli Strains Isolated from Human and Animal Wastewater. *Res. Microbiol.* **2008**, *159*, 288–293. [CrossRef]
160. Da Costa, P.M.; Vaz-Pires, P.; Bernardo, F. Antimicrobial Resistance in Enterococcus Spp. Isolated in Inflow, Effluent and Sludge from Municipal Sewage Water Treatment Plants. *Water Res.* **2006**, *40*, 1735–1740. [CrossRef] [PubMed]
161. da Costa, P.M.; Oliveira, M.; Bica, A.; Vaz-Pires, P.; Bernardo, F. Antimicrobial Resistance in Enterococcus Spp. and Escherichia Coli Isolated from Poultry Feed and Feed Ingredients. *Vet. Microbiol.* **2007**, *120*, 122–131. [CrossRef] [PubMed]
162. Mao, D.; Yu, S.; Rysz, M.; Luo, Y.; Yang, F.; Li, F.; Hou, J.; Mu, Q.; Alvarez, P.J.J. Prevalence and Proliferation of Antibiotic Resistance Genes in Two Municipal Wastewater Treatment Plants. *Water Res.* **2015**, *85*, 458–466. [CrossRef] [PubMed]
163. Cacace, D.; Fatta-Kassinos, D.; Manaia, C.M.; Cytryn, E.; Kreuzinger, N.; Rizzo, L.; Karaolia, P.; Schwartz, T.; Alexander, J.; Merlin, C.; et al. Antibiotic Resistance Genes in Treated Wastewater and in the Receiving Water Bodies: A Pan-European Survey of Urban Settings. *Water Res.* **2019**, *162*, 320–330. [CrossRef]
164. Lien, L.; Lan, P.; Chuc, N.; Hoa, N.; Nhung, P.; Thoa, N.; Diwan, V.; Tamhankar, A.; Stålsby Lundborg, C. Antibiotic Resistance and Antibiotic Resistance Genes in Escherichia Coli Isolates from Hospital Wastewater in Vietnam. *Int. J. Environ. Res. Public Health* **2017**, *14*, 699. [CrossRef]
165. Lundborg, C.S.; Tamhankar, A.J. Antibiotic Residues in the Environment of South East Asia. *BMJ* **2017**, *358*, 42–45. [CrossRef]
166. Selvarajan, R.; Sibanda, T.; Pandian, J.; Mearns, K. Taxonomic and Functional Distribution of Bacterial Communities in Domestic and Hospital Wastewater System: Implications for Public and Environmental Health. *Antibiotics* **2021**, *10*, 1059. [CrossRef]
167. Kunhikannan, S.; Thomas, C.J.; Franks, A.E.; Mahadevaiah, S.; Kumar, S.; Petrovski, S. Environmental Hotspots for Antibiotic Resistance Genes. *Microbiologyopen* **2021**, *10*, e1197. [CrossRef]
168. Rozman, U.; Duh, D.; Cimerman, M.; Turk, S.Š. Hospital Wastewater Effluent: Hot Spot for Antibiotic Resistant Bacteria. *J. Water Sanit. Hyg. Dev.* **2020**, *10*, 171–178. [CrossRef]
169. Wang, Q.; Wang, P.; Yang, Q. Occurrence and Diversity of Antibiotic Resistance in Untreated Hospital Wastewater. *Sci. Total Environ.* **2018**, *621*, 990–999. [CrossRef]
170. Obayiuwana, A.; Ibekwe, A.M. Antibiotic Resistance Genes Occurrence in Wastewaters from Selected Pharmaceutical Facilities in Nigeria. *Water* **2020**, *12*, 1897. [CrossRef]
171. Zhang, S.; Huang, J.; Zhao, Z.; Cao, Y.; Li, B. Hospital Wastewater as a Reservoir for Antibiotic Resistance Genes: A Meta-Analysis. *Front. Public Health* **2020**, *8*, 574968. [CrossRef] [PubMed]

172. Obinwanne, C.; Nyaruaba, R.; Ekeng, R.; Okon, U.; Izuma, C.; Ebido, C.C.; Oluwole, A.; Sunday, E.; Ikechukwu, K. Antibiotic Resistance in the Aquatic Environment: Analytical Techniques and Interactive Impact of Emerging Contaminants. *Environ. Toxicol. Pharmacol.* **2022**, *96*, 103995. [CrossRef]
173. Baquero, F.; Martínez, J.L.; Cantón, R. Antibiotics and Antibiotic Resistance in Water Environments. *Curr. Opin. Biotechnol.* **2008**, *19*, 260–265. [CrossRef] [PubMed]
174. Wang, R.; Ji, M.; Zhai, H.; Guo, Y.; Liu, Y. Science of the Total Environment Occurrence of Antibiotics and Antibiotic Resistance Genes in WWTP Ef Fl Uent-Receiving Water Bodies and Reclaimed Wastewater Treatment Plants. *Sci. Total Environ.* **2021**, *796*, 148919. [CrossRef]
175. Park, J.C.; Lee, J.C.; Oh, J.Y.; Jeong, Y.W.; Cho, J.W.; Joo, H.S.; Lee, W.K.; Lee, W.B. Antibiotic Selective Pressure for the Maintenance of Antibiotic Resistant Genes in Coliform Bacteria Isolated from the Aquatic Environment. *Water Sci. Technol.* **2003**, *47*, 249–253. [CrossRef]
176. Zhu, B. Abundance Dynamics and Sequence Variation of Neomycin Phosphotransferase Gene (NptII) Homologs in River Water. *Aquat. Microb. Ecol.* **2007**, *48*, 131–140. [CrossRef]
177. Mohapatra, H.; Mohapatra, S.S.; Mantri, C.K.; Colwell, R.R.; Singh, D. V Vibrio Cholerae Non-O1, Non-O139 Strains Isolated before 1992 from Varanasi, India Are Multiple Drug Resistant, Contain IntSXT, Dfr18 and AadA5 Genes. *Environ. Microbiol.* **2008**, *10*, 866–873. [CrossRef]
178. Pei, R.; Kim, S.-C.; Carlson, K.H.; Pruden, A. Effect of River Landscape on the Sediment Concentrations of Antibiotics and Corresponding Antibiotic Resistance Genes (ARG). *Water Res.* **2006**, *40*, 2427–2435. [CrossRef]
179. Mukherjee, S.; Chakraborty, R. Incidence of Class 1 Integrons in Multiple Antibiotic-Resistant Gram-Negative Copiotrophic Bacteria from the River Torsa in India. *Res. Microbiol.* **2006**, *157*, 220–226. [CrossRef]
180. Bergeron, S.; Boopathy, R.; Nathaniel, R.; Corbin, A.; LaFleur, G. Presence of Antibiotic Resistant Bacteria and Antibiotic Resistance Genes in Raw Source Water and Treated Drinking Water. *Int. Biodeterior. Biodegrad.* **2015**, *102*, 370–374. [CrossRef]
181. Vulliet, E.; Cren-olivé, C. Screening of Pharmaceuticals and Hormones at the Regional Scale, in Surface and Groundwaters Intended to Human Consumption. *Environ. Pollut.* **2011**, *159*, 2929–2934. [CrossRef] [PubMed]
182. Kaiser, R.A.; Polk, J.S.; Datta, T.; Parekh, R.R.; Agga, G.E. Occurrence of Antibiotic Resistant Bacteria in Urban Karst Groundwater Systems. *Water* **2022**, *14*, 960. [CrossRef]
183. Andrade, L.; Kelly, M.; Hynds, P.; Weatherill, J.; Majury, A.; Dwyer, O. Groundwater Resources as a Global Reservoir for Antimicrobial-Resistant Bacteria. *Water Res.* **2020**, *170*, 115360. [CrossRef]
184. Zou, H.Y.; He, L.Y.; Gao, F.Z.; Zhang, M.; Chen, S.; Wu, D.L.; Liu, Y.S.; He, L.X.; Bai, H.; Ying, G.G. Antibiotic Resistance Genes in Surface Water and Groundwater from Mining Affected Environments. *Sci. Total Environ.* **2021**, *772*, 145516. [CrossRef]
185. Kampouris, I.D.; Alygizakis, N.; Klümper, U.; Agrawal, S.; Lackner, S.; Cacace, D.; Kunze, S.; Thomaidis, N.S.; Slobdonik, J.; Berendonk, T.U. Elevated Levels of Antibiotic Resistance in Groundwater during Treated Wastewater Irrigation Associated with Infiltration and Accumulation of Antibiotic Residues. *J. Hazard. Mater.* **2022**, *423*, 127155. [CrossRef]
186. Murphy, H.M.; Prioleau, M.D.; Borchardt, M.A.; Hynds, P.D. Epidemiological Evidence of Groundwater Contribution to Global Enteric Disease, 1948–2015. *Hydrogeol. J.* **2017**, *25*, 981–1001. [CrossRef]
187. Hatosy, S.M.; Martiny, A.C. The Ocean as a Global Reservoir of Antibiotic Resistance Genes. *Appl. Environ. Microbiol.* **2015**, *81*, 7593–7599. [CrossRef]
188. Habibi, N.; Uddin, S.; Lyons, B.; Al-Sarawi, H.A.; Behbehani, M.; Shajan, A.; Razzack, N.A.; Zakir, F.; Alam, F. Antibiotic Resistance Genes Associated with Marine Surface Sediments: A Baseline from the Shores of Kuwait. *Sustainability* **2022**, *14*, 8029. [CrossRef]
189. Feng-xia, Y.; Da-qing, M.A.O.; Yi, L.U.O.; Qing, W.; Quan-Hua, M.U. Horizontal Transfer of Antibiotic Resistance Genes in the Environment. *Yingyong Shengtai Xuebao* **2013**, *24*, 2993–3002.
190. Song, L.; Li, L.; Yang, S.; Lan, J.; He, H.; McElmurry, S.P.; Zhao, Y. Sulfamethoxazole, Tetracycline and Oxytetracycline and Related Antibiotic Resistance Genes in a Large-Scale Landfill, China. *Sci. Total Environ.* **2016**, *551*, 9–15. [CrossRef] [PubMed]
191. Xu, J.; Xu, Y.; Wang, H.; Guo, C.; Qiu, H.; He, Y.; Zhang, Y.; Li, X.; Meng, W. Occurrence of Antibiotics and Antibiotic Resistance Genes in a Sewage Treatment Plant and Its Effluent-Receiving River. *Chemosphere* **2015**, *119*, 1379–1385. [CrossRef] [PubMed]
192. Zou, S.; Xu, W.; Zhang, R.; Tang, J.; Chen, Y.; Zhang, G. Occurrence and Distribution of Antibiotics in Coastal Water of the Bohai Bay, China: Impacts of River Discharge and Aquaculture Activities. *Environ. Pollut.* **2011**, *159*, 2913–2920. [CrossRef] [PubMed]
193. Lin, Z.; Yuan, T.; Zhou, L.; Cheng, S.; Qu, X.; Lu, P.; Feng, Q. Impact Factors of the Accumulation, Migration and Spread of Antibiotic Resistance in the Environment. *Environ. Geochem. Health* **2021**, *43*, 1741–1758. [CrossRef]
194. Seiler, C.; Berendonk, T.U. Heavy Metal Driven Co-Selection of Antibiotic Resistance in Soil and Water Bodies Impacted by Agriculture and Aquaculture. *Front. Microbiol.* **2012**, *3*, 399. [CrossRef]
195. Qiu, Z.; Shen, Z.; Qian, D.; Jin, M.; Yang, D.; Wang, J.; Zhang, B.; Yang, Z.; Chen, Z.; Wang, X. Effects of Nano-TiO2 on Antibiotic Resistance Transfer Mediated by RP4 Plasmid. *Nanotoxicology* **2015**, *9*, 895–904. [CrossRef]
196. Wang, X.; Yang, F.; Zhao, J.; Xu, Y.; Mao, D.; Zhu, X.; Luo, Y.; Alvarez, P.J.J. Bacterial Exposure to ZnO Nanoparticles Facilitates Horizontal Transfer of Antibiotic Resistance Genes. *NanoImpact* **2018**, *10*, 61–67. [CrossRef]
197. Qiu, X.; Zhou, G.; Wang, H. Nanoscale Zero-Valent Iron Inhibits the Horizontal Gene Transfer of Antibiotic Resistance Genes in Chicken Manure Compost. *J. Hazard. Mater.* **2022**, *422*, 126883. [CrossRef]

198. Imran, M.; Das, K.R.; Naik, M.M. Co-Selection of Multi-Antibiotic Resistance in Bacterial Pathogens in Metal and Microplastic Contaminated Environments: An Emerging Health Threat. *Chemosphere* **2019**, *215*, 846–857. [CrossRef]
199. Bondarczuk, K.; Markowicz, A.; Piotrowska-Seget, Z. The Urgent Need for Risk Assessment on the Antibiotic Resistance Spread via Sewage Sludge Land Application. *Environ. Int.* **2016**, *87*, 49–55. [CrossRef]
200. Yang, Y.; Xu, C.; Cao, X.; Lin, H.; Wang, J. Antibiotic Resistance Genes in Surface Water of Eutrophic Urban Lakes Are Related to Heavy Metals, Antibiotics, Lake Morphology and Anthropic Impact. *Ecotoxicology* **2017**, *26*, 831–840. [CrossRef] [PubMed]
201. Andersson, D.I.; Balaban, N.Q.; Baquero, F.; Courvalin, P.; Glaser, P.; Gophna, U.; Kishony, R.; Molin, S.; Tønjum, T. Antibiotic Resistance: Turning Evolutionary Principles into Clinical Reality. *FEMS Microbiol. Rev.* **2020**, *44*, 171–188. [CrossRef] [PubMed]
202. Baker-Austin, C.; Wright, M.S.; Stepanauskas, R.; McArthur, J.V. Co-Selection of Antibiotic and Metal Resistance. *Trends Microbiol.* **2006**, *14*, 176–182. [CrossRef] [PubMed]
203. Ouvrard, S.; Barnier, C.; Bauda, P.; Beguiristain, T.; Biache, C.; Bonnard, M.; Caupert, C.; Cebron, A.; Cortet, J.; Cotelle, S.; et al. In Situ Assessment of Phytotechnologies for Multicontaminated Soil Management. *Int. J. Phytoremediation* **2011**, *13*, 245–263. [CrossRef] [PubMed]
204. Sun, R.; He, L.; Li, T.; Dai, Z.; Sun, S.; Ren, L.; Liang, Y.-Q.; Zhang, Y.; Li, C. Impact of the Surrounding Environment on Antibiotic Resistance Genes Carried by Microplastics in Mangroves. *Sci. Total Environ.* **2022**, *837*, 155771. [CrossRef]
205. Aslam, B.; Wang, W.; Arshad, M.I.; Khurshid, M.; Muzammil, S.; Rasool, M.H.; Nisar, M.A.; Alvi, R.F.; Aslam, M.A.; Qamar, M.U.; et al. Antibiotic Resistance: A Rundown of a Global Crisis. *Infect. Drug Resist.* **2018**, *11*, 1645. [CrossRef] [PubMed]
206. Aydin, S.; Ünlü, İ.D.; Arabacı, D.N.; Duru, Ö.A. Evaluating the Effect of Microalga Haematococcus Pluvialis Bioaugmentation on Aerobic Membrane Bioreactor in Terms of Performance, Membrane Fouling and Microbial Community Structure. *Sci. Total Environ.* **2022**, *807*, 149908. [CrossRef] [PubMed]
207. Pu, M.; Ailijiang, N.; Mamat, A.; Chang, J.; Zhang, Q.; Liu, Y.; Li, N. Occurrence of Antibiotics in the Different Biological Treatment Processes, Reclaimed Wastewater Treatment Plants and Effluent-Irrigated Soils. *J. Environ. Chem. Eng.* **2022**, *10*, 107715. [CrossRef]
208. Munir, M.; Wong, K.; Xagoraraki, I. Release of Antibiotic Resistant Bacteria and Genes in the Effluent and Biosolids of Five Wastewater Utilities in Michigan. *Water Res.* **2010**, *45*, 681–693. [CrossRef]
209. Yan, Q.; Xu, Y.; Chen, L.; Cao, Z.; Shao, Y.; Xu, Y.; Yu, Y.; Fang, C.; Zhu, Z.; Feng, G.; et al. Irrigation with Secondary Municipal-Treated Wastewater: Potential Effects, Accumulation of Typical Antibiotics and Grain Quality Responses in Rice (*Oryza Sativa* L.). *J. Hazard. Mater.* **2021**, *410*, 124655. [CrossRef]
210. Dungan, R.S.; Strausbaugh, C.A.; Leytem, A.B. Survey of Selected Antibiotic Resistance Genes in Agricultural and Non-Agricultural Soils in South-Central Idaho. *FEMS Microbiol. Ecol.* **2019**, *95*, fiz071. [CrossRef] [PubMed]
211. Bougnom, B.P.; Thiele-Bruhn, S.; Ricci, V.; Zongo, C.; Piddock, L.J.V. Raw Wastewater Irrigation for Urban Agriculture in Three African Cities Increases the Abundance of Transferable Antibiotic Resistance Genes in Soil, Including Those Encoding Extended Spectrum β-Lactamases (ESBLs). *Sci. Total Environ.* **2020**, *698*, 134201. [CrossRef] [PubMed]
212. Szczepanowski, R.; Linke, B.; Krahn, I.; Gartemann, K.-H.; Guetzkow, T.; Eichler, W.; Pühler, A.; Schlueter, A. Detection of 140 Clinically Relevant Antibiotic-Resistance Genes in the Plasmid Metagenome of Wastewater Treatment Plant Bacteria Showing Reduced Susceptibility to Selected Antibiotics. *Microbiology* **2009**, *155*, 2306–2319. [CrossRef] [PubMed]
213. Gudda, F.O.; Waigi, M.G.; Odinga, E.S.; Yang, B.; Carter, L.; Gao, Y. Antibiotic-Contaminated Wastewater Irrigated Vegetables Pose Resistance Selection Risks to the Gut Microbiome. *Environ. Pollut.* **2020**, *264*, 114752. [CrossRef] [PubMed]
214. Onalenna, O.; Rahube, T.O. Assessing Bacterial Diversity and Antibiotic Resistance Dynamics in Wastewater Effluent-Irrigated Soil and Vegetables in a Microcosm Setting. *Heliyon* **2022**, *8*, e09089. [CrossRef]
215. Sun, C.; Zhang, B.; Ning, D.; Zhang, Y.; Dai, T.; Wu, L.; Li, T.; Liu, W.; Zhou, J.; Wen, X. Seasonal Dynamics of the Microbial Community in Two Full-Scale Wastewater Treatment Plants: Diversity, Composition, Phylogenetic Group Based Assembly and Co-Occurrence Pattern. *Water Res.* **2021**, *200*, 117295. [CrossRef] [PubMed]
216. Abdalla, S.E.; Abia, A.L.K.; Amoako, D.G.; Perrett, K.; Bester, L.A.; Essack, S.Y. From Farm-to-Fork: E. Coli from an Intensive Pig Production System in South Africa Shows High Resistance to Critically Important Antibiotics for Human and Animal Use. *Antibiotics* **2021**, *10*, 178. [CrossRef]
217. Molechan, C.; Amoako, D.G.; Abia, A.L.K.; Somboro, A.M.; Bester, L.A.; Essack, S.Y. Molecular Epidemiology of Antibiotic-Resistant Enterococcus Spp. from the Farm-to-Fork Continuum in Intensive Poultry Production in KwaZulu-Natal, South Africa. *Sci. Total Environ.* **2019**, *692*, 868–878. [CrossRef]
218. Chereau, F.; Opatowski, L.; Tourdjman, M.; Vong, S. Risk Assessment for Antibiotic Resistance in South East Asia. *BMJ* **2017**, *358*, j3393. [CrossRef]
219. Fatoba, D.O.; Abia, A.L.K.; Amoako, D.G.; Essack, S.Y. Rethinking Manure Application: Increase in Multidrug-Resistant Enterococcus Spp. in Agricultural Soil Following Chicken Litter Application. *Microorganisms* **2021**, *9*, 885. [CrossRef]
220. Zhang, L.; Li, L.; Sha, G.; Liu, C.; Wang, Z.; Wang, L. Aerobic Composting as an Effective Cow Manure Management Strategy for Reducing the Dissemination of Antibiotic Resistance Genes: An Integrated Meta-Omics Study. *J. Hazard. Mater.* **2020**, *386*, 121895. [CrossRef] [PubMed]
221. Skandalis, N.; Maeusli, M.; Papafotis, D.; Miller, S.; Lee, B.; Theologidis, I.; Luna, B. Environmental Spread of Antibiotic Resistance. *Antibiotics* **2021**, *10*, 640. [CrossRef] [PubMed]
222. Chen, X.; Du, Z.; Guo, T.; Wu, J.; Wang, B.; Wei, Z.; Jia, L.; Kang, K. Effects of Heavy Metals Stress on Chicken Manures Composting via the Perspective of Microbial Community Feedback. *Environ. Pollut.* **2022**, *294*, 118624. [CrossRef]

223. Mu, M.; Yang, F.; Han, B.; Tian, X.; Zhang, K. Manure Application: A Trigger for Vertical Accumulation of Antibiotic Resistance Genes in Cropland Soils. *Ecotoxicol. Environ. Saf.* **2022**, *237*, 113555. [CrossRef] [PubMed]
224. Peng, S.; Zhang, H.; Song, D.; Chen, H.; Lin, X.; Wang, Y.; Ji, L. Distribution of Antibiotic, Heavy Metals and Antibiotic Resistance Genes in Livestock and Poultry Feces from Different Scale of Farms in Ningxia, China. *J. Hazard. Mater.* **2022**, *440*, 129719. [CrossRef] [PubMed]
225. Patricia Macías Farrera, G.; Tenorio Borroto, E.; Rivera Ramírez, F.; Vázquez Chagoyán, J.; Talavera Rojas, M.; Yong Angel, G.; Montes de Oca Jimenez, R. Detection of Quinolone Resistance in Salmonella Typhimurium Pig Isolates Determined by GyrA Gene Mutation Using PCR-and Sequence-Based Techniques within the GyrA Gene. *Curr. Pharm. Des.* **2016**, *22*, 5079–5084. [CrossRef] [PubMed]
226. Ramakrishnan, B.; Venkateswarlu, K.; Sethunathan, N.; Megharaj, M. Local Applications but Global Implications: Can Pesticides Drive Microorganisms to Develop Antimicrobial Resistance? *Sci. Total Environ.* **2019**, *654*, 177–189. [CrossRef]
227. Xing, Y.; Herrera, D.; Zhang, S.; Kang, X.; Men, Y. Site-Specific Target-Modification Mutations Exclusively Induced by the Coexposure to Low Levels of Pesticides and Streptomycin Caused Strong Streptomycin Resistance in Clinically Relevant Escherichia Coli. *J. Hazard. Mater. Adv.* **2022**, *7*, 100141. [CrossRef]
228. Shahid, M.; Khan, M.S. Tolerance of Pesticides and Antibiotics among Beneficial Soil Microbes Recovered from Contaminated Rhizosphere of Edible Crops. *Curr. Res. Microb. Sci.* **2022**, *3*, 100091. [CrossRef]
229. Komijani, M.; Shamabadi, N.S.; Shahin, K.; Eghbalpour, F.; Tahsili, M.R.; Bahram, M. Heavy Metal Pollution Promotes Antibiotic Resistance Potential in the Aquatic Environment. *Environ. Pollut.* **2021**, *274*, 116569. [CrossRef]
230. Wang, Y.; Lu, S.; Liu, X.; Chen, J.; Han, M.; Wang, Z.; Guo, W. Profiles of Antibiotic Resistance Genes in an Inland Salt-Lake Ebinur Lake, Xinjiang, China: The Relationship with Antibiotics, Environmental Factors, and Microbial Communities. *Ecotoxicol. Environ. Saf.* **2021**, *221*, 112427. [CrossRef] [PubMed]
231. Gupta, S.; Sreekrishnan, T.R.; Ahammad, S.Z. Effects of Heavy Metals on the Development and Proliferation of Antibiotic Resistance in Urban Sewage Treatment Plants. *Environ. Pollut.* **2022**, *308*, 119649. [CrossRef] [PubMed]
232. Shi, L.; Zhang, J.; Lu, T.; Zhang, K. Metagenomics Revealed the Mobility and Hosts of Antibiotic Resistance Genes in Typical Pesticide Wastewater Treatment Plants. *Sci. Total Environ.* **2022**, *817*, 153033. [CrossRef] [PubMed]
233. Liu, Y.; Cheng, D.; Xue, J.; Feng, Y.; Wakelin, S.A.; Weaver, L.; Shehata, E.; Li, Z. Fate of Bacterial Community, Antibiotic Resistance Genes and Gentamicin Residues in Soil after Three-Year Amendment Using Gentamicin Fermentation Waste. *Chemosphere* **2022**, *291*, 132734. [CrossRef] [PubMed]
234. Niu, Q.; Li, K.; Yang, H.; Zhu, P.; Huang, Y.; Wang, Y.; Li, X.; Li, Q. Exploring the Effects of Heavy Metal Passivation under Fenton-like Reaction on the Removal of Antibiotic Resistance Genes during Composting. *Bioresour. Technol.* **2022**, *359*, 127476. [CrossRef] [PubMed]
235. Huang, J.; Zhu, J.; Liu, S.; Luo, Y.; Zhao, R.; Guo, F.; Li, B. Estuarine Salinity Gradient Governs Sedimentary Bacterial Community but Not Antibiotic Resistance Gene Profile. *Sci. Total Environ.* **2022**, *806*, 151390. [CrossRef]
236. Manaia, C.M.; Rocha, J.; Scaccia, N.; Marano, R.; Radu, E.; Biancullo, F.; Cerqueira, F.; Fortunato, G.; Iakovides, I.C.; Zammit, I.; et al. Antibiotic Resistance in Wastewater Treatment Plants: Tackling the Black Box. *Environ. Int.* **2018**, *115*, 312–324. [CrossRef]
237. Li, Z.; Sun, A.; Liu, X.; Chen, Q.-L.; Bi, L.; Ren, P.-X.; Shen, J.-P.; Jin, S.; He, J.-Z.; Hu, H.-W.; et al. Climate Warming Increases the Proportions of Specific Antibiotic Resistance Genes in Natural Soil Ecosystems. *J. Hazard. Mater.* **2022**, *430*, 128442. [CrossRef]
238. Schmeisser, C.; Steele, H.; Streit, W.R. Metagenomics, Biotechnology with Non-Culturable Microbes. *Appl. Microbiol. Biotechnol.* **2007**, *75*, 955–962. [CrossRef]
239. Liu, H.; Taylor, T.H.; Pettus, K.; Johnson, S.; Papp, J.R.; Trees, D. Comparing the Disk-Diffusion and Agar Dilution Tests for Neisseria Gonorrhoeae Antimicrobial Susceptibility Testing. *Antimicrob. Resist. Infect. Control.* **2016**, *5*, 46. [CrossRef]
240. Kuchibiro, T.; Komatsu, M.; Yamasaki, K.; Nakamura, T.; Niki, M.; Nishio, H.; Kida, K.; Ohama, M.; Nakamura, A.; Nishi, I. Evaluation of the VITEK2 AST—XN17 Card for the Detection of Carbapenemase—Producing Enterobacterales in Isolates Primarily Producing Metallo β—Lactamase. *Eur. J. Clin. Microbiol. Infect. Dis.* **2022**, *41*, 723–732. [CrossRef] [PubMed]
241. Zaheer, R.; Noyes, N.; Ortega Polo, R.; Cook, S.R.; Marinier, E.; Van Domselaar, G.; Belk, K.E.; Morley, P.S.; McAllister, T.A. Impact of Sequencing Depth on the Characterization of the Microbiome and Resistome. *Sci. Rep.* **2018**, *8*, 5890. [CrossRef] [PubMed]
242. He, Y.; Zhou, X.; Chen, Z.; Deng, X.; Gehring, A.; Ou, H.; Zhang, L.; Shi, X. PRAP: Pan Resistome Analysis Pipeline. *BMC Bioinform.* **2020**, *21*, 20. [CrossRef]
243. Zhuang, M.; Achmon, Y.; Cao, Y.; Liang, X.; Chen, L.; Wang, H.; Siame, B.A.; Leung, K.Y. Distribution of Antibiotic Resistance Genes in the Environment. *Environ. Pollut.* **2021**, *285*, 117402. [CrossRef] [PubMed]
244. Perry, J.A.; Wright, G.D. Forces Shaping the Antibiotic Resistome. *BioEssays* **2014**, *36*, 1179–1184. [CrossRef] [PubMed]
245. Dos Santos, D.F.K.; Istvan, P.; Quirino, B.F.; Kruger, R.H. Functional Metagenomics as a Tool for Identification of New Antibiotic Resistance Genes from Natural Environments. *Microb. Ecol.* **2017**, *73*, 479–491. [CrossRef] [PubMed]
246. Liu, M.; Feng, M.; Yang, K.; Cao, Y.; Zhang, J.; Xu, J.; Hernández, S.H.; Wei, X.; Fan, M. Transcriptomic and Metabolomic Analyses Reveal Antibacterial Mechanism of Astringent Persimmon Tannin against Methicillin-Resistant Staphylococcus Aureus Isolated from Pork. *Food Chem.* **2020**, *309*, 125692. [CrossRef] [PubMed]
247. Yu, K.; Zhang, T. Metagenomic and Metatranscriptomic Analysis of Microbial Community Structure and Gene Expression of Activated Sludge. *PLoS ONE* **2012**, *7*, e38183. [CrossRef]

248. Su, C.; Lei, L.; Duan, Y.; Zhang, K.Q.; Yang, J. Culture-Independent Methods for Studying Environmental Microorganisms: Methods, Application, and Perspective. *Appl. Microbiol. Biotechnol.* **2012**, *93*, 993–1003. [CrossRef]
249. Martinez, J.L. Environmental Pollution by Antibiotics and by Antibiotic Resistance Determinants. *Environ. Pollut.* **2009**, *157*, 2893–2902. [CrossRef]
250. Brain, R.A.; Hanson, M.L.; Solomon, K.R.; Brooks, B.W. Aquatic Plants Exposed to Pharmaceuticals: Effects and Risks. *Rev. Environ. Contam. Toxicol.* **2008**, *192*, 67–115. [PubMed]
251. Jechalke, S.; Heuer, H.; Siemens, J.; Amelung, W.; Smalla, K. Fate and Effects of Veterinary Antibiotics in Soil. *Trends Microbiol.* **2014**, *22*, 536–545. [CrossRef] [PubMed]
252. Boxall, A.B.A.; Rudd, M.A.; Brooks, B.W.; Caldwell, D.J.; Choi, K.; Hickmann, S.; Innes, E.; Ostapyk, K.; Staveley, J.P.; Verslycke, T.; et al. Pharmaceuticals and Personal Care Products in the Environment: What Are the Big Questions? *Environ. Health Perspect.* **2012**, *120*, 1221–1229. [CrossRef] [PubMed]
253. Murray, C.J.; Ikuta, K.S.; Sharara, F.; Swetschinski, L.; Robles Aguilar, G.; Gray, A.; Han, C.; Bisignano, C.; Rao, P.; Wool, E.; et al. Global Burden of Bacterial Antimicrobial Resistance in 2019: A Systematic Analysis. *Lancet* **2022**, *399*, 629–655. [CrossRef]
254. Gentilini, F.; Turba, M.E.; Pasquali, F.; Mion, D.; Romagnoli, N.; Zambon, E.; Terni, D.; Peirano, G.; Pitout, J.D.D.; Parisi, A.; et al. Hospitalized Pets as a Source of Carbapenem-Resistance. *Front. Microbiol.* **2018**, *9*, 2872. [CrossRef] [PubMed]
255. Köck, R.; Daniels-Haardt, I.; Becker, K.; Mellmann, A.; Friedrich, A.W.; Mevius, D.; Schwarz, S.; Jurke, A. Carbapenem-Resistant Enterobacteriaceae in Wildlife, Food-Producing, and Companion Animals: A Systematic Review. *Clin. Microbiol. Infect.* **2018**, *24*, 1241–1250. [CrossRef] [PubMed]
256. Poirel, L.; Berçot, B.; Millemann, Y.; Bonnin, R.A.; Pannaux, G.; Nordmann, P. Carbapenemaseproducing Acinetobacter Spp. in Cattle, France. *Emerg. Infect. Dis.* **2012**, *18*, 523–525. [CrossRef]
257. Jansen, K.U.; Knirsch, C.; Anderson, A.S. The Role of Vaccines in Preventing Bacterial Antimicrobial Resistance. *Nat. Med.* **2018**, *24*, 10–19. [CrossRef]
258. Van Boeckel, T.; Pires, J.; Silvester, R.; Zhao, C.; Song, J.; Criscuolo, N.; Gilbert, M.; Bonhoeffer, S.; Laxminarayan, R. Global Trends in Antimicrobial Resistance in Animals in Low-and Middle-Income Countries. *Int. J. Infect. Dis.* **2020**, *101*, 19. [CrossRef]
259. Marshall, B.M.; Levy, S.B. Food Animals and Antimicrobials: Impacts on Human Health. *Clin. Microbiol. Rev.* **2011**, *24*, 718–733. [CrossRef]
260. Renault, V.; Humblet, M.F.; Saegerman, C. Biosecurity Concept: Origins, Evolution and Perspectives. *Animals* **2022**, *12*, 63. [CrossRef] [PubMed]
261. Callaway, T.R.; Lillehoj, H.; Chuanchuen, R.; Gay, C.G. Erratum: Callaway et Al. Alternatives to Antibiotics: A Symposium on the Challenges and Solutions for Animal Health and Production. *Antibiotics* **2021**, *10*, 1024. [CrossRef] [PubMed]
262. Holmes, A.H.; Moore, L.S.P.; Sundsfjord, A.; Steinbakk, M.; Regmi, S.; Karkey, A.; Guerin, P.J.; Piddock, L.J. V Understanding the Mechanisms and Drivers of Antimicrobial Resistance. *Lancet* **2016**, *387*, 176–187. [CrossRef] [PubMed]
263. World Health Organization. *Antibacterial Agents in Clinical Development: An Analysis of the Antibacterial Clinical Development Pipeline*; WHO: Geneva, Switzerland, 2019.

antibiotics

MDPI

Perspective

Antimicrobial Resistance in the Environment: Towards Elucidating the Roles of Bioaerosols in Transmission and Detection of Antibacterial Resistance Genes

Paul B. L. George [1,2], Florent Rossi [2,3], Magali-Wen St-Germain [2,4], Pierre Amato [3], Thierry Badard [5], Michel G. Bergeron [6], Maurice Boissinot [6], Steve J. Charette [2,7], Brenda L. Coleman [8], Jacques Corbeil [1,6], Alexander I. Culley [2,7], Marie-Lou Gaucher [9], Matthieu Girard [10], Stéphane Godbout [11,12], Shelley P. Kirychuk [13], André Marette [4,14], Allison McGeer [8,15], Patrick T. O'Shaughnessy [16], E. Jane Parmley [17,18], Serge Simard [4], Richard J. Reid-Smith [18,19], Edward Topp [20,21], Luc Trudel [2], Maosheng Yao [22], Patrick Brassard [12], Anne-Marie Delort [3], Araceli D. Larios [11,23], Valérie Létourneau [4], Valérie E. Paquet [2,7], Marie-Hélène Pedneau [4], Émilie Pic [6], Brooke Thompson [13], Marc Veillette [4], Mary Thaler [2,7], Ilaria Scapino [1,4], Maria Lebeuf [4], Mahsa Baghdadi [2,4], Alejandra Castillo Toro [13], Amélia Bélanger Cayouette [2,4], Marie-Julie Dubois [4,14], Alicia F. Durocher [2,4,7], Sarah B. Girard [2,7], Andrea Katherín Carranza Diaz [11,12], Asmaâ Khalloufi [2,9], Samantha Leclerc [2,4], Joanie Lemieux [2,4,6], Manuel Pérez Maldonado [18], Geneviève Pilon [4,15], Colleen P. Murphy [19], Charly A. Notling [13], Daniel Ofori-Darko [19], Juliette Provencher [2,7], Annabelle Richer-Fortin [2,4], Nathalie Turgeon [4] and Caroline Duchaine [2,4,*]

check for updates

Citation: George, P.B.L.; Rossi, F.; St-Germain, M.-W.; Amato, P.; Badard, T.; Bergeron, M.G.; Boissinot, M.; Charette, S.J.; Coleman, B.L.; Corbeil, J.; et al. Antimicrobial Resistance in the Environment: Towards Elucidating the Roles of Bioaerosols in Transmission and Detection of Antibacterial Resistance Genes. *Antibiotics* **2022**, *11*, 974. https://doi.org/10.3390/antibiotics11070974

Academic Editors: Akebe Luther King Abia and Carlos M. Franco

Received: 30 May 2022
Accepted: 15 July 2022
Published: 19 July 2022

1 Département de Médecine Moléculaire, Université Laval, Quebec City, QC G1V 0A6, Canada; paul.george@bcm.ulaval.ca (P.B.L.G.); jacques.corbeil@fmed.ulaval.ca (J.C.); ilaria.scapino.1@ulaval.ca (I.S.)
2 Département de Biochimie, de Microbiologie et de Bio-Informatique, Université Laval, Quebec City, QC G1V 0A6, Canada; florent.rossi@uca.fr (F.R.); magali-wen.st-germain.1@ulaval.ca (M.-W.S.-G.); steve.charette@bcm.ulaval.ca (S.J.C.); alexander.culley@bcm.ulaval.ca (A.I.C.); luc.trudel@bcm.ulaval.ca (L.T.); valerie.paquet.2@ulaval.ca (V.E.P.); mary.thaler.1@ulaval.ca (M.T.); mahsa.baghdadi.1@ulaval.ca (M.B.); amelia.belanger-cayouette.1@ulaval.ca (A.B.C.); alicia.durocher.1@ulaval.ca (A.F.D.); sarah.girard.7@ulaval.ca (S.B.G.); asmaa.khalloufi@umontreal.ca (A.K.); samantha.leclerc.3@ulaval.ca (S.L.); joanie.lemieux.2@ulaval.ca (J.L.); juliette.provencher.1@ulaval.ca (J.P.); annabelle.richer-fortin.1@ulaval.ca (A.R.-F.)
3 Institut de Chimie de Clermont-Ferrand, SIGMA Clermont, CNRS, Université Clermont-Auvergne, 63178 Clermont-Ferrand, France; pierre.amato@uca.fr (P.A.); a-marie.delort@uca.fr (A.-M.D.)
4 Centre de Recherche de L'Institut Universitaire de Cardiologie et de Pneumologie de Québec, Quebec City, QC G1V 4G5, Canada; andre.marette@criucpq.ulaval.ca (A.M.); serge.simard@criucpq.ulaval.ca (S.S.); valerie.letourneau@criucpq.ulaval.ca (V.L.); marie-helene.pedneau@mat.ulaval.ca (M.-H.P.); marc.veillette@criucpq.ulaval.ca (M.V.); maria.lebeuf.1@ulaval.ca (M.L.); marie-julie.dubois@criucpq.ulaval.ca (M.-J.D.); genevieve.pilon@criucpq.ulaval.ca (G.P.); nathalie.turgeon@criucpq.ulaval.ca (N.T.)
5 Centre de Recherche en Données et Intelligence Géospatiales (CRDIG), Quebec City, QC G1V 0A6, Canada; thierry.badard@scg.ulaval.ca
6 Centre de Recherche en Infectiologie, Centre de Recherche du CHU de Québec-Université Laval, Axe Maladies Infectieuses et Immunitaires, Quebec City, QC G1V 4G2, Canada; michel.g.bergeron@crchudequebec.ulaval.ca (M.G.B.); maurice.boissinot@crchudequebec.ulaval.ca (M.B.); emilie.pic@crchudequebec.ulaval.ca (É.P.)
7 Institut de Biologie Intégrative et des Systèmes, Université Laval, Quebec City, QC G1V 0A6, Canada
8 Dalla Lana School of Public Health, University of Toronto, Toronto, ON M5T 3M7, Canada; brenda.coleman@sinaihealth.ca (B.L.C.); allison.mcgeer@sinaihealth.ca (A.M.)
9 Research Chair in Meat Safety, Département de Pathologie et Microbiologie, Université de Montréal, Saint-Hyacinthe, QC J2S 2M2, Canada; marie-lou.gaucher@umontreal.ca
10 Agrivitia Canada, Saskatoon, SK S7N 2Z4, Canada; matthieu.girard@usask.ca
11 Institut de Recherche et de Développement en Agroenvironnement (IRDA), Quebec City, QC G1P 3W8, Canada; stephane.godbout@irda.qc.ca (S.G.); dalila.larios@irda.qc.ca (A.D.L.); andrea-katherin.carranza-diaz.1@ulaval.ca (A.K.C.D.)
12 Département des Sols et de Génie Agroalimentaire, Université Laval, Quebec City, QC G1V 0A6, Canada; patrick.brassard@irda.qc.ca
13 Department of Medicine, University of Saskatchewan, Saskatoon, SK S7N 0X8, Canada; shelley.kirychuk@usask.ca (S.P.K.); brooke.thompson@usask.ca (B.T.); alejandracastillo@javeriana.edu.co (A.C.T.); can291@mail.usask.ca (C.A.N.)

[14] Institut sur la Nutrition et les Aliments Fonctionnels, Université Laval, Quebec City, QC G1V 0A6, Canada
[15] Department of Laboratory Medicine and Pathobiology, University of Toronto, Toronto, ON M5S 1A8, Canada
[16] Department of Occupational and Environmental Health, The University of Iowa, Iowa City, IA 52246, USA; patrick-oshaughnessy@uiowa.edu
[17] Canadian Wildlife Health Cooperative, University of Guelph, Guelph, ON N1G 2W1, Canada; jparmley@uoguelph.ca
[18] Department of Population Medicine, University of Guelph, Guelph, ON N1G 2W1, Canada; richard.reid-smith@phac-aspc.gc.ca (R.J.R.-S.); mperezma@uoguelph.ca (M.P.M.)
[19] Centre for Foodborne, Environmental and Zoonotic Infectious Diseases, Public Health Agency of Canada, Guelph, ON N1G 3W4, Canada; colleen.murphy@phac-aspc.gc.ca (C.P.M.); daniel.ofori-darko@phac-aspc.gc.ca (D.O.-D.)
[20] Agriculture and Agri-Food Canada, London Research and Development Centre, London, ON N5V 4T3, Canada; ed.topp@agr.gc.ca
[21] Department of Biology, The University of Western Ontario, London, ON N6A 5B7, Canada
[22] State Key Joint Laboratory of Environmental Simulation and Pollution Control, College of Environmental Sciences and Engineering, Peking University, Beijing 100871, China; yao@pku.edu.cn
[23] Tecnológico Nacional de México/ITS de Perote, Perote 91270, Mexico
* Correspondence: caroline.duchaine@bcm.ulaval.ca

Abstract: Antimicrobial resistance (AMR) is continuing to grow across the world. Though often thought of as a mostly public health issue, AMR is also a major agricultural and environmental problem. As such, many researchers refer to it as the preeminent One Health issue. Aerial transport of antimicrobial-resistant bacteria via bioaerosols is still poorly understood. Recent work has highlighted the presence of antibiotic resistance genes in bioaerosols. Emissions of AMR bacteria and genes have been detected from various sources, including wastewater treatment plants, hospitals, and agricultural practices; however, their impacts on the broader environment are poorly understood. Contextualizing the roles of bioaerosols in the dissemination of AMR necessitates a multidisciplinary approach. Environmental factors, industrial and medical practices, as well as ecological principles influence the aerial dissemination of resistant bacteria. This article introduces an ongoing project assessing the presence and fate of AMR in bioaerosols across Canada. Its various sub-studies include the assessment of the emissions of antibiotic resistance genes from many agricultural practices, their long-distance transport, new integrative methods of assessment, and the creation of dissemination models over short and long distances. Results from sub-studies are beginning to be published. Consequently, this paper explains the background behind the development of the various sub-studies and highlight their shared aspects.

Keywords: antibiotic resistance genes; large-scale monitoring; one Health; culturomics; DNA sequencing; quantitative PCR; bioaerosols

1. Introduction

Rising levels of antimicrobial resistance (AMR) have caused great concern amongst policymakers, doctors, and governments in recent years. In 2019, an estimated 4.95 million deaths were associated with AMR globally, of which approximately 1.27 million were directly attributable to resistant bacteria [1]. These data likewise revealed stark geographic trends, with the greatest number of deaths due to AMR found in sub-Saharan Africa and south Asia, whereas the fewest were observed in Australasia [1]. Unfortunately, this number is expected to increase, and consequently, so will healthcare and economic costs. In Canada, AMR could reduce GDP projections by 13–21 billion CAD by 2050, with an increase in associated healthcare costs from 1.4 billion CAD in 2018 to 8 billion CAD in 2050 [2]. The knock-on effects of the SARS-CoV2 pandemic exemplify the extent to which novel or re-emerging pathogens pressure economic [3] and healthcare systems [4]. Yet the problem of AMR represents a convergence of many factors, such as antimicrobial overuse and misuse, pollution [5], and natural coevolution dynamics [6], and requires a multidisciplinary approach to mitigate adverse outcomes.

This reality has led scientists and policymakers to consider AMR as the preeminent One Health question [7]. Much attention has been directed to studying the spread of AMR—particularly antimicrobial resistance genes (ARGs)—in the environment reviewed in [5]. To date, most work focused on ARGs in the broader environment has been conducted in soils, water bodies, or wildlife [5,8]. For example, animal production is the leading consumer of antimicrobial agents globally [9], accounting for ~78% of agents used in Canada in 2018 [10]. Run-off from manure application or livestock barns introduces unprocessed antimicrobial compounds and resistant organisms to soils and watercourses, allowing ARGs to spread to populations of naïve microbes via horizontal gene transfer [5]. However, airborne ARG dispersal is increasingly recognized as an important, though severely understudied, route for disseminating AMR in the environment [5,11,12].

Indeed, Huijbers and collaborators [8] reported 157 studies of AMR bacteria in the environment as of 2014. Only 5 of these studies (3%) looked at bioaerosols or settled dust, compared to 25 for soil, 56 for water, and 71 for wildlife. In the intervening years, there has been a marked increase in the number of studies assessing airborne ARGs in the environment. Notably, bioaerosols are known to influence the dispersal of resistant microorganisms through wildlife, domestic animals, soil, water, and humans [8]. Studies have reported ARG-laden bioaerosols detected approximately 2 km from agricultural buildings [13] and projected dispersal footprints of up to 10 km [14]. This is of great concern as bioaerosol emissions are challenging to control.

Understanding the role bioaerosols play in ARG transmission is critical to addressing AMR in the environment. Yet this requires a multidisciplinary approach that can integrate data from diverse systems, including indoor (i.e., wastewater treatment, livestock buildings) and outdoor environments (i.e., agricultural fields, urban air) or remote areas (i.e., clouds, Canadian North, overseas) and produce data that can be integrated into the current understanding of AMR. To this end, we have launched a multi-year research program dedicated to the airborne dissemination of ARGs. The project is funded by a Natural Sciences and Engineering Research Council of Canada (NSERC) Discovery Frontiers opportunity, specifically targeting AMR in the environment (2019 competition), as a major research topic of the Canada Research Chair on Bioaerosols and a network of Canadian and international collaborators. Here, we outline the rationale for this undertaking and describe the ongoing research topics. The purpose of this article is to present (i) the current knowledge gaps in the roles of bioaerosols in AMR; (ii) our ongoing work to address them; (iii) stimulating discussion and interest amongst the broader scientific community to further shed light on the roles of bioaerosols in disseminating ARGs; and (iv) open doors for new collaborations.

2. Bioaerosols

Bioaerosols are particles suspended in the air upon which, microorganisms, living or dead, microbial fragments, and viruses may be found. Such biological material can be transported over many kilometres in the environment. Bioaerosols are defined as particles of less than 100 μm and may remain airborne indefinitely, depending on air currents and turbulence [15]. The aerial microbial community has been studied for over 150 years, notably heralded by Pasteur's observations of airborne bacteria [16]. Sources of bioaerosol emissions are now well known and include natural and stochastic events (wind, raindrops) and anthropogenic-associated ones, such as wastewater treatment and agricultural practices [17]. Much of the literature on bioaerosols has focused on disease propagation [18,19] and food production processes like brewing [20]. Increasingly, occupational, industrial, and agricultural bioaerosols have been studied, providing a better understanding of their ecology and biodiversity. However, a recent synthesis by Šantl-Temkiv and colleagues highlighted significant gaps in our understanding of outdoor bioaerosols [21]. In particular, they highlighted an absence of knowledge surrounding airborne communities in natural and built environments, their emission rates in natural environments, and the impacts of anthropogenic change on airborne microorganisms. Addressing these knowledge gaps requires new and integrative methodological approaches.

Bioaerosols are representative of their sources and together form a combined sample of multiple origins, although a recent hypothesis tends to support the existence of a specific atmospheric microbiota [22]. Following transport by bioaerosols, microorganisms can colonize depositional environments, cause infections, or simply decay after settling; additionally, their genetic material (free or within cells) can be transferred throughout the environment. Despite the heavy research focus on human-associated bioaerosols, most bioaerosols are derived from plants, soil [23,24], and natural bodies of water [25]. Increasingly, researchers have attempted to track the fate of bioaerosols from anthropogenic sources [11,13,14].

Often researchers rely on modeling approaches or database references to infer the source community of bioaerosols [26]. Since viable microorganisms can travel thousands of kilometres by air [27], the role of bioaerosols as a vector for the dissemination of ARGs is an increasingly important area of research. These organisms may exhibit AMR, making their aerial transport a significant health concern. Many studies have detected potentially pathogenic taxa from the air, such as *Legionella* [28,29] and *Staphylococcus* [14,30] using DNA-based methods and culturomics—the use of multiple media and growth conditions to better facilitate the isolation of bacteria under controlled conditions.

Bioaerosols may play an active role in the dissemination of ARGs in the environment. In Colorado, concentrated animal feeding operations were shown to emit ARGs detectable over 2 km from buildings [13]. Furthermore, non-agricultural indoor environments such as clinics and homeless shelters were found to be a source of ARG in the broader environment [13]. The richness of ARG types in urban smog exposed to pharmaceutical pollution is higher than in wastewater or sludge [31]. The high taxonomic and genetic bacterial diversity of outdoor environments indicates that bioaerosols are a vast reservoir of ARGs with the potential to be transferred to pathogenic agents.

Particulate matter (PM) present in pollution events harbours ARGs in greater concentrations than under ambient conditions [31]. Several studies have revealed the presence of ARGs in PM in urban areas [31–33] of various cities and the air is now a suspected transmission route for AMR bacteria from point sources such as wastewater treatment plants. A recent study assessed the distribution of ARGs worldwide using automobile cabin filters and found marked geographical variations [33]. Additionally, laboratory studies have shown that compounds found in vehicle exhaust stimulate bacterial stress responses, including promoting the expression of plasmid transfer genes, potentially accelerating ARG transfer in urban air [34].

Recent research has shown that ARGs are present in the indoor air of wastewater treatment facilities [35] and livestock buildings [14,36,37]. It is expected that ventilation will expel high concentrations of ARG-laden bioaerosols into the environment. Other activities, such as manure application, generate bioaerosols that may contain medically important bacteria or functional genes over wide areas [38]. It is unknown whether occupational exposure to these organisms in outdoor environments poses health risks. ARG transfer from the environment to humans is poorly understood, though limited evidence has found that specific pathways, mainly via water, are viable [39]. Further work is needed to integrate ambient bioaerosols into exposure models.

Nevertheless, the above examples provide evidence that a significant number of ARGs are present in bioaerosols. For instance, in their worldwide sampling of dust collected from vehicle air filters, Li et al. detected ARGs against aminoglycosides, beta-lactams, macrolides, quinolones, sulfonamides, tetracyclines, and vancomycin [33]. Bioaerosols containing tetracycline ARGs have been observed in many different locations worldwide [33]; specific genes such as *tetM* and *tetO* have been found in the air of agricultural buildings and farms [14,37]. Furthermore, in healthcare settings, the *tetW* gene was common in health clinics and a homeless shelter in Colorado, USA [13]. In a South Carolina, USA wastewater treatment plants, macrolide resistance genes *ermB* and *ermC* were highly abundant [35]. Yet, there is still much work to be carried out to identify ARGs in bioaerosols and link them to source locations.

3. The Frontiers Project

3.1. Project Members

Dr. Caroline Duchaine has spearheaded a multi-year project funded by an NSERC Discovery Frontiers program to study ARGs in bioaerosols to address these fundamental questions. The overarching project incorporates studies of indoor environments, their emissions into the environment and their long-distance transport, novel ARG tracking and surveillance methods, selective culture approaches, and animal models that can be incorporated into exposure and risk assessment models (Figure 1). The aspects of each sub-study can be categorized into several topical areas but at this stage can be best summarized by methodological approaches and study environments. All aspects of the project follow a One Health approach. Table 1 presents a summary of all types of samples collected, sampling sites, number of samples, and expected outcomes.

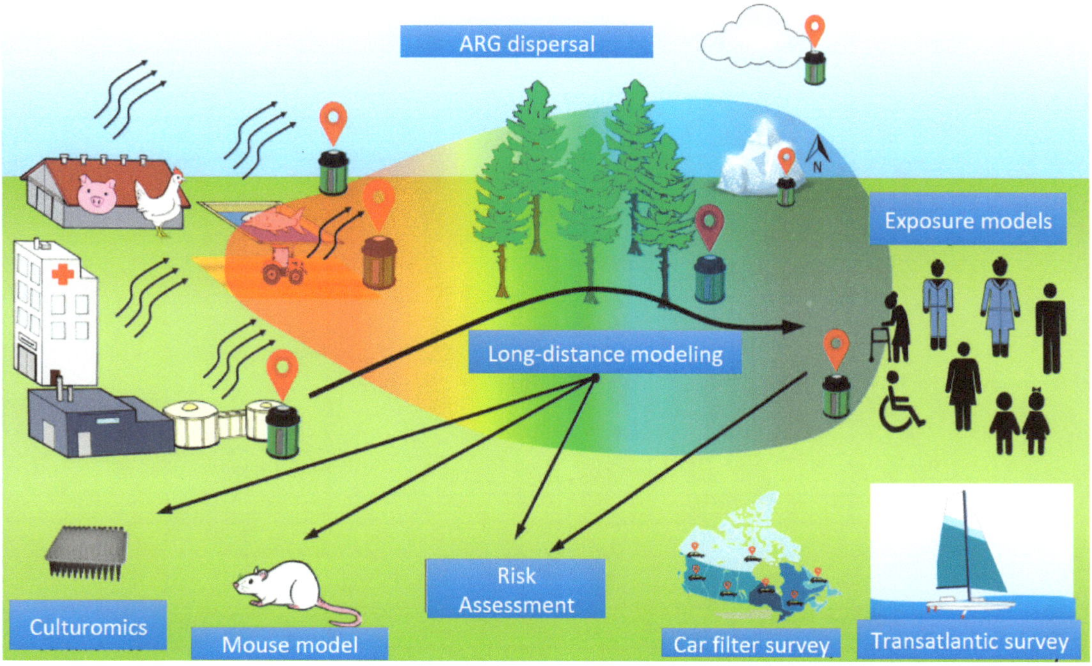

Figure 1. Graphical summary of the research program. Depicted are representations of the environments and objectives of the overarching project. Samples from human-associated sampling environments include livestock buildings, fish farms, arable fields, hospitals, and wastewater treatment plants to investigate ARG emissions. Environmental samples will also be taken from clouds, the Canadian North, a transatlantic survey, vehicle filters collected from sites across Canada, and conifer needles to inform the long-distance dispersal of ARGs. The data generated in these projects will inform culturomics and enrichment experiments, in vivo ARG transfer studies in animal models, and exposure models in humans. Finally, selected data will be used to inform risk assessment models.

Table 1. Summary of sampling sites, number of samples, type of analysis, and outcomes.

Aims	Sampling Sites or Sample Type	Number of Samples	Analyses	Expected Outcome
1	Vehicle cabin filters	478 AC filters	qPCR total bacteria qPCR ARG panel DNA sequencing (subset)	Relative abundance of ARGs/bacteria Network analyses Mapping ARGs throughout Canada
2	Hospitals	100 air samples	DNA sequencing Culture	Network analyses Genomic and ARG profiles ARG enrichment-culturomics
	Wastewater treatment plants	100 air samples from beside aeration tanks (outdoor) or in the ventilation exit (indoor)	Meteorological data qPCR total bacteria qPCR ARG panel Culture DNA sequencing (subset)	Relative abundance of ARG/bacteria ARG transfer in animal model ARG enrichment-culturomics Network analyses
	Fish farm	24 indoor 24 outdoor 24 downwind 24 upwind	Meteorological data qPCR fish pathogen and mobile genetic elements in air, water, and sediments qPCR ARG panel	Relative abundance of ARG/bacteria Detection of mobile genetic elements
	Aquatic Containment Level 2 facility (LARSEM)	18	qPCR fish pathogen and mobile genetic elements	Transmission of ARGs in controlled setup
	Swine and poultry farms in depth analyses	2 swine barns 2 poultry barns (Quebec)	Meteorological data DNA sequencing qPCR ARG panel qPCR total bacteria Building ventilation properties	Relative abundance of ARG/bacteria Network analyses Emission rates Transport models ARG transfer in animal model ARG enrichment-culturomics Provincial and climatic variations
		2 swine barns 2 poultry barns (Saskatchewan)		
	Swine and poultry farms modest analyses	15 swine barns 8 poultry barns 1 poultry abattoir 1 swine abattoir (Quebec)	Meteorological data qPCR ARG panel	Seasonal variations Variation in emission rates of ARGs
		8 swine barns 8 poultry barns 1 poultry abattoir 1 swine abattoir (Saskatchewan)	qPCR total bacteria Building ventilation properties (estimation with CO_2)	Transport models Province and climate variations
	Manure spreading	108 Swine slurries 36 Chicken manures with bedding 36 Chicken manures without bedding	Moisture content Meteorological data qPCR ARG panel DNA sequencing (subset) Geolocation and perception survey	Relative abundance of ARG/bacteria Network analyses Variation in emission rates of ARG Impact of spreading material and method Geolocation and perception model Transport models
3	In vitro ARG transfer study using samples from wastewater treatment plants and swine and poultry farms			
	Animal model of ARG transfer using samples from aims wastewater treatment plants and swine and poultry farms			
4	Conifer needles	Sampling gradient from known source Source sampling	qPCR total bacteria qPCR ARG panel	Proof of concept Transport model validation
4	Northern Canada	Ellesmere Island, Nunavut (50 samples) Resolute Bay, Nunavut (50 samples)	qPCR total bacteria qPCR ARG panel DNA sequencing (subset)	Long distance transport of ARGs Characterize Arctic resistome Transport model validation
4	Clouds	Puy-de-Dôme, France (15 samples)	qPCR total bacteria qPCR ARG panel DNA sequencing (subset)	Long distance transport of ARGs Describe remote spreading of ARGs Transport model validation
	Transatlantic	Transatlantic air samples (30 samples)		
	Precipitation	Opme meteo station (15 samples)		
4	Dispersion model using data from aims 2 and 3			
5	Integrated assessment model using data collected throughout the research program			

This project is led by the Canada Research Chair in Bioaerosols based in the bioaerosol laboratory, *Institut Universitaire de Cardiologie et Pneumologie de Québec*, Université Laval in Quebec City, QC, Canada. A multidisciplinary team of collaborators at Université Laval, across Canada (University of Saskatchewan, Université de Montréal, University of Guelph, Western University, Public Health Agency of Canada, Agriculture and Agri-Food Canada, Mount Sinai Research Institute) and internationally (Université Clermont Auvergne, France; University of Iowa, IA, USA; Peking University, China) are participating in the project. They bring expertise in human, veterinary and aquacultural disease, antibiotics, virology, bioaerosols, culture approaches, geography, modeling, bioinformatics, and artificial intelligence.

Together, our team proposes to estimate the contribution of agricultural and sanitation activities to ARG dispersal across Canada and the potential for long-distance transfers through a program addressing the following objectives: (i) assess ARG dispersion and associated bacterial diversity across Canada and their relationships to land use via vehicle cabin filters; (ii) assess ARG dispersion and associated bacterial diversity of bioaerosols in representative source locations by using high-volume air samplers; (iii) determine the subsequent fate of airborne ARGs; (iv) determine the potential for long-distance transport of ARGs; and (v) adding the role of bioaerosols to an integrated assessment model on AMR. The findings will significantly enhance the understanding of ARGs in bioaerosols and provide a framework for future research. It is hoped that the project will stimulate other researchers to pursue interdisciplinary approaches to studying bioaerosols.

3.2. Bioaerosol Sampling

3.2.1. Short Distance Air Sampling and Local Emission Sources Determination

Evaluating the contributions of various bioaerosol sources is key to exposure and mitigation strategies. Hospitals, wastewater treatment plants, fish farms, livestock barns — particularly those of swine and poultry—and manure spreading are being evaluated in this research. Assessing the emissions of bioaerosols within and around these locations requires the use of multiple sampling methodologies involving a range of air samplers (Table 2). These instruments physically collect air and concentrate PM either through filtration or via gravitational forces reviewed in [40]. Air samples will be collected at multiple locations: inside buildings and both up- and downwind of emission sources. Active high-volume air sampling will be performed using a wide range of air samplers (Table 2) to evaluate bacterial diversity and ARG profile up- and downwind from source locations. Upwind samples are collected to establish an ambient profile of airborne organisms to which inputs from source locations can be compared.

While frequently used in indoor environments, the deployment of such samplers outdoors presents challenges. Decisions in deployment location (both on the ground and at height) and duration may introduce sampling biases into collection. Sampling is also limited to relatively short periods, which may not align with ideal weather conditions for bioaerosol collection. Standardized sampling approaches have been implemented by all investigators to reduce bias throughout the project. The SASS3100 (Research International, Seattle, WA, USA) electret sampler is part of most of the sampling campaigns. However, it is unsuitable for culture techniques and does not maintain microbial viability. For culture and viability purposes, liquid samplers will be added to protocols, such as the SASS2300 and Coriolis μ (Bertin-Instruments, Montigny-le-Bretonneux, France), where appropriate.

In terms of study locations, these sampling campaigns will be undertaken in several locations across the Canadian provinces of Quebec, Ontario, and Saskatchewan. Several wastewater treatment plants have been selected for study. The presence of ARGs in bioaerosols was shown by previous work from our research team in swine barns [36,41] and poultry barns [42,43] in Quebec and Saskatchewan. However, the emissions of ARGs from these buildings, their subsequent local dispersion and their contribution to the long-range exposure are not well documented. To that end, comparisons will be drawn from farms in these two provinces, where intensive agriculture is common, as well as between conventional and antibiotic-free farms. Impacts of various manure spreading techniques on bioaerosol formation and composition are underway at the *Institut de Recherche et de Développement en Agroenvironnement* (IRDA) farm at Saint-Lambert-de-Lauzon, Quebec. Several Quebec fish farms, including the *Laboratoire Aquatique de Recherche enSsciences Environnementales et Médicales* (LARSEM) will also be studied. Air will be sampled in hospitals in Toronto, ON, Canada.

Table 2. Air extractors selected for aims 2 and 4.

Air Sampler	Type	Flow Rate (L/min)	Air Volume (m^3)	Type of Analysis	Indoor/ Outdoor	Sites
SASS 3100	Electret filter	300	10	Molecular biology	I/O	Hospitals Wastewater treatment plants Fish farms Livestock buildings Manure spreading
SASS 4100	Electret filter + Virtual impactor	4000	100	Molecular biology	O	Northern Canada Fish farms
SASS 2300	Liquid cyclone	325	10	Molecular biology and culture	O	Hospitals Wastewater treatment plants Livestock buildings Manure spreading
Coriolis μ	Liquid cyclone	300	6	Molecular biology and culture	I/O	Hospitals Wastewater treatment plants Livestock buildings Manure spreading
High Flow Rate Impinger	Liquid impaction	530	100	Molecular biology and culture	O	Puy-de-Dôme, France

3.2.2. Long-Distance ARG Transport

Assessing the long-distance transport of ARGs is a critical objective of this project. We will address this question using a variety of complementary approaches. The aerial microbiome of remote locations in the Canadian North will be characterized. Arctic bioaerosols are a critical blind spot in our understanding of airborne biodiversity [21], which experience a pronounced set of environmental pressures from a warming climate and changing population demographics. Losses of polar ice and permafrost may increase aerosolization rates of particulate matter [44] and, thereby augment the polar bioaerosol community. Bioaerosols of pristine sites (Ward Hunt Island, Nunavut, Canada) and an Inuit community (Resolute Bay, Nunavut, Canada) will be collected. Bioaerosols are expected to be very diluted in these areas, so a complementary approach using a large volume concentrator (SASS4100) and small volume extractors (i.e., SASS3100) will be used to maximize sampling potential.

The resistome of clouds will also be characterized. Clouds can be considered as an oases for microorganisms, providing them with more favourable conditions such as water or shading against UV radiation [22]. Such situations can potentially affect their atmospheric transport and, therefore, facilitate the atmospheric dispersion of ARGs worldwide. This project will undertake cloud samplings at the Puy-de-Dôme meteorological station in Clermont-Ferrand, France (1465 m elevation). Here the continuous collection of multiple physical and meteorological parameters is undertaken by a team of atmospheric microbiologists. Bacterial community and ARG content in cloud water will be assessed and related to the geographical origin of air masses and their physical and chemical features. Clouds have been sampled using cloud droplet impactors [45] to allow for the characterization of cloud water chemical properties. In parallel, recently developed high flow rate impingers filled with a nucleic acid preservative solution will be used [46] for the molecular monitoring of ARGs.

The potential for long-distance transport of ARGs will be complemented by a 15-day low altitude transatlantic survey of airborne bioaerosols aboard a sailboat. Monitoring ARGs at sea constitutes a novel and innovative approach to better characterize ARG transport and identify the marine contribution to ARG emission worldwide. The campaign will be performed with the collaboration of the Blue Observer organization (www.blue-observer.com). It will consist of a 7000 km trip from Brest, France to Woods Hole, MA, USA, with daily air sampling using two different types of air collectors. A SASS3100 extractor will be mounted on the mast of a sailing ship (8–10 m high) and deployed daily for 1 h each night and each day. In parallel, three filter holders connected to individual pumps (7 L min^{-1}) will be deployed continuously to perform 24 h sampling.

3.2.3. Integrative Sampling Methods

In addition to using complementary methods and experimental designs, aspects of this project will incorporate and assess relatively novel methods that integrate air sampling with the realities and pressures introduced by anthropogenic changes to the environment. These integrative methods include the study the ARGs present in vehicle cabin air filters and on the conifer needle phyllosphere as proxies for long-term air sampling. Specifically, a modified version of the vehicle cabin filter method pioneered by Li and colleagues [33] and a new approach using the conifer needle phyllosphere as a biomonitor of airborne ARGs following Galés and colleagues [47]. These methods will allow for monitoring ARGs over longer temporal and geographic scales. Vehicle air filters have been collected from every province and territory of Canada and analyses are underway. To our knowledge, this method has only been performed once before [34]. However, it holds tremendous potential as the vehicle filters can construct an aggregate PM sample of a wide area at annual or biannual scales. It will be used to look for regional differences in airborne ARGs that could be linked to geographical or socioeconomic factors, such as landscape, land use, or population demographics.

The phyllosphere—referring to the cumulative aboveground plant biomass—is one of the largest biomes on Earth, 10^8 km^2 [48] supporting an estimated 10^7 microbial cells cm^{-2} [49]. Phyllosphere microbial communities are strongly influenced by anthropogenic activities that emit microbes or alter deposition patterns [50,51]. Indeed, differences in ARG diversity of leaf-associated bacteria have been observed between agricultural and forest plants [51]. A pilot study on the efficacy of conifer needles as biomonitors of airborne ARGs has recently been published [52]. Briefly, conifer needles were collected near swine barns and in the farming community as well as the boreal forest to observe the diversity of ARGs in the phyllosphere from different environments. The needles were homogenized using a Stomacher (Aes Laboritoire, Bruz, France) and differentially centrifuged to generate pellets for DNA extraction. Differences were observed between the Boreal forest samples and those associated with human activities. This method holds great promise and will be expanded upon in upcoming experiments.

3.3. ARG Detection and Quantification

Determining the presence of ARGs in our diverse range of samples requires standardized methods. A shared ARG panel has been developed for qPCR analyses (Table 3). It is designed to capture a wide range of AMR. Since this type of nationwide project has not been previously undertaken in Canada, the panel was designed to be comparable to previous studies worldwide. The ARGs of interest were primarily selected from an array proposed by Stedfeldt and colleagues [53], but other genes were included at the suggestion of collaborators. For example, the colistin resistance gene *mcr-1* [54] was included due to its recent detection in swine feces in Québec [55]. A marker for the 16S rRNA gene will be used to provide biomass values and a reference point for ARG analyses [56]. We are employing a Takara SmartChip high-throughput qPCR system (TakaraBio USA, San Jose, CA, USA) to expedite sample processing using the shared ARG panel, in addition to validation using standard qPCR methods. For instance, bacterial biomass will be assessed via qPCR using the 16S rRNA marker gene.

Table 3. List of shared gene targets and primers used for qPCR analyses. Genes noted by * used a FAM probe all others used SYBR Green fluorescence.

Gene	Gene Type	Primer Sequence	Ref.
16S rRNA *	rRNA gene—used here for biomass and reference	**F:** GGTAGTCYAYGCMSTAAACG **R:** GACARCCATGCASCACCTG **P:**TKCGCGTTGCDTCGAATTAAWCCAC-BHQ	[56]
aac(6′)-II	Aminoglycoside resistance	**F:** CGACCCGACTCCGAACAA **R:** CGACCCGACTCCGAACAA	[53]
aac(6′)-Ib	Aminoglycoside resistance	**F:** CGTCGCCGAGCAACTTG **R:** CGGTACCTTGCCTCTCAAACC	[53]
aac(3)-iid_iii_iif_iia_iie	Aminoglycoside resistance	**F:** CGATGGTCGCGGTTGGTC **R:** TCGGCGTAGTGCAATGCG	[53]
blaCMY2	Beta-lactam resistance	**F:** AAAGCCTCATGGGTGCATAAA **R:** ATAGCTTTTGTTTGCCAGCATCA	[53]
blaCTX-M-1,3,15 *	Beta-lactam resistance	**F:** CGTACCGAGCCGACGTTAA **R:** CAACCCAGGAAGCAGGCA **P:** CCARCGGGCZENGCAGYTGGTGAC	[57]
blaGES	Beta-lactam resistance	**F:** GCAATGTGCTCAACGTTCAAG **R:** GTGCCTGAGTCAATTCTTTCAAAG	[53]
blaOXA	Beta-lactam resistance	**F:** CGACCGAGTATGTACCTGCTTC **R:** TCAAGTCCAATACGACGAGCTA	[53]
blaMOX/blaCMY	Beta-lactam resistance	**F:** CTATGTCAATGTGCCGAAGCA **R:** GGCTTGTCCTCTTTCGAATAGC	[53]
blaSHV-11	Beta-lactam resistance	**F:** TTGACCGCTGGGAAACGG **R:** TCCGGTCTTATCGGCGATAAAC	[53]
blaTEM	Beta-lactam resistance	**F:** AGCATCTTACGGATGGCATGA **R:** TCCTCCGATCGTTGTCAGAAGT	[53]
blaVEB	Beta-lactam resistance	**F:** CCCGATGCAAAGCGTTATG **R:** GAAAGATTCCCTTTATCTATCTCAGACAA	[53]
blaVIM	Beta-lactam resistance	**F:** GCACTTCTCGCGGAGATTG **R:** CGACGGTGATGCGTACGTT	[53]
erm(35)	Macrolide resistance	**F:** CCTTCAGTCAGAACCGGCAA **R:** GCTGATTTGACAGTTGGTGGTG	[53]
ermB	Macrolide resistance	**F:** GAACACTAGGGTTGTTCTTGCA **R:** CTGGAACATCTGTGGTATGGC	[53]
ermF	Macrolide resistance	**F:** CAGCTTTGGTTGAACATTTACGAA **R:** AAATTCCTAAAATCACAACCGACAA	[53]
ermT	Macrolide resistance	**F:** GTTCACTAGCACTATTTTTAATGACAGAAGT **R:** GAAGGGTGTCTTTTTAATACAATTAACGA	[53]
ermX	Macrolide resistance	**F:** GCTCAGTGGTCCCCATGGT **R:** ATCCCCCCGTCAACGTT	[53]
imp-marko	Beta-lactam resistance	**F:** GGAATAGAGTGGCTTAATTC **R:** GGTTTAACAAAACAACCACC	[53]
int1-a-marko	Mobile genetic element	**F:** CGAAGTCGAGGCATTTCTGTC **R:** GCCTTCCAGAAAACCGAGGA	[53]
is26	Mobile genetic element	**F:** ATGGATGAAACCTACGTGAAGGTC **R:** CGGTACTTAATCTGTCGGTGTTCA	[53]
mcr-1 *	Colistin resistance	**F:** CACATCGACGGCGTATTCTG **R:** CAACGAGCATACCGACATCG	[54]
qepA	Quinolone resistance	**F:** GGGCATCGCGCTGTTC **R:** GCGCATCGGTGAAGCC **P:** CTACAGACCZENGACCAAGCCGA	[53]

Table 3. *Cont.*

Gene	Gene Type	Primer Sequence	Ref.
qnrB	Quinolone resistance	**F:** TCACCACCCGCACCTG **R:** GGATATCTAAATCGCCCAGTTCC	[53]
sul1	Sulfonamide resistance	**F:** GCCGATGAGATCAGACGTATTG **R:** CGCATAGCGCTGGGTTTC	[53]
sul2	Sulfonamide resistance	**F:** TCATCTGCCAAACTCGTCGTTA **R:** GTCAAAGAACGCCGCAATGT	[53]
tet32	Tetracycline resistance	**F:** CCATTACTTCGGACAACGGTAGA **R:** CAATCTCTGTGAGGGCATTTAACA	[53]
tetA	Tetracycline resistance	**F:** CTCACCAGCCTGACCTCGAT **R:** CACGTTGTTATAGAAGCCGCATAG	[53]
tetC	Tetracycline resistance	**F:** ACTGGTAAGGTAAACGCCATTGTC **R:** ATGCATAAACCAGCCATTGAGTAAG	[53]
tetL	Tetracycline resistance	**F:** ATGGTTGTAGTTGCGCGCTATAT **R:** ATCGCTGGACCGACTCCTT	[53]
tetM	Tetracycline resistance	**F:**GGAGCGATTACAGAATTAGGAAGC **R:** TCCATATGTCCTGGCGTGTC	[53]
tetO	Tetracycline resistance	**F:** CAACATTAACGGAAAGTTTATTGTATACCA **R:** TTGACGCTCCAAATTCATTGTATC	[54]
tetQ	Tetracycline resistance	**F:** CGCCTCAGAAGTAAGTTCATACACTAAG **R:**TCGTTCATGCGGATATTATCAGAAT	[54]
tetS	Tetracycline resistance	**F:** TTAAGGACAAACTTTCTGACGACATC **R:** TGTCTCCCATTGTTCTGGTTCA	[54]
tetW	Tetracycline resistance	**F:** ATGAACATTCCCACCGTTATCTTT **R:** ATATCGGCGGAGAGCTTATCC	[54]
tetX	Tetracycline resistance	**F:** AAATTTGTTACCGACACGGAAGTT **R:** CATAGCTGAAAAAATCCAGGACAGTT	[54]
tnpA	Mobile genetic element	**F:** AATTGATGCGGACGGCTTAA **R:**TCACCAAACTGTTTATGGAGTCGTT	[54]
vanA	Vancomycin resistance	**F:** GGGCTGTGAGGTCGGTTG **R:** TTCAGTACAATGCGGCCGTTA	[54]
vanB	Vancomycin resistance	**F:** TTGTCGGCGAAGTGGATCA **R:** AGCCTTTTTCCGGCTCGTT	[54]
vanRA	Vancomycin resistance	**F:** CCCTTACTCCCACCGAGTTTT **R:** TTCGTCGCCCCATATCTCAT	[54]
vanSA	Vancomycin resistance	**F:** CGCGTCATGCTTTCAAAATTC **R:** TCCGCAGAAAGCTCAATTTGTT	[54]

Note: F indicates forward primer sequences; P indicates reverse primer sequences; P indicates FAM probe sequences.

3.4. Identification of Antimicrobial Resistant Bacteria

A selective culture approach with antibiotics will be used to target airborne antibiotic-resistant bacteria (ARB) carrying ARGs. Culture can retrieve less abundant bacteria which is one of the major biases of culture-independent methods [58]. This is the reason why air samples in the present work will be plated directly on solid agar media as well as inoculated in broths to enrich specific genera and/or specific types of ARB. Incubation in different atmospheres will allow the isolation of aerobic, micro-aerophilic, and anaerobic bacteria. All plates and broths will be supplemented with antibiotics, those of which will be chosen after known ARGs found in the type of environments studied, clinical isolates and for enrichment and inhibitory purposes. Isolated and purified colonies will be identified using MALDI-TOF mass spectrometry and DNA sequencing. Bacterial species will be further analyzed by antibiotic susceptibility testing against commonly used antibiotics, as previously described [59]. Whole-genome sequencing will permit species taxonomic assignation and detection of ARGs and their associated mobile genetic elements (MGEs) [60]. A shared DNA sequencing pipeline for metagenomics analyses will be developed and a suite of powerful tools for genome assembly, including Ray [61], Ray Meta for metagenome assembly [62], and Ray Surveyor for comparing metagenomes [63] will be deployed. Moreover, co-investigators have created machine-learning algorithms, such as KOVER [64], that can investigate important sequence features that can be associated with specific phenotypes including ARGs. Selective culture approaches will be performed on specific samples from hospitals, wastewater treatment plants, and livestock farms (Table 2).

Understanding the fate of ARGs and potential risks to human health is a key to this project. However, bacterial communities are shaped by a complex array of evolutionary, ecological, and environmental factors. As such, it is difficult to predict the fate of ARGs in environmental samples. The lack of functional demonstrations for ARGs in environmental metagenomes is a considerable limitation when characterizing the environmental resistome and assessing of its clinical relevance. Therefore, a selective culture approach will be employed to enrich bacterial species from selected samples collected at emission sources (i.e., hospitals, farms, wastewater treatment plants). The ARGs and or MGEs present in these isolates will be analyzed.

Furthermore, animal models will be developed to assess the risk of ARG transfer in vivo. Briefly, C57BL/6 mice will be treated with a mixture of antibiotics to perturb their gut microbiota over a period of five days. Liquid cultures of sorbitol peptone broth and bile salts media derived from air samples from selected environments will be introduced to the mouse gut once daily over the course of the eight-week experiment to mimic chronic exposure to potentially harmful bioaerosols. Faecal samples will be collected before, during, and after this process. DNA will be extracted from these samples and will be processed through the metagenomics pipeline described earlier.

3.5. Modeling

An atmospheric pollutant dispersion model will evaluate the dispersion and fate of bioaerosols and ARGs emitted from specific activities. Atmospheric dispersion models have been used extensively for both research and regulatory purposes. Previous research demonstrates the efficacy of dispersion models to estimate the risk of infection from bioaerosol exposure for residents near manure application sites [65]. Given the difficulty and expense of obtaining ambient air pollutant measurements over a large region, plume dispersion modeling is an effective alternative for assessing the impacts of bioaerosol sources on air quality in surrounding areas. The AERMOD [66] dispersion model will be used to determine the spatial distribution of bioaerosols and ARGs in proximity to their potential sources. AERMOD is approved for regulatory purposes by the U.S. Environmental Protection Agency and incorporates the Gaussian-plume modeling approach; a plume emanating from a source is considered to disperse in a manner analogous to the Gaussian distribution in both the y (lateral) and z (vertical) directions, whereas pollutants move by advection (wind transport) in the x (downwind) direction. AERMOD treats a pollutant as a non-reactive contaminant. It requires three fundamental inputs: the source type, the emission rate of the source, and local meteorological information to assess the emissions, and resulting downwind concentrations of bioaerosols from continuous emitters.

Maps of ARG and bacterial concentrations will also be produced to provide examples of plume development in a given direction to demonstrate how concentrations are reduced with distance away from sources. The same concentration maps will also be used to evaluate dispersion from short-term emissions, for example, from manure spreading. Results from this aspect of this research project will contribute to the development of information to inform policy decisions regarding safe distances from ARG sources to prevent their transmission to humans and domestic animals.

The roles of exposure pathways, bacterial relationships, co-selective pressures, ARG transmission, and the combined and cumulative effects of antimicrobial use need to be brought together in a One Health context. The One Health ethos posits that the interconnectedness of human, animal, and environmental activities are so great that they must be addressed together in an interdisciplinary manner to ensure health across systems and scales [67]. Integrated assessment models (IAM), developed for dealing with complex issues such as climate change, are a framework for organizing and processing evidence and uncertainties for complex systems in a complex manner, yet are still easily interpreted, ordered, and computationally efficient manner. An IAM specific to AMR in Canada (iAM.AMR) has been under development since 2015 [68]. The iAM.AMR quantitatively characterizes multiple linked transmission pathways of dissemination of AMR among humans, animals, and the environment. It uses a branching tree probability approach to modify the baseline probability of AMR using measures of association and the frequency of factor occurrence.

To date, the iAM.AMR framework has been populated with a significant body of information on AMR and antimicrobial use from the scientific literature and surveillance data. Model development has focused on specific antimicrobial/bacteria/pathway combinations related to the food chain, particularly the poultry, swine, and beef production chains [68]. Our results will be added to the existing iAM.AMR framework to include AMR dissemination through bioaerosols in environmental pathways. This process will incorporate data from short and long-distance ARG transport models, as well as in vivo transfer in animal models. Ultimately, the aerosolized ARG transmission from multiple sources will assess the relative contributions of total transmission throughout the food chain, healthcare settings, watershed, and other systems, in order to identify optimal intervention points for AMR mitigation strategies (Figure 2).

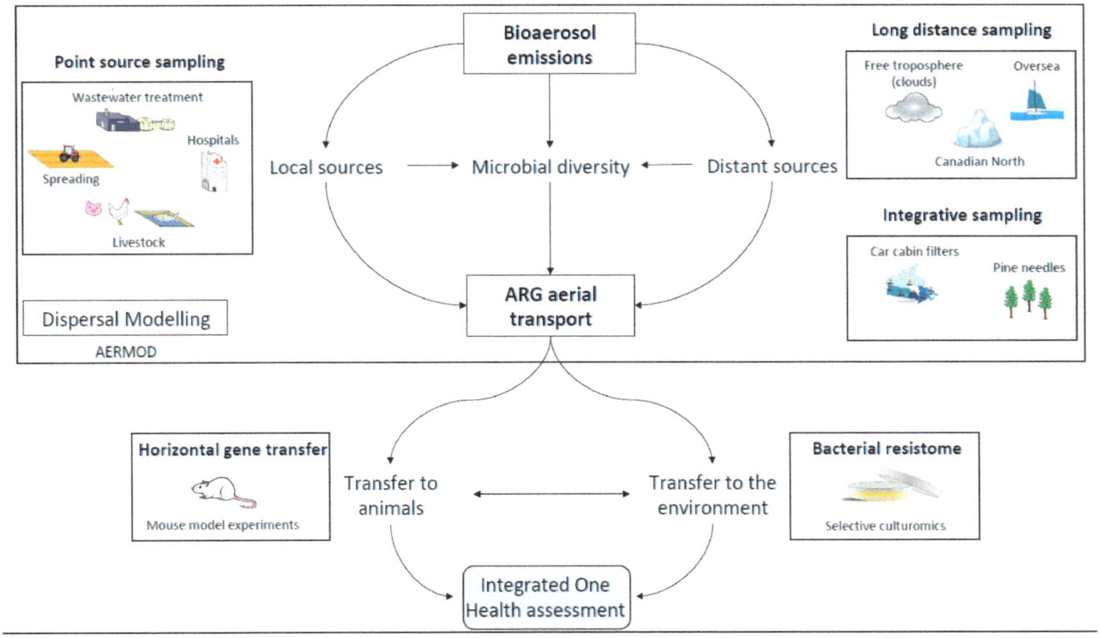

Figure 2. Conceptual diagram showing the creation of ARG risk assessment models. Data collected from the various study sites will be assembled to assess ARG emissions at point sources and over long distances. These will in turn inform ARG transfer studies in animal models and transport modeling. Together, these data will be used in an integrative ARG health risk assessment model. Ultimately this model aims to incorporate all relevant data to provide information to policymakers to make informed decisions to address the antibacterial resistance crisis.

3.6. Data Management

Given the interdisciplinary nature of this project, shared data collection and management practices must be implemented. The project will use a shared ARG panel (Table 3) and metagenomics pipeline. The limited selection of air samplers and standardized sampling design allows for uniform sampling techniques regardless of location, thus improving comparability of results from different locations and environments across Canada.

All researchers will upload their data to a secure, shared data portal. Data entry will conform to a standardized format to be accessible for all team members. This shared format will also permit the integration of different sampling campaigns into model design. These data can be selected or removed from models as needed by the lead statisticians without lengthy delays in contacting researchers for their data and reformatting them for specific uses.

4. Conclusions

Presently, the spread of ARGs in bioaerosols is not understood. This research program has the power to change paradigms by comprehensively addressing ARG emissions, exposure, and risk models, to inform policy for antimicrobial management and address AMR in the context of the environment. Antibiotic use and association with bioaerosols and geographical distribution of ARG across landscapes will be important knowledge produced from this work. Proof-of-concept for developing surveillance networks in natural and man-made environments using new rapid detection systems will be presented. Modeling will allow activity-based estimations of distribution. In addition, studying the contribution of ARG sources in bioaerosols will better contextualize our understanding of the contributions of activities to ARGs. The potential routes for transmission of antimicrobial-resistant bacteria and AMR genes between animals and people are complex and include many environmental routes beyond direct contact and the food chain. Thus, all data generated in this project will be made available to inform and expand an integrated exposure model on AMR.

The scientific data and models produced in this project will be accessible. This way, it is hoped our designs may be applicable to other countries and climates. The program addresses the complete ARG transport chain from sources, emissions, dispersal, and long-distance transport to models of exposure potential and risk in humans and animal models to elucidate the roles of bioaerosols in their transmission and detection of ARGs. These results have the potential for a far-reaching impact across Canada and internationally through collaborative team efforts, developing expertise and promoting the study of airborne ARGs to other anthropogenic and natural activities. Results will be important to policymakers, stakeholders, and communities to understand and develop strategies for mitigating ARG emissions. Ultimately, it is hoped that this project will serve as a blueprint for developing strategies to study bioaerosols and address AMR in the environment.

Author Contributions: P.B.L.G., F.R., N.T. and C.D. conceptualized this paper; they also wrote the first draft with contributions from T.B., M.G.B., M.B. (Maurice Boissinot), S.J.C., B.L.C., J.C., A.I.C., M.-L.G., M.G., S.G., S.P.K., A.M. (André Marette), A.M. (Allison McGeer), P.T.O., E.J.P., R.J.R.-S., E.T., A.D.L., É.P., B.T., M.T., I.S., A.F.D., A.K.C.D., A.K., J.L. and C.P.M. regarding their specific projects. C.D., P.A., S.J.C., S.P.K., J.C., A.I.C., E.T., T.B., M.G.B., M.G., M.-L.G., P.T.O., R.J.R.-S., A.-M.D., M.B. (Maurice Boissinot), M.Y., B.L.C. and A.M. (Allison McGeer), secured funding for this project. P.B.L.G., F.R., E.J.P., S.S., A.-M.D., M.Y., L.T., P.B., A.D.L., V.L., V.E.P., M.-H.P., É.P., B.T., M.V., M.T., I.S., M.L., M.B. (Mahsa Baghdadi), A.C.T., A.B.C., M.-J.D., A.F.D., S.B.G., A.K.C.D., A.K., S.L., J.L., M.P.M., G.P., C.P.M., C.A.N., D.O.-D., J.P., A.R.-F. and N.T. are responsible for data collection, analyses, and interpretation for their respective projects. M.-W.S.-G. and F.R. developed the conceptual diagrams. All authors have read and agreed to the published version of the manuscript.

Funding: The authors wish to acknowledge the support of NSERC through the Frontiers Grant (GRANT No. 539024-2019) awarded to CD and co-investigators (TB, MGB, SJC, JC, AIC, MLG, MG, SPK, AM, and ET), which in turn funds many students and research professionals. Aspects of this research were funded by NSERC, *Fonds de Recherche du Québec–Nature et technologies*, the Networks of Centres of Excellence program, ArcticNet, and the Sentinelle Nord program at Université Laval (Canada First Research Excellence Fund). Core and key pathway development of the iAM.AMR is supported by the Genomics Research and Development Initiative Shared Priority Project on Antimicrobial Resistance 2 (GRDI-AMR 2) and the Alberta Major Innovation Fund Grant RCP-19-

003-MIF and was previously supported by GRDI-AMR 1 and the Ontario Ministry of Agriculture Food and Rural Affairs New Directions Research Grant ND2013-1967. PBLG is supported by a Sentinelle Nord Postdoctoral Fellowship. M-WS-G is supported by funds from the *Centre de Recherche en Infectiologie Porcine et Avicole* (CRIPA) and *l'Institut de Recherché Robert-Sauvé en Santé et en Sécurité du Travail.* CD holds a Tier 1 Canada Research Chair in Bioaerosols. JC holds a Tier 1 Canada Research Chair in Medical Genomics. IS is supported by a training program scholarship from the *Institut sur la Nutrition et les Aliments Fonctionnels.* VEP is supported by a grant from the LARSEM facility. AFD is supported by *Fonds de Recherche du Québec – Santé* (FRQ-S) and NSERC scholarships. MB Is supported by a CRIPA graduate scholarship. JL is supported by an FRQ-S scholarship. JP was supported by the Northern Scientific Training Program. MPM is supported by an International Doctoral Tuition Scholarship (University of Guelph and Ontario Veterinary College).

Acknowledgments: We thank the Polar Continental Shelf Program (Natural Resources Canada) and Parks Canada for logistical and in-kind support. High-performance computing is conducted through Compute Canada and Calcul Québec, We thank Scott McEwan for his contributions towards securing the NSERC Frontiers Grant. We thank all collaborating organizations for their support in site access and sample collection.

Conflicts of Interest: The authors have no conflict of interest to declare.

References

1. Murray, C.J.; Ikuta, K.S.; Sharara, F.; Swetschniski, L.; Aguilar, G.R.; Gray, A.; Han, C.; Bisignano, P.; Rao, P.; Wool, E.; et al. Global burden of bacterial antimicrobial resistance in 2019: A systemic analysis. *Lancet* **2022**, *399*, 629–655. [CrossRef]
2. Finlay, B.B.; Conly, J.; Coyte, P.C.; Dillon, J.-A.R.; Douglas, G.; Goddard, E.; Greco, L.; Nicolle, L.E.; Patrick, D.; Prescott, J.F. When Antibiotics Fail: The Expert Panel on the Potential Socio-Economic Impacts of Antimicrobial Resistance in Canada. 2019. Available online: https://cca-reports.ca/reports/the-potential-socio-economic-impacts-of-antimicrobial-resistance-in-canada/ (accessed on 4 March 2022).
3. Bonaccorsi, G.; Pierri, F.; Cinelli, M.; Flori, A.; Galeazzi, A.; Porcelli, F.; Schmidt, A.L.; Valensise, C.M.; Scala, A.; Quattrociocchi, W.; et al. Economic and Social Consequences of Human Mobility Restrictions under COVID-19. *Proc. Natl. Acad. Sci. USA* **2020**, *117*, 15530–15535. [CrossRef] [PubMed]
4. Edoka, I.; Fraser, H.; Jamieson, L.; Meyer-Rath, G.; Mdewa, W. Inpatient Care Costs of COVID-19 in South Africa's Public Healthcare System. *Int. J. Health Policy Manag.* **2021**, 1–8. [CrossRef] [PubMed]
5. Singer, A.C.; Shaw, H.; Rhodes, V.; Hart, A. Review of Antimicrobial Resistance in the Environment and Its Relevance to Environmental Regulators. *Front. Microbiol.* **2016**, *7*, 1728. [CrossRef]
6. Larsen, J.; Raisen, C.L.; Ba, X.; Sadgrove, N.J.; Padilla-González, G.F.; Simmonds, M.S.J.; Loncaric, I.; Kerschner, H.; Apfalter, P.; Hartl, R.; et al. Emergence of Methicillin Resistance Predates the Clinical Use of Antibiotics. *Nature* **2022**, *602*, 135–141. [CrossRef]
7. Robinson, T.P.; Bu, D.P.; Carrique-Mas, J.; Fèvre, E.M.; Gilbert, M.; Grace, D.; Hay, S.I.; Jiwakanon, J.; Kakkar, M.; Kariuki, S.; et al. Antibiotic Resistance Is the Quintessential One Health Issue. *Trans. R. Soc. Trop. Med. Hyg.* **2016**, *110*, 377–380. [CrossRef]
8. Huijbers, P.M.C.; Blaak, H.; de Jong, M.C.M.; Graat, E.A.M.; Vandenbroucke-Grauls, C.M.J.E.; de Roda Husman, A.M.E. Role of the environment in the transmission of antimicrobial resistance to humans: A review. *Environ. Sci. Technol.* **2015**, *49*, 11993–12004. [CrossRef]
9. Van Boeckel, T.P.; Brower, C.; Gilbert, M.; Grenfell, B.T.; Levin, S.A.; Robinson, T.P.; Teillant, A.; Laxminarayan, R. Global Trends in Antimicrobial Use in Food Animals. *Proc. Natl. Acad. Sci. USA* **2015**, *112*, 5649–5654. [CrossRef]
10. Government of Canada. *Canadian Integrated Program for Antimicrobial Resistance Surveillance (CIPARS) 2018: Integrated Findings 2020*; Public Health Agency of Canada: Guelph, ON, Canada, 2020.
11. Ginn, O.; Lowry, S.; Brown, J. A Systematic Review of Enteric Pathogens and Antibiotic Resistance Genes in Outdoor Urban Aerosols. *Environ. Res.* **2022**, *212*, 113097. [CrossRef]
12. Gwenzi, W.; Shamsizadeh, Z.; Gholipour, S.; Nikaeen, M. The Air-Borne Antibiotic Resistome: Occurrence, Health Risks, and Future Directions. *Sci. Total Environ.* **2022**, *804*, 150154. [CrossRef]
13. Ling, A.L.; Pace, N.R.; Hernandez, M.T.; LaPara, T.M. Tetracycline Resistance and Class 1 Integron Genes Associated with Indoor and Outdoor Aerosols. *Environ. Sci. Technol.* **2013**, *47*, 4046–4052. [CrossRef] [PubMed]
14. Bai, H.; He, L.-Y.; Wu, D.-L.; Gao, F.-Z.; Zhang, M.; Zou, H.-Y.; Yao, M.-S.; Ying, G.-G. Spread of Airborne Antibiotic Resistance from Animal Farms to the Environment: Dispersal Pattern and Exposure Risk. *Environ. Int.* **2022**, *158*, 106927. [CrossRef] [PubMed]
15. Milton, D.K.A. Rosetta Stone for Understanding Infectious Drops and Aerosols. *J. Pediatr. Infect. Dis. Soc.* **2020**, *9*, 413–415. [CrossRef]
16. Pasteur, L. Mémoire sur les corpuscules organisés qui existent dans l'atmosphère, examen de la doctrine des générations spontanées. *Ann. Sci. Nat. Zoo.* **1861**, *16*, 5–98.
17. Wéry, N.; Galès, A.; Brunet, Y. Bioaerosols Sources. In *Microbiology of Aerosols*; Delort, A.-M., Amato, P., Eds.; John Wiley & Sons Inc.: Hoboken, NJ, USA, 2018; pp. 117–136.

18. Fiegel, J.; Clarke, R.; Edwards, D.A. Airborne Infectious Disease and the Suppression of Pulmonary Bioaerosols. *Drug Discov.* **2006**, *11*, 51–57. [CrossRef]
19. Mack, S.M.; Madl, A.K.; Pinkerton, K.E. Respiratory Health Effects of Exposure to Ambient Particulate Matter and Bioaerosols. In *Comprehensive Physiology*; Terjung, R., Ed.; Wiley: Hoboken, NJ, USA, 2019; pp. 1–20. [CrossRef]
20. Dysvik, A.; La Rosa, S.L.; De Rouck, G.; Rukke, E.-O.; Westereng, B.; Wicklund, T. Microbial Dynamics in Traditional and Modern Sour Beer Production. *Appl. Environ. Microbiol.* **2020**, *86*, e00566-20. [CrossRef]
21. Šantl-Temkiv, T.; Sikoparija, B.; Maki, T.; Carotenuto, F.; Amato, P.; Yao, M.; Morris, C.E.; Schnell, R.; Jaenicke, R.; Pöhlker, C.; et al. Bioaerosol Field Measurements: Challenges and Perspectives in Outdoor Studies. *Aerosol Sci. Technol.* **2020**, *54*, 520–546. [CrossRef]
22. Šantl-Temkiv, T.; Amato, P.; Casamayor, E.O.; Lee, P.K.H.; Pointing, S.B. Microbial Ecology of the Atmosphere. *FEMS Microbiol. Rev.* **2022**, fuac009. [CrossRef] [PubMed]
23. Barberán, A.; Ladau, J.; Leff, J.W.; Pollard, K.S.; Menninger, H.L.; Dunn, R.R.; Fierer, N. Continental-Scale Distributions of Dust-Associated Bacteria and Fungi. *Proc. Natl. Acad. Sci. USA* **2015**, *112*, 5756–5761. [CrossRef]
24. Fröhlich-Nowoisky, J.; Pickersgill, D.A.; Després, V.R.; Pöschl, U. High Diversity of Fungi in Air Particulate Matter. *Proc. Natl. Acad. Sci. USA* **2009**, *106*, 12814–12819. [CrossRef]
25. de Leeuw, G.; Andreas, E.L.; Anguelova, M.D.; Fairall, C.W.; Lewis, E.R.; O'Dowd, C.; Schulz, M.; Schwartz, S.E. Production Flux of Sea Spray Aerosol. *Rev. Geophys.* **2011**, *49*, RG2001. [CrossRef]
26. Xie, W.; Li, Y.; Bai, W.; Hou, J.; Ma, T.; Zeng, X.; Zhang, L.; An, T. The Source and Transport of Bioaerosols in the Air: A Review. *Front. Environ. Sci. Eng.* **2021**, *15*, 44. [CrossRef] [PubMed]
27. Griffin, D.W. Atmospheric Movement of Microorganisms in Clouds of Desert Dust and Implications for Human Health. *Clin. Microbiol. Rev.* **2007**, *20*, 459–477. [CrossRef] [PubMed]
28. Nhu Nguyen, T.M.; Ilef, D.; Jarraud, S.; Rouil, L.; Campese, C.; Che, D.; Haeghebaert, S.; Ganiayre, F.; Marcel, F.; Etienne, J.; et al. Community-Wide Outbreak of Legionnaires Disease Linked to Industrial Cooling Towers—How Far Can Contaminated Aerosols Spread? *J. Infect. Dis.* **2006**, *193*, 102–111. [CrossRef] [PubMed]
29. Bonifait, L.; Marchand, G.; Veillette, M.; M'Bareche, H.; Dubuis, M.-E.; Pépin, C.; Cloutier, Y.; Bernard, Y.; Duchaine, C. Workers' Exposure to Bioaerosols from Three Different Types of Composting Facilities. *J. Occup. Environ. Hyg.* **2017**, *14*, 815–822. [CrossRef] [PubMed]
30. Degois, J.; Simon, X.; Clerc, F.; Bontemps, C.; Leblond, P.; Duquenne, P. One-Year Follow-up of Microbial Diversity in Bioaerosols Emitted in a Waste Sorting Plant in France. *Waste Manag.* **2021**, *120*, 257–268. [CrossRef]
31. Pal, C.; Bengtsson-Palme, J.; Kristiansson, E.; Larsson, D.G.J. The Structure and Diversity of Human, Animal and Environmental Resistomes. *Microbiome* **2016**, *4*, 54. [CrossRef]
32. Hu, J.; Zhao, F.; Zhang, X.-X.; Li, K.; Li, C.; Ye, L.; Li, M. Metagenomic Profiling of ARGs in Airborne Particulate Matters during a Severe Smog Event. *Sci. Total Environ.* **2018**, *615*, 1332–1340. [CrossRef]
33. Xie, J.; Jin, L.; He, T.; Chen, B.; Luo, X.; Feng, B.; Huang, W.; Li, J.; Fu, P.; Li, X. Bacteria and Antibiotic Resistance Genes (ARGs) in $PM_{2.5}$ from China: Implications for Human Exposure. *Environ. Sci. Technol.* **2019**, *53*, 963–972. [CrossRef]
34. Li, J.; Cao, J.; Zhu, Y.; Chen, Q.; Shen, F.; Wu, Y.; Xu, S.; Fan, H.; Da, G.; Huang, R.; et al. Global Survey of Antibiotic Resistance Genes in Air. *Environ. Sci. Technol.* **2018**, *52*, 10975–10984. [CrossRef]
35. Zhang, Y.; Gu, A.Z.; Cen, T.; Li, X.; Li, D.; Chen, J. Petrol and Diesel Exhaust Particles Accelerate the Horizontal Transfer of Plasmid-Mediated Antimicrobial Resistance Genes. *Environ. Int.* **2018**, *114*, 280–287. [CrossRef] [PubMed]
36. Gaviria-Figueroa, A.; Preisner, E.C.; Hoque, S.; Feigley, C.E.; Norman, R.S. Emission and Dispersal of Antibiotic Resistance Genes through Bioaerosols Generated during the Treatment of Municipal Sewage. *Sci. Total Environ.* **2019**, *686*, 402–412. [CrossRef] [PubMed]
37. Pilote, J.; Létourneau, V.; Girard, M.; Duchaine, C. Quantification of Airborne Dust, Endotoxins, Human Pathogens and Antibiotic and Metal Resistance Genes in Eastern Canadian Swine Confinement Buildings. *Aerobiologia* **2019**, *35*, 283–296. [CrossRef]
38. Song, L.; Wang, C.; Jiang, G.; Ma, J.; Li, Y.; Chen, H.; Guo, J. Bioaerosol Is an Important Transmission Route of Antibiotic Resistance Genes in Pig Farms. *Environ. Int.* **2021**, *154*, 106559. [CrossRef] [PubMed]
39. Jahne, M.A.; Rogers, S.W.; Holsen, T.M.; Grimberg, S.J. Quantitative Microbial Risk Assessment of Bioaerosols from a Manure Application Site. *Aerobiologia* **2015**, *31*, 73–87. [CrossRef]
40. Laurens, C.; Jean-Pierre, H.; Licznar-Fajardo, P.; Hantova, S.; Godreuil, S.; Martinez, O.; Jumas-Bilak, E. Transmission of IMI-2 Carbapenemase-Producing Enterobacteriaceae from River Water to Human. *J. Glob. Antimicrob. Resist.* **2018**, *15*, 88–92. [CrossRef]
41. M'bareche, H.; Brisebois, E.; Veillette, M.; Duchaine, C. Bioaerosol Sampling and Detection Methods Based on Molecular Approaches: No Pain No Gain. *Sci. Total Environ.* **2017**, *599–600*, 2095–2104. [CrossRef]
42. Létourneau, V.; Nehmé, B.; Mériaux, A.; Massé, D.; Cormier, Y.; Duchaine, C. Human Pathogens and Tetracycline-Resistant Bacteria in Bioaerosols of Swine Confinement Buildings and in Nasal Flora of Hog Producers. *Int. J. Hyg. Environ. Health* **2010**, *213*, 444–449. [CrossRef]
43. Just, N.A.; Létourneau, V.; Kirychuk, S.P.; Signh, B.; Duchaine, C. Potentially Pathogenic Bacteria and Antimicrobial Resistance in Bioaerosols from Cage-Housed and Floor-Housed Poultry Operations. *Ann. Occup. Hyg.* **2012**, *56*, 440–449. [CrossRef]

44. Boy, M.; Thomson, E.S.; Acosta Navarro, J.-C.; Arnalds, O.; Batchvarova, E.; Bäck, J.; Berninger, F.; Bilde, M.; Brasseur, Z.; Dagsson-Waldhauserova, P.; et al. Interactions between the Atmosphere, Cryosphere, and Ecosystems at Northern High Latitudes. *Atmos. Chem. Phys.* **2019**, *19*, 2015–2061. [CrossRef]
45. Šantl-Temkiv, T.; Amato, P.; Gosewinkel, U.; Thyrhaug, R.; Charton, A.; Chicot, B.; Finster, K.; Bratbak, G.; Löndahl, J. High-Flow-Rate Impinger for the Study of Concentration, Viability, Metabolic Activity, and Ice-Nucleation Activity of Airborne Bacteria. *Environ. Sci. Technol.* **2017**, *51*, 11224–11234. [CrossRef] [PubMed]
46. Amato, P.; Besaury, L.; Joly, M.; Penaud, B.; Deguillaume, L.; Delort, A.-M. Metatranscriptomic Exploration of Microbial Functioning in Clouds. *Sci. Rep.* **2019**, *9*, 4383. [CrossRef] [PubMed]
47. Galès, A.; Latrille, E.; Wéry, N.; Steyer, J.-P.; Godon, J.-J. Needles of *Pinus Halepensis* as Biomonitors of Bioaerosol Emissions. *PLoS ONE* **2014**, *9*, e112182. [CrossRef]
48. Morris, C.; Kinkel, L. Fifty years of phyllosphere microbiology: Significant contributions to research in related fields. In *Phyllosphere Microbiology*; Lindow, S., Hecht-Poinar, E., Elliott, V., Eds.; APS Press: St. Paul, MN, USA, 2002; pp. 365–375.
49. Lindow, S.E.; Leveau, J.H.J. Phyllosphere Microbiology. *Curr. Opin. Biotechnol.* **2002**, *13*, 238–243. [CrossRef]
50. Smets, W.; Wuyts, K.; Oerlemans, E.; Wuyts, S.; Denys, S.; Samson, R.; Lebeer, S. Impact of Urban Land Use on the Bacterial Phyllosphere of Ivy (*Hedera* sp.). *Atmos. Environ.* **2016**, *147*, 376–383. [CrossRef]
51. Xiang, Q.; Zhu, D.; Giles, M.; Neilson, R.; Yang, X.-R.; Qiao, M.; Chen, Q.-L. Agricultural Activities Affect the Pattern of the Resistome within the Phyllosphere Microbiome in Peri-Urban Environments. *J. Hazard. Mate.* **2020**, *382*, 121068. [CrossRef]
52. George, P.B.L.; Leclerc, S.; Turgeon, N.; Veillette, M.; Duchaine, C. Conifer needles as passive monitors of bioareosolised antibiotic resistance genes. *Antibiotics* **2022**, *11*, 907. [CrossRef]
53. Stedtfeld, R.D.; Guo, X.; Stedtfeld, T.M.; Sheng, H.; Williams, M.R.; Hauschild, K.; Gunturu, S.; Tift, L.; Wang, F.; Howe, A.; et al. Primer Set 2.0 for Highly Parallel QPCR Array Targeting Antibiotic Resistance Genes and Mobile Genetic Elements. *FEMS Microbiol. Ecol.* **2018**, *94*, fiy130. [CrossRef]
54. Nijuis, R.H.T.; Veldman, K.T.; Schelfaut, J.; Van Essen-Zandbergen, A.; Wessels, E.; Claas, E.C.J.; Gooskens, J. Detection of the Plasmid-Mediated Colistin-Resistance Gene Mcr-1 in Clinical Isolates and Stool Specimens Obtained from Hospitalized Patients Using a Newly Developed Real-Time PCR Assay. *J. Antimicrob. Chemother.* **2016**, *71*, 2344–2346. [CrossRef]
55. Rhouma, M.; Thériault, W.; Rabhi, N.; Duchaine, C.; Quessy, S.; Fravalo, P. First Identification of Mcr-1/Mcr-2 Genes in the Fecal Microbiota of Canadian Commercial Pigs during the Growing and Finishing Period. *Vet. Med Res. Rep.* **2019**, *10*, 65–67. [CrossRef]
56. Bach, H.-J.; Tomanova, J.; Schloter, M.; Munch, J.C. Enumeration of Total Bacteria and Bacteria with Genes for Proteolytic Activity in Pure Cultures and in Environmental Samples by Quantitative PCR Mediated Amplification. *J. Microbiol. Methods* **2002**, *49*, 235–245. [CrossRef]
57. Roschanski, N.; Fischer, J.; Guerra, B.; Roesler, U. Development of a real-time PCR for the rapid detection of the predominant beta-lactamase genes CTX-M, SHV, TEM and CIT-Type AmpCs in Enterobacteriaceae. *PLoS ONE* **2014**, *9*, e100956. [CrossRef] [PubMed]
58. Zhang, M.; Zuo, J.; Yu, X.; Shi, X.; Chen, L.; Li, Z. Quantification of Multi-Antibiotic Resistant Opportunistic Pathogenic Bacteria in Bioaerosols in and around a Pharmaceutical Wastewater Treatment Plant. *J. Environ. Sci. (China)* **2018**, *72*, 53–63. [CrossRef] [PubMed]
59. Lagier, J.-C.; Dubourg, G.; Million, M.; Cadoret, F.; Bilen, M.; Fenollar, F.; Levasseur, A.; Rolain, J.-M.; Fournier, P.-E.; Raoult, D. Culturing the Human Microbiota and Culturomics. *Nat. Rev. Microbiol.* **2018**, *16*, 540–550. [CrossRef]
60. Raymond, F.; Boissinot, M.; Ouameur, A.A.; Déraspe, M.; Plante, P.-L.; Kpanou, S.R.; Bérubé, È.; Huletsky, A.; Roy, P.H.; Ouellette, M.; et al. Culture-Enriched Human Gut Microbiomes Reveal Core and Accessory Resistance Genes. *Microbiome* **2019**, *7*, 56. [CrossRef]
61. Boisvert, S.; Laviolette, F.; Corbeil, J. Ray: Simultaneous Assembly of Reads from a Mix of High-Throughput Sequencing Technologies. *J. Comput. Biol.* **2010**, *17*, 1519–1533. [CrossRef]
62. Boisvert, S.; Raymond, F.; Godzaridis, É.; Laviolette, F.; Corbeil, J. Ray Meta: Scalable de Novo Metagenome Assembly and Profiling. *Genome Biol.* **2012**, *13*, R122. [CrossRef]
63. Déraspe, M.; Raymond, F.; Boisvert, S.; Culley, A.; Roy, P.H.; Laviolette, F.; Corbeil, J. Phenetic Comparison of Prokaryotic Genomes Using K-Mers. *Mol. Biol. Evol.* **2017**, *34*, 2716–2729. [CrossRef]
64. Drouin, A.; Giguère, S.; Déraspe, M.; Marchand, M.; Tyers, M.; Loo, V.G.; Bourgault, A.-M.; Laviolette, F.; Corbeil, J. Predictive Computational Phenotyping and Biomarker Discovery Using Reference-Free Genome Comparisons. *BMC Genom.* **2016**, *17*, 754. [CrossRef]
65. Van Leuken, J.P.G.; Swart, A.N.; Havelaar, A.H.; Van Pul, A.; Van der Hoek, W.; Heederik, D. Atmospheric Dispersion Modelling of Bioaerosols That Are Pathogenic to Humans and Livestock—A Review to Inform Risk Assessment Studies. *Microb. Risk Anal.* **2016**, *1*, 19–39. [CrossRef]
66. Cimorelli, A.J.; Perry, S.G.; Venkatram, A.; Weil, J.C.; Paine, R.J.; Wilson, R.B.; Lee, R.F.; Peters, W.D.; Brode, R.W.; Paumier, J.O.; et al. *AERMOD: Model Formulation and Evaluation Results*; National Exposure Research Laboratory, Office of Research and Development: Research Triangle Park, NC, USA, 2021.

67. Destoumieux-Garzón, D.; Mavingui, P.; Boetsch, G.; Bossier, J.; Darriet, F.; Duboz, P.; Fritsch, C.; Giraudoux, P.; Le Roux, F.; Morand, S.; et al. The One Health Concept: 10 Years Old and a Long Road Ahead. *Front. Vet. Sci.* **2018**, *5*, 14. [CrossRef] [PubMed]
68. Murphy, C.P.; Carson, C.; Smith, B.A.; Chapman, B.; Marrotte, J.; McCann, M.; Primeau, C.; Sharma, P.; Parmley, E.J. Factors Potentially Linked with the Occurrence of Antimicrobial Resistance in Selected Bacteria from Cattle, Chickens and Pigs: A Scoping Review of Publications for Use in Modelling of Antimicrobial Resistance (IAM.AMR Project). *Zoonoses Public Health* **2018**, *65*, 957–971. [CrossRef] [PubMed]

antibiotics

MDPI

Article

Formulating a Community-Centric Indicator Framework to Quantify One Health Drivers of Antibiotic Resistance: A Preliminary Step towards Fostering 'Antibiotic-Smart Communities'

Philip Mathew [1], Sujith J. Chandy [2], Satya Sivaraman [1], Jaya Ranjalkar [1,*], Hyfa Mohammed Ali [1] and Shruthi Anna Thomas [1]

[1] ReAct Asia Pacific, Department of Pharmacology and Clinical Pharmacology, Christian Medical College, Vellore 632002, Tamil Nadu, India; philipmathewrap@gmail.com (P.M.); satyasagar@gmail.com (S.S.); hyfarap@gmail.com (H.M.A.); shruthiannarap@gmail.com (S.A.T.)
[2] Department of Pharmacology and Clinical Pharmacology, Christian Medical College, Vellore 632002, Tamil Nadu, India; sjchandy@cmcvellore.ac.in
* Correspondence: drjayarap@gmail.com

Abstract: Antibiotic resistance (ABR) is increasing the mortality and morbidity associated with infectious diseases, besides increasing the cost of healthcare, saturating health system capacity, and adversely affecting food security. Framing an appropriate narrative and engaging local communities through the 'One Health' approach is essential to complement top-down measures. However, the absence of objective criteria to measure the performance of ABR interventions in community settings makes it difficult to mobilize interest and investment for such interventions. An exercise was therefore carried out to develop an indicator framework for this purpose. A comprehensive list of indicators was developed from experiences gathered through community engagement work in a local *panchayat* (small administrative area) in Kerala, India and a consultative process with health, veterinary, environment, and development experts. A prioritization exercise was carried out by global experts on ABR, looking at appropriateness, feasibility, and validity. A 15-point indicator framework was designed based on the prioritization process. The final set of indicators covers human health, animal health, environment management, and Water Sanitation and Hygiene (WASH) domains. The indicator framework was piloted in the *panchayat* (located in Kerala), which attained a score of 34 (maximum 45). The score increased when interventions were implemented to mitigate the ABR drives, indicating that the framework is sensitive to change. The indicator framework was tested in four sites from three other Indian states with different socioeconomic and health profiles, yielding different scores. Those collecting the field data were able to use the framework with minimal training. It is hoped that, this indicator framework can help policymakers broadly understand the factors contributing to ABR and measure the performance of interventions they choose to implement in the community as part of National Action Plan on AMR.

Keywords: antimicrobial resistance; National Action Plans; AMR; WASH; IPC; One Health; ASC

Citation: Mathew, P.; Chandy, S.J.; Sivaraman, S.; Ranjalkar, J.; Ali, H.M.; Thomas, S.A. Formulating a Community-Centric Indicator Framework to Quantify One Health Drivers of Antibiotic Resistance: A Preliminary Step towards Fostering 'Antibiotic-Smart Communities'. *Antibiotics* **2024**, *13*, 63. https://doi.org/10.3390/antibiotics13010063

Academic Editor: Akebe Luther King Abia

Received: 28 November 2023
Revised: 28 December 2023
Accepted: 2 January 2024
Published: 8 January 2024

1. Introduction

Antibiotic resistance (ABR) was associated with 4.95 million deaths and was the attributable cause of 1.27 million deaths in 2019 [1]. This is much higher than the previous estimate of 700,000 deaths per year [2]. The projected cost of ABR is also high, with the World Bank estimating a 1.1% loss in the global Gross Domestic Product (GDP) by 2050 and an annual reduction of USD 1 trillion per year beyond 2030 in the best-case scenario [3]. The burden of ABR is expected to be much higher in Lower–Middle-Income Countries (LMICs) due to their dysfunctional health systems, poor agricultural production practices, and sub-optimal environmental management [4]. Additionally, antibiotic consumption is increasing rapidly in many LMICs, thereby increasing ABR [5]. Therefore, action to contain ABR should be a priority for the public health system, especially in low-resource settings.

The global efforts made to tackle ABR have been anchored in the Global Action Plan on Antimicrobial Resistance (GAP-AMR) adopted by the World Health Assembly in 2015 [6]. Since then, most countries have adopted their own action plans, but very few of them have been funded and fully operationalized [7]. The Inter-Agency Coordination Group on AMR (IACG-AMR) submitted its report to the United Nations Secretary-General on a globally coordinated response and called for a systematic and meaningful engagement of all stakeholders at global, regional, national, and local levels. The report conveyed the need for contextualized interventions based on locally generated data and insights rather than on a uniform strategy [8]. Engaging local organizations and governance structures for broad-basing ABR containment efforts has been a consistent recommendation in several documents since the Jim O'Neill report was released. All of these documents also call for the engagement of communities in a meaningful and systematic manner [8]. Framing the right narrative for ABR at the ground level to engage local communities and creating a bottom-up process to supplement national and sub-national action plans have been challenging [9]. Studies have shown that there are also language and perceptional issues associated with ABR [10].

Recently, studies have shown that community-based interventions could be beneficial in reducing inappropriate antibiotic use [11]. Community engagement interventions could also facilitate ABR behavior change, specifically in LMICs, because they employ a contextualized approach that supports communities to develop locally relevant and viable solutions [12]. For successful community engagement in ABR it is important to understand the local context, develop relationships with key stakeholders, build motivation and trust, and engage with them on the topic of antibiotics and ABR [13].

While there are some examples of community engagement in ABR, our literature review did not yield any attempts to quantify ABR at the community level. It was therefore deemed important to conceptualize a community-centric indicator framework that could help policymakers (both nationally and locally), local government officials, and other relevant stakeholders to establish a baseline, understand the issues and factors contributing to ABR, as well as measure the impact of the interventions they choose to implement in that community. This paper is therefore a description of such a framework and the multi-stage process we undertook in its development, so that others may also be able to use this framework in similar low-resource settings.

In addition, the framework could also be used to aim for 'antibiotic-smart communities'. Antibiotic smartness can be explained as the preparedness of a community to effectively and sustainably tackle ABR by addressing the drivers of ABR with a One Heath lens such as by taking measures to prevent infections, improve awareness, and promote the rational use of antibiotics.

2. Methods

ReAct is part of an independent science, policy, and advocacy-based network that has been working on antibiotic resistance since 2005. ReAct Asia Pacific (RAP) is one of the regional nodes of ReAct. RAP started working on the concept of an 'antibiotic-smart communities' with the hypothesis that the activities for ABR containment are predominantly at the national and subnational level, and community-level focus on ABR was inadequate. Developing an indicator framework was meant to help plug this gap.

We selected Kerala as it was the first state to adopt a sub-national action plan on AMR. Kerala is an Indian state with high levels of literacy and education and a high human development index [14]. Kerala has a robust collectivist culture that fosters social cohesiveness and an ingroup aim [15,16]. In addition, Kerala's strong local governance has engaged itself in managing and abating the impact of multiple health issues, including the provision of palliative care services and a decentralized response to COVID-19 rooted in the grassroots [17,18]. In this context, the investigators chose Kerala as the site to pilot the indicator framework since the setting is ideal for community engagement projects. Kerala's state government is also supportive of community engagement initiatives given its history of community engagement [19,20]. This exploratory project was undertaken in a panchayat in the state of Kerala, India. A 'panchayat' is the smallest administrative unit in India's three-tier local self-governance system, though the size and functions of a panchayat may vary widely between states. We selected Mallapuzhasserry, a panchayat with a population of 11,000 (as per the data from the last national census in India, conducted in 2011) and spread over a total area of 15 square kilometers. The project took place from 2018 to 2022. The steps in the project are summarized below in Figure 1.

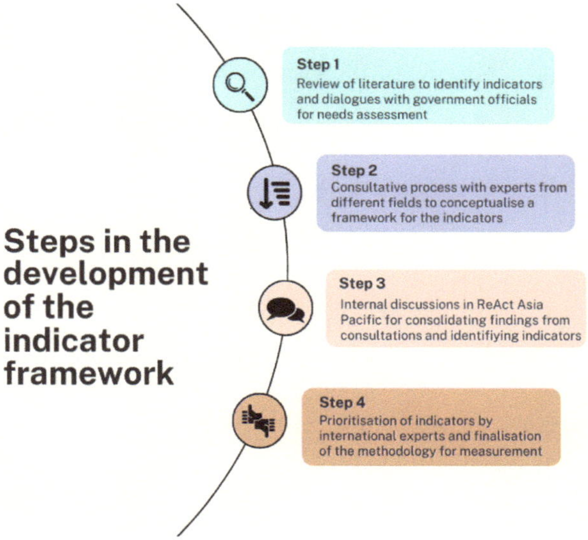

Figure 1. Steps in the process of the development of an indicator framework.

Step 1: Literature review and needs assessment: As a first step, a literature review was undertaken in 2018 to identify existing frameworks. Dialogues were held with local government officials and other key stakeholders to identify their priorities concerning antimicrobial resistance. To gain access and build confidence, we used a healthcare delivery project managed by a local medical school and a community organization for piggybacking. These interactions gave an overview of ABR in the community and helped to draw a baseline narrative regarding existing efforts to combat ABR.

Step 2: Meeting with experts from public/human health, animal health, environment, and agriculture: After the literature review, three consultation meetings were held in 2019, with experts from different sectors to conceptualize a framework for assessing different ABR drivers and their components. The experts deliberated on the need for a framework, what a hypothetical framework should contain, and possible principles that such a framework should entail to support the bottom-up approach for the development and implementation of state and national action plans. SDG indicators were used as a starting point for such discussions. The experts suggested that the framework should reflect drivers from ABR-specific and ABR-sensitive areas and capture the deficiencies in the system that influence these drivers. Figure 2 shows the conceptual framework used for developing the antibiotic-smart communities.

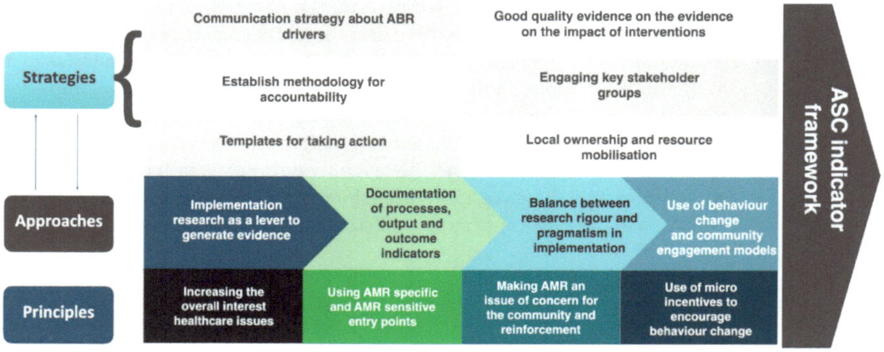

Figure 2. Conceptual framework used for developing the antibiotic-smart communities. Legend: ABR: Antibiotic Resistance; ASCs': Antibiotic-Smart Communities; AMR: Antimicrobial Resistance.

Step 3: Following the consultative meetings, the findings were consolidated and discussed internally (within ReAct Asia Pacific). Based on the suggestions from the consultation meetings and internal discussions, an initial set of 34 indicators was identified. A preliminary method of measurement for each of these indicators at the community level and the rationale for their inclusion were also drafted. This exercise was done keeping in mind that the framework will not always be used by research or academic entities but should be user-friendly for local self-governments and community-based organizations.

The refining of the indicator framework and the prioritization exercise (Step 3 and Step 4) was conducted between March 2020 and September 2021.

Step 4: Following this internal exercise, 30 international ABR experts were identified across intergovernmental agencies, academic entities, and civil societies. Twenty of them responded and agreed to assist in the prioritization. The initial set of 34 indicators, the proposed methodology for the data collection for each of these indicators, the rationale for their inclusion, and the methodology for data collection for each one of these indicators were sent over to these experts for prioritization using Google Formsxx over email. The experts were asked to prioritize the indicators based on three different criteria:

1. Appropriateness of the indicator in measuring ABR-specific/sensitive activities at the community level in local communities;
2. Feasibility of measurement in LMIC contexts;
3. Validity of the indicator in detecting changes in response to the intervention on the ground.

The experts were asked to score each indicator from 1 to 5 after carefully assessing the framing, measurement methodology, and reason for inclusion. Experts provided qualitative feedback that was used to draw up criteria for assigning these scores (1–3) to each indicator. In addition to the conceptual framework and the criteria for assigning scores, the data collection methodology drawn up by ReAct Asia Pacific was further refined based on the feedback obtained from the experts. The scores assigned by the experts while evaluating each indicator ranged from 1 to 5. In contrast, each indicator in the framework during data collection were assigned scores of 1 to 3.

Based on the scoring and prioritization given by the experts, 15 indicators were chosen for the final framework. While all indicators were assigned equal weights in the conceptual framework, each indicator can be assigned a minimum score of 1 and a maximum score of 3 depending on the level of progress made by the community in these respective domains.

3. Results

Throughout the process, both community stakeholders and experts from different sectors mentioned the need for a framework that can quantify the burden of ABR drivers.

The literature review yielded different models of community engagement for ABR, but there were no publications on metrics to quantify ABR drivers or progress made during the 2019–2021 period when this study was carried out. The dialogues with local government suggested the need for a framework that could help identify AMR drivers simultaneously and allocate local resources.

During the consultation meetings in 2019, experts pointed out that the framework should be specifically intended for low resource settings where there are gaps in WASH, access to medicines, and other challenges and take a holistic One Health perspective. The experts suggested that the number of indicators should be manageable for measurement by communities and local government structures. The results of the prioritisation exercise (Step 4) are given in Table 1.

Table 1. Scores assigned by the international experts after assessment of each indicator with due consideration of method of measurement and its feasibility, appropriateness, and validity.

Indicator	Total Score Appropriateness (Out of 100)	Total Score Feasibility (Out of 100)	Total Score Validity (Out of 100)	Mean Total Score (Out of 100)
1. Awareness about antibiotic use and antibiotic resistance among general public	77	75	70	74.0
2. Over-the-counter availability of antibiotics in retail pharmacies in the area	85	85	73	81.0 #
3. Proportion of healthcare facilities that have implemented a written Infection Prevention and Control (IPC) plan	65	80	60	68.3
4. Proportion of population using safely managed drinking water services	85	80	82	82.3 #
5. Proportion of healthcare facilities with a written antibiotic protocol for at least three disease/syndrome conditions caused by bacteria	78	80	80	79.3 #
6. Percentage of access antibiotics (as per AWaRe classification of WHO) in total antibiotics dispensed in out-patient settings at healthcare facilities	92	83	83	86.0 #
7. Proportion of healthcare facilities which are accredited by any standard agency (government/private) for quality assurance in delivery of services	77	75	70	74.0
8. Percentage of suspected urinary tract infections (community- or healthcare-associated) being subjected to culture and sensitivity testing	77	67	73	72.3
9. Prevalence of stunting (height for age < -2 standard deviation from the median of the World Health Organization (WHO) Child Growth Standards)	48	67	48	54.3
10. Average under-5 mortality rate (number of deaths among children under 5 years of age compared to number of live births) in the area for the past 3 years	72	83	63	72.6
11. Average out-of-pocket expenditure on healthcare by households in the area	62	68	60	63.3
12. Access to healthcare	70	68	65	67.6

Table 1. *Cont.*

Indicator	Total Score Appropriateness (Out of 100)	Total Score Feasibility (Out of 100)	Total Score Validity (Out of 100)	Mean Total Score (Out of 100)
13. Coverage for pediatric vaccines listed in the immunization schedule published by the competent national authority	90	87	88	88.3 #
14. Availability of laboratory services in healthcare facilities within the community	75	78	75	76.0
15. Hygiene facilities in primary and secondary schools in the community	90	87	92	89.6 #
16. Educational initiatives in the past one year to increase awareness about antibiotic or biocide use among farmers	80	80	70	76.6 #
17. Use of highest priority critically important antibiotics in agriculture	88	80	85	84.3 #
18. Regulatory oversight regarding best farm management practices and biosecurity measures	78	78	70	75.3
19. Presence of veterinary health facilities in the community	78	80	75	77.6 #
20. Vaccination coverage for farm animals in the community	82	75	72	76.3
21. Government subsidies or incentives for infrastructural improvement in farms for better infection control practices	70	78	65	71.0
22. Availability of veterinary laboratory services for disease diagnostics	85	83	82	83.3 #
23. Incentive system for farmers who make products without routine use of antibiotics	80	70	73	74.3
24. Presence of schemes to promote local or household-based production of food	63	73	63	66.3
25. Proportion of wastewater treated using any established wastewater treatment technologies, as per WHO's guidelines on sanitation and health (2019)	80	77	80	79.0 #
26. Biomedical waste management system in healthcare facilities	92	83	82	85.6 #
27. System for disposal of antibiotics and other medicinal waste generated from households	85	65	75	75.0
28. Use of chemical/synthetic pesticides, herbicides, and other biocides in farms	83	72	82	79.0 #
29. Farm waste contaminating water resources in the community	87	70	80	79.0 #
30. Proportion of households having access to Individual Household Latrine (IHHL) with water supply within the premises of their houses	88	87	55	76.6 #

Table 1. *Cont.*

Indicator	Total Score Appropriateness (Out of 100)	Total Score Feasibility (Out of 100)	Total Score Validity (Out of 100)	Mean Total Score (Out of 100)
31. Proportion of population covered by at least one social insurance or assurance schemes for health protection	62	70	58	63.3
32. Proportion of population below the nationally accepted poverty line	68	78	65	70.3
33. Proportion of children between ages 5 and 14 receiving nutritional support from government	68	78	68	71.3
34. Female literacy rate	72	77	80	76.3

Legend: # indicates the final indicator.

The final set of 15 indicators (see Table 2 below) covered human health, animal health, Agriculture, environment management, and trans-sectoral domains.

Table 2. Final list of 15 indicators after prioritization exercise.

1	Hygiene facilities in primary and secondary schools in the community
2	Access to Individual Household Latrine (IHHL) with water supply in households
3	Coverage for pediatric vaccines as per the national immunization schedule
4	Percentage of access antibiotics (as per AWaRe classification of WHO) in total antibiotics dispensed in outpatient settings at healthcare facilities
5	Antibiotic protocols in healthcare facilities
6	Over-the-counter (OTC) availability of antibiotics in retail pharmacies in the area
7	Access to safely managed drinking water services
8	Use of highest priority critically important antibiotics in agriculture
9	Presence of functional veterinary health facilities and services in the community
10	Veterinary laboratory services for disease diagnostics
11	Educational initiatives on antibiotic use among farmers
12	Biomedical waste management system in healthcare facilities
13	Treatment of wastewater generated in households
14	Use of chemical/synthetic pesticides, herbicides, and other biocides in farms
15	Farm waste contaminating water resources in the community

As seen from Table 2, the indicators use a 'One-Health' approach.

The selection of indicators was based on the scores during the prioritization exercise, no other criterion was applied, and stratification was not carried out. Some of the indicators, such as the 'over-the-counter' availability of antibiotics, are specific drivers of the ABR problem in the communities. However, some others, such as the 'Proportion of households having access to Individual Household Latrine (IHHL) with water supply within the premises of their house', are linked to systemic capacities to reduce the load of infections in the community and thereby limit the use of antibiotics.

Piloting the indicator framework: The indicator framework was piloted in the community that we were working with to assess its ease of application and feasibility of obtaining information from relevant stakeholder groups. A facilitator from the ReAct Asia Pacific team trained a field worker on the data collection methods using a handbook prepared on data collon. A single trained field worker was employed for data collection after the necessary permissions were obtained from the local self-government body and other concerned institutions.

The piloting of the indicator framework was carried out from October to December 2021 in the selected community in the state of Kerala, India. The ease of application and data availability during the data collection process were optimal. The trained field worker was able to successfully undertake the data collection, and 5% of the collected data were validated through phone calls and in-person visits. In addition, the validity of the data was checked by comparing it with publicly available datasets like the National Family Health Survey. The final results from the piloting process are shown in Table 3.

Table 3. Results of the piloting of the indicator framework carried out in a selected community in India.

Indicator	Performance of the Community			Score
Hygiene facilities in primary and secondary schools in the community	Good	Reasonable	Inadequate	3
Access to Individual Household Latrine (IHHL) with water supply in households	All	Most	Some	3
Coverage for pediatric vaccines as per the national immunization schedule	High	Reasonable	Low	3
Percentage of access antibiotics (as per AWaRe classification of WHO) in total antibiotics dispensed in outpatient settings at healthcare facilities	High	Reasonable	Low	2
Antibiotic protocols in healthcare facilities	All	Some	None	2
Over-the-counter (OTC) availability of antibiotics in retail pharmacies in the area	Poor OTC availability	Partial OTC availability	Free OTC availability	1
Access to safely managed drinking water services	All	Most	Some	3
Use of highest priority critically important antibiotics in agriculture	None	Some	High	2
Presence of functional veterinary services, health facilities, and services in the community	Fully functional	Semi-functional	Not functional	3
Veterinary laboratory services for disease diagnostics	Fully functional	Semi-functional	Not functional	2
Educational initiatives on antibiotic use among farmers	Fully functional	Semi-functional	Not functional	1
Biomedical waste management system in healthcare facilities	All	Some	None	2
Treatment of wastewater generated in households	All	Most	Some	2
Use of chemical/synthetic pesticides, herbicides, and other biocides in farms	Low	Significant	High	2
Farm waste contaminating water resources in the community	High	Some	None	3
Final score				34/45

To test the sensitivity of the indicators to measure change in One Health ABR drivers, targeted context-specific activities were undertaken in the community over a period of six months in collaboration with the community members and local self-government in 2022.

A re-assessment that was undertaken following the intervention showed an improvement in the score. The score increased from 34/45 to 38/45. The framework not only aided the research team in considering drawing up an action agenda to address multiple ABR drivers, but it also acted as an entry point for action in the community.

To check the ease of application and validity of the ASC framework, the ASC indicator framework was piloted in four other communities in India in 2022. The four sites were situated in Himachal Pradesh, Bihar, and Assam. The collaborators and local field workers were trained using the standardized data collection handbook. All of these sites successfully piloted the framework, yielding varying scores.

4. Discussion

The iterative process to design an indicator framework was based on a shared understanding of the need to engage communities on the ABR issue and to create greater local ownership and sustainable resource mobilization. In the past, there have been attempts in low-resource settings to use performance appraisal frameworks and systematic accountability frameworks to achieve specific programmatic outcomes in the implementation of vertical health programs [21,22]. This approach to mobilize communities has been used in health program implementation in the past with good success [21]. Such measurement frameworks can also provide robust data to funders, program managers, and researchers to assess the real impact of their interventions and help them in prioritizing activities for ABR containment [23]. The authors of this work focused on emulating the success of these approaches/frameworks for ABR, measuring the 'antibiotic smartness' of a community through the Antibiotic Smart Communities' project. Such indicator frameworks can be used for advocacy by comparing the performance of similarly placed regions or local contexts. Since ABR can be considered as an issue with systemic drivers, the containment efforts should be able to reflect the need for systemic changes on the ground [24]. Engaging local communities may be essential for increasing the local ownership of ABR interventions, enhance accountability in implementing machinery, robustly mobilizing resources, and improving the general understanding of the issue [25]. Additionally, it has been demonstrated that community-level behavioral change efforts can be more successful when the relevant local stakeholder groups are fully involved in the efforts [26]. Such a framework which we are proposing can therefore also be a tool for local engagement with the ABR issue and a self-assessment of where the local community stands.

While drafting the methodology of data collection for the indicator framework, the researchers and the experts involved have emphasized the feasibility of collecting data. Therefore, the data collection methodology was made as simple as possible to ensure that trained field workers could collect data in a short duration of time. Some of the piloting data generated using the indicator framework was cross-verified with reports such as the National Family Health Survey 5 (NFHS) [27]. There were no discrepancies between the piloting data and the data gathered through larger and more intensive surveys such as the NFHS. However, the NFHS does not capture data on all indicators in the ASC indicator framework.

One limitation of this indicator framework is that it was developed based on a conceptual framework, which is focused on low-resource settings and not applicable for high-resource settings. The utilization of a consultative process to select and refine the indicators, instead of standard statistical methods, is another limitation. However, the authors have followed the criteria laid down by Statistics New Zealand to select the indicators to overcome the issue of not using statistical techniques (Good Practice Guidelines for Indicator Development and Reporting) [28]. Another limitation was that a cut-off of 15 was chosen, considering that feasibility and other frameworks adopt similar cutoffs and are not analyzed on the basis of scores [28,29].

5. Conclusions

The Antibiotic-Smart Communities indicator framework is meant to be a measurement and advocacy tool that can help mobilize local communities in LMICs. An analysis of some of the existing national action plans on antimicrobial resistance has shown gaps in accountability, sustainability, behavioral economics, and local community engagement. This tool can serve to address these gaps, and provide policymakers a way to improve the situation on the ground through appropriate interventions towards optimizing and implementing their national action plans on AMR.

Author Contributions: Conceptualization: P.M., S.J.C. and S.S.; data curation: P.M., S.J.C., J.R., S.S., H.M.A. and S.A.T.; formal analysis: P.M., S.J.C., S.S. and J.R.; investigation: P.M., H.M.A. and S.A.T.; methodology: P.M., H.M.A., S.A.T., S.J.C., S.S. and J.R.; validation: P.M., H.M.A. and S.A.T.; project administration: P.M.; writing—original draft: P.M.; writing—review and editing: S.J.C., J.R. and S.S.; inputs to final version: H.M.A. and S.A.T.; funding acquisition: S.J.C.; supervision: S.J.C. All authors have read and agreed to the published version of the manuscript.

Funding: This project was part of ReAct Asia Pacific project. ReAct Asia Pacific is funded by a grant from the Swedish International Development Cooperation Agency (SIDA) through the ReAct project.

Institutional Review Board Statement: This study was conducted in accordance with the Declaration of Helsinki. Ethics committee approval was obtained from the Puspagiri Institute of Medical Sciences and Research Centre (through IRB study reference number 07/08/2022).

Informed Consent Statement: Not applicable.

Data Availability Statement: The handbook for data collection will be published online on the ReAct tool box. ReAct Toolbox for Action on Antibiotic Resistance. Available online: https://www.reactgroup.org/toolbox/ (accessed on 28 December 2023).

Acknowledgments: The authors would like to thank the ReAct members and all of the experts who helped to refine and prioritize the indicator framework. We also acknowledge Thomas Mathew (project assistant, ReAct Asia Pacific) for his assistance during the data collection as a part of piloting. The authors would also like to acknowledge Raghini Ranganathan (Consultant, ReAct Asia Pacific) for her valuable inputs on the final version of the manuscript.

Conflicts of Interest: The authors declare no conflicts of interest.

References

1. Murray, C.J.; Ikuta, K.S.; Sharara, F.; Swetschinski, L.; Aguilar, G.R.; Gray, A.; Han, C.; Bisignano, C.; Rao, P.; Wool, E.; et al. Global Burden of Bacterial Antimicrobial Resistance in 2019: A Systematic Analysis. *Lancet* **2022**, *399*, 629–655. [CrossRef] [PubMed]
2. *AMR Review Paper—Tackling a Crisis for the Health and Wealth of Nations_1.Pdf. Antimicrobial Resistance: Tackling a Crisis for the Health and Wealth of Nations/the Review on Antimicrobial Resistance Chaired by Jim O'Neill. Attribution 4.0 International (CC BY 4.0)*; Wellcome Collection Musuem and Library: London, UK, 2014; Available online: https://wellcomecollection.org/works/rdpck35v (accessed on 24 November 2023).
3. Jonas, O.B.; Irwin, A.; Berthe, F.C.J.; Le Gall, F.G.; Marquez, P.V. Drug-Resistant Infections: A Threat to Our Economic Future (Vol. 2): Final Report. Available online: https://documents.worldbank.org/en/publication/documents-reports/documentdetail/323311493396993758/final-report (accessed on 24 November 2023).
4. Ayukekbong, J.A.; Ntemgwa, M.; Atabe, A.N. The Threat of Antimicrobial Resistance in Developing Countries: Causes and Control Strategies. *Antimicrob. Resist. Infect. Control* **2017**, *6*, 47. [CrossRef] [PubMed]
5. Global Antibiotic Consumption and Usage in Humans, 2000–2018: A Spatial Modelling Study—The Lancet Planetary Health. Available online: https://www.thelancet.com/journals/lanplh/article/PIIS2542-5196(21)00280-1/fulltext (accessed on 24 November 2023).
6. Global Action Plan on Antimicrobial Resistance. Available online: https://www.who.int/publications-detail-redirect/9789241509763 (accessed on 9 November 2022).
7. Target Global Database for the Tripartite Antimicrobial Resistance (AMR) Country Self-Assessment Survey (TrACSS). Available online: http://amrcountryprogress.org/ (accessed on 21 August 2022).
8. No Time to Wait: Securing the Future from Drug-Resistant Infections. Available online: https://www.who.int/publications-detail-redirect/no-time-to-wait-securing-the-future-from-drug-resistant-infections (accessed on 15 November 2022).
9. Mathew, P.; Sivaraman, S.; Chandy, S. Communication Strategies for Improving Public Awareness on Appropriate Antibiotic Use: Bridging a Vital Gap for Action on Antibiotic Resistance. *J. Fam. Med. Prim. Care* **2019**, *8*, 1867. [CrossRef]

10. Wind, L.L.; Briganti, J.S.; Brown, A.M.; Neher, T.P.; Davis, M.F.; Durso, L.M.; Spicer, T.; Lansing, S. Finding What Is Inaccessible: Antimicrobial Resistance Language Use among the One Health Domains. *Antibiotics* **2021**, *10*, 385. [CrossRef] [PubMed]
11. Ghiga, I.; Sidorchuk, A.; Pitchforth, E.; Stålsby Lundborg, C.; Machowska, A. 'If You Want to Go Far, Go Together'-Community-Based Behaviour Change Interventions to Improve Antibiotic Use: A Systematic Review of Quantitative and Qualitative Evidence. *J. Antimicrob. Chemother.* **2023**, *78*, 1344–1353. [CrossRef]
12. Mitchell, J.; Cooke, P.; Ahorlu, C.; Arjyal, A.; Baral, S.; Carter, L.; Dasgupta, R.; Fieroze, F.; Fonseca-Braga, M.; Huque, R.; et al. Community Engagement: The Key to Tackling Antimicrobial Resistance (AMR) across a One Health Context? *Glob. Public Health* **2022**, *17*, 2647–2664. [CrossRef]
13. Cai, H.T.N.; Tran, H.T.; Nguyen, Y.H.T.; Vu, G.Q.T.; Tran, T.P.; Bui, P.B.; Nguyen, H.T.T.; Pham, T.Q.; Lai, A.T.; Van Nuil, J.I.; et al. Challenges and Lessons Learned in the Development of a Participatory Learning and Action Intervention to Tackle Antibiotic Resistance: Experiences From Northern Vietnam. *Front. Public Health* **2022**, *10*, 822873. [CrossRef] [PubMed]
14. Shukla, S. Kerala: India's Highest HDI, a Testament to Economic Advancement. *Medium* **2023**.
15. Triandis, H.C. Individualism-Collectivism and Personality—PubMed. *J. Pers.* **2001**, *69*, 907–924. [CrossRef]
16. Meyer, H.-D. Framing Disability: Comparing Individualist and Collectivist Societies. *Comp. Sociol.* **2010**, *9*, 165–181. [CrossRef]
17. Babu, M.G.S.; Ghosh, D.; Gupte, J.; Raza, M.A.; Kasper, E.; Mehra, P. *Kerala's Grass-Roots-Led Pandemic Response: Deciphering the Strength of Decentralisation*; Institute of Development Studies (IDS): Brighton, UK, 2021.
18. Azeez, E.P.A.; Anbuselvi, G. Is the Kerala Model of Community-Based Palliative Care Operations Sustainable? Evidence from the Field. *Indian J. Palliat. Care* **2021**, *27*, 18–22. [CrossRef]
19. Benny, G.; Joseph, J.; Surendran, S.; Nambiar, D. On the Forms, Contributions and Impacts of Community Mobilisation Involved with Kerala's COVID-19 Response: Perspectives of Health Staff, Local Self Government Institution and Community Leaders. *PLoS ONE* **2023**, *18*, e0285999. [CrossRef] [PubMed]
20. Thomas, V. Kerala's Resilience Comes from Community Participation in Policies ... Besides High Investments in Health and Education. *Times of India*, 18 May 2021.
21. Noorihekmat, S.; Rahimi, H.; Mehrolhassani, M.H.; Chashmyazdan, M.; Haghdoost, A.A.; Ahmadi Tabatabaei, S.V.; Dehnavieh, R. Frameworks of Performance Measurement in Public Health and Primary Care System: A Scoping Review and Meta-Synthesis. *Int. J. Prev. Med.* **2020**, *11*, 165. [CrossRef]
22. Tegegne, S.G.; MKanda, P.; Yehualashet, Y.G.; Erbeto, T.B.; Touray, K.; Nsubuga, P.; Banda, R.; Vaz, R.G. Implementation of a Systematic Accountability Framework in 2014 to Improve the Performance of the Nigerian Polio Program. *J. Infect. Dis.* **2016**, *213* (Suppl. S3), S96–S100. [CrossRef]
23. Karris, M.Y.; Dubé, K.; Moore, A.A. What Lessons It Might Teach Us? Community Engagement in HIV Research. *Curr. Opin. HIV AIDS* **2020**, *15*, 142–149. [CrossRef] [PubMed]
24. Cars, O.; Chandy, S.J.; Mpundu, M.; Peralta, A.Q.; Zorzet, A.; So, A.D. Resetting the Agenda for Antibiotic Resistance through a Health Systems Perspective. *Lancet Glob. Health* **2021**, *9*, e1022–e1027. [CrossRef] [PubMed]
25. Haldane, V.; Chuah, F.L.H.; Srivastava, A.; Singh, S.R.; Koh, G.C.H.; Seng, C.K.; Legido-Quigley, H. Community Participation in Health Services Development, Implementation, and Evaluation: A Systematic Review of Empowerment, Health, Community, and Process Outcomes. *PLoS ONE* **2019**, *14*, e0216112. [CrossRef] [PubMed]
26. Boaz, A.; Hanney, S.; Borst, R.; O'Shea, A.; Kok, M. How to Engage Stakeholders in Research: Design Principles to Support Improvement. *Health Res. Policy Syst.* **2018**, *16*, 60. [CrossRef]
27. National Family Health Survey. Available online: http://rchiips.org/nfhs/kerala.shtml (accessed on 24 November 2023).
28. OECD. Available online: https://www.oecd.org/site/progresskorea/43586563.pdf (accessed on 24 November 2023).
29. Papageorgiou, A.; Henrysson, M.; Nuur, C.; Sinha, R.; Sundberg, C.; Vanhuyse, F. Mapping and Assessing Indicator-Based Frameworks for Monitoring Circular Economy Development at the City-Level. *Sustain. Cities Soc.* **2021**, *75*, 103378. [CrossRef]

MDPI AG
Grosspeteranlage 5
4052 Basel
Switzerland
Tel.: +41 61 683 77 34

Antibiotics Editorial Office
E-mail: antibiotics@mdpi.com
www.mdpi.com/journal/antibiotics

www.ingramcontent.com/pod-product-compliance
Lightning Source LLC
LaVergne TN
LVHW072347090526
838202LV00019B/2496

* 9 7 8 3 7 2 5 8 3 0 4 6 6 *